T0210579

Medical Education, Politics and Social Justice

This book critically analyses how politics and power affect the ways that medicine is taught and learned. Challenging society's historic reluctance to connect the realm of politics to the realm of medicine, *Medical Education, Politics and Social Justice: The Contradiction Cure* emphasizes the need for medical students to engage with social justice issues, including global health crises resulting from the climate emergency, and the health implications of widening social inequality.

Arguing for an increased focus on community-based learning rather than acute care, this innovative text maps the territory of medicine's contradictory engagement with politics as a springboard for creative curriculum design. It demonstrates why the socially disempowered – such as political and climate refugees, the homeless or those without health insurance – should be primary subjects of attention for medical students, while exploring how political engagement can be refined, sharp, cultivated and creative, engaging imagination and demanding innovation.

Exploring how the medical humanities can promote engagement with politics to improve medical education, this book is a ground-breaking and inspiring contribution. It is an essential read for all those with a focus on medical education and medical humanities, as well as medical and healthcare students with an interest in the social determinants of health.

Alan Bleakley is Life Emeritus Professor of Medical Education and Medical Humanities at Plymouth Peninsula School of Medicine, Faculty of Health. He is an internationally acclaimed figure in the fields of medical education and medical humanities, with a strong profile of research grants, keynote conference talks, peer-reviewed publications, book chapters and books. He has an academic background in zoology, psychology, psychoanalytic psychotherapy and education, and has been instrumental in developing the medical humanities in medical education internationally, including organizing international conferences. He is past president of the Association for Medical Humanities and founding fellow of the Academy of Medical Educators. Alan is also a widely published poet with four collections, and a keen, longstanding surfer. He lives in the far west of Cornwall – where granite coast meets the, often wild, Atlantic – with his wife Sue, who is a visual artist.

Routledge Advances in the Medical Humanities

For more information about this series visit: www.routledge.com/Routledge-Advances-in-the-Medical-Humanities/book-series/RAMH

Medical Education, Politics and Social Justice
The Contradiction Cure

Alan Bleakley

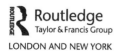
Routledge
Taylor & Francis Group

LONDON AND NEW YORK

First published 2021

by Routledge
2 Park Square, Milton Park, Abingdon, Oxon OX14 4RN

and by Routledge
52 Vanderbilt Avenue, New York, NY 10017

Routledge is an imprint of the Taylor & Francis Group, an informa business

© 2021 Alan Bleakley

British Library Cataloguing-in-Publication Data
A catalogue record for this book is available from the British Library

Library of Congress Cataloging-in-Publication Data
Names: Bleakley, Alan (Alan Douglas), author.
Title: Medical education, politics and social justice : the contradiction cure / Alan Bleakley.
Description: Milton Park, Abingdon, Oxon ; New York, NY : Routledge, 2021. | Series: Routledge advances in medical humanities | Includes bibliographical references and index. |
Identifiers: LCCN 2020039049 (print) | LCCN 2020039050 (ebook) | ISBN 9780367567132 (hardback) | ISBN 9781003099093 (ebook)
Subjects: LCSH: Medical education. | Medical education--Political aspects. | Social justice.
Classification: LCC R737 .B564 2021 (print) | LCC R737 (ebook) | DDC 610.71/1--dc23
LC record available at https://lccn.loc.gov/2020039049
LC ebook record available at https://lccn.loc.gov/2020039050

ISBN: 978-0-367-56713-2 (hbk)
ISBN: 978-1-003-09909-3 (ebk)

Typeset in Goudy
By Deanta Global Publishing Services, Chennai, India

Dedicated to my loving family, as always. They give unconditional humour, warmth and hope for the future. Particularly to Sue – without whose love and creativity my life would be hollowed out.

Contents

Figures

Tables

Foreword *by Professor*
Yrjö Engeström

In this book, Alan Bleakley invites us to embrace and work with dialectical contradictions. This is an invitation to start nourishing and cultivating a mindset radically different from the safe and yet devastatingly destructive logic of non-contradiction. But this is also a very practical invitation, close to the daily, lived reality of any professional who retains a willingness to feel and explore the discomfort of the dualities of practice.

> The doctor who buys a practice in some little provincial place may be very seriously trying to reduce his fellow citizens' suffering from illness, and may see his calling in just that. He must, however, want the number of the sick to increase, because his life and practical opportunity to follow his calling depend on that.
>
> This dualism distorts man's most elementary feelings. Even love proves capable of acquiring the most ugly forms, not to mention love of money, which can become a veritable passion.
>
> The penetration of these relations into consciousness also finds psychological reflection in a "disintegration" of its general structure characterized by the rise of an estrangement between the senses and meanings in which the world around man and his own life are refracted for him.
>
> Whatever concrete, historical feature of man's psyche under the dominance of private property relations that we take (whether thought, interests, or feelings), it inevitably bears the impress of this structure of consciousness and can only be properly understood from its peculiarities. To ignore these peculiarities and remove them from the context of psychological research is to deprive psychology of historical concreteness, converting it into a science solely of the psyche of an abstract man, of "man in general".
>
> (Leont'ev 1981: 255)

Leont'ev's observation pertains to the primary contradiction of medical work and medical learning in capitalism: the unavoidable duality of serving both the generation of use value (health, wellbeing) and the generation of privately appropriated exchange value (money, profit, cost-cutting). There is no way to select just one and abandon the other. A true dialectical contradiction, the two poles both require and repel one another.

Leont'ev's example of a village doctor needs to be translated into the complex organizational fields of today's medicine. Take the Covid-19 pandemic and the race to produce a viable vaccine. On July 25, 2020, *The New York Times* published an article titled *Corporate Insiders Pocket $1 Billion in Rush for Coronavirus Vaccine* (Gelles and Drucker 2020). Here are small excerpts from the article:

Executives at a long list of companies have reaped seven- or eight-figure profits thanks to their work on coronavirus vaccines and treatments. Shares of Regeneron, a biotech company in Tarrytown, N.Y., have climbed nearly 80 percent since early February, when it announced a collaboration with the Department of Health and Human Services to develop a Covid-19 treatment. Since then, the company's top executives and board members have sold nearly $700 million in stock. The chief executive, Leonard Schleifer, sold $178 million of shares on a single day in May.

Moderna, a 10-year-old vaccine developer based in Cambridge, Mass., that has never brought a product to market, announced in late January that it was working on a coronavirus vaccine. It has issued a stream of news releases hailing its vaccine progress, and its stock has more than tripled, giving the company a market value of almost $30 billion.

Moderna insiders have sold about $248 million of shares since that January announcement, most of it after the company was selected in April to receive federal funding to support its vaccine efforts.

Also, a dissenting voice was reported:

It is inappropriate for drug company executives to cash in on a crisis," said Ben Wakana, executive director of Patients for Affordable Drugs, a non-profit advocacy group. "Every day, Americans wake up and make sacrifices during this pandemic. Drug companies see this as a payday.

Can contradictions be turned into a cure? An aggravated contradiction is experienced as a conflict of motives, often paralysing in its impact, as evidenced in a conversation between home care managers in Helsinki, Finland, in our own research:

Home care manager 5: Last week I participated in a home visit to a client who is, who lies in bed and receives 80 hours a week personal assistant service, plus another similar number of hours of our services. And his needs are just enormous. Even what he now gets is not nearly sufficient. You know the case.

Home care manager 8: Yes, I have also visited his home. *Home care manager 5:* And the situation has been terribly aggravated for a long time. Negotiations have been conducted for a long time, I've been involved. And now we were there, the chief physician, and the social worker, and me, and the responsible home care nurse, and the home care supervisor, and we are sitting around his bed, thinking about this client's […] quite concretely, what does he want and what do we have, what do we have to give. And as I am myself competent in the substance [of nursing], having been there in the field, I have a terrible agony, about having to be a sort of a policeman and gatekeeper: "no we cannot", "no we cannot", "no we cannot", "unfortunately this will be terminated", "and this […] and this, and this, and this". We cannot provide. I don't know. This client's need is completely absurd, what he would want. And I understand it. That is somehow it. And our workers are in panic because they cannot respond to the need. And they have to say "no, we cannot" all the time, and they feel awfully bad about it. They want me to come and say that "no, we cannot", so that they get someone to take the load off their shoulders, that they cannot meet the need. I mean, it is somehow extremely difficult to bring this up, I mean the client's need and our need, and what is actually the object. I at least can ponder, what is our object. (Engeström and Sannino 2011: 381)

Here, the mechanism of double stimulation steps into focus. In the study from which the above excerpt is taken, the home care managers' shared conflict of motives (being a caregiver *vs.* being a policeman and gatekeeper), seemingly an iron cage, was cracked open by constructing and putting into use a "service palette". In the service palette brochure, the services offered to the patients by home care were explained and made available for negotiation with the patients. This had not been done before. As one of the home care managers pointed out, the elderly home care patients were expected to take what was given, sort of like we would go to a pizzeria and instead of being given a menu to consider, we would be required to eat whatever the pizzeria decided. The service palette was a second stimulus that enabled the home care workers to switch from "doing for" to "doing with". This meant much more than acquiring a new skill – it meant generating *will*, transformative agency in everyday actions. The second stimulus became a "warping anchor" (Sannino 2020) with which the practitioners and their patients could pull their activity out of the paralysis.

The service palette is an example of a move towards an equitable and dialogical relationship between the professional caregivers and the patients. This is one of the foundational characteristics of medical humanities as proposed and elaborated upon by Alan Bleakley in the present ground-breaking book. Medical humanities are here seen as a comprehensive and flexible second stimulus, an instrumentality for the entire process of medical education. This is a bold initiative, visionary but also solidly grounded in already tested and stabilized practices in innovative institutions of medical education.

What makes the medical humanities uniquely powerful is that they bring together arts and aesthetics on the one hand – often regarded as the typical "soft stuff" of humanities – and radical politics of equity, justice and sustainability on the other hand. The latter is not soft stuff. It requires taking a stand against commoditization and acting to create and sustain alternatives to neo-liberal capitalism in the practice and learning of medicine.

Eloquent, deeply learned and analytically razor-sharp, this book charts the contours of an emerging zone of proximal development for medical learning. It is an exciting first leg of a journey we need to embark on. As Bleakley himself concludes: "There is much work to be done".

References

Engeström Y, Sannino A. Discursive Manifestations of Contradictions in Organizational Change Efforts. *Journal of Organizational Change Management.* 2011; 24: 368–87.

Gelles D, Drucker J. Corporate Insiders Pocket $1 Billion in Rush for Coronavirus Vaccine. *The New York Times*, 25 July 2020

Leont'ev AN. 1981. *Problems of the Development of the Mind.* Moscow: Progress.

Sannino A. 2020. Transformative Agency as Warping: How Collectives Accomplish Change Amidst Uncertainty. *Pedagogy, Culture & Society.* Published online 18 August 2020. DOI: 10.1080/14681366.2020.1805493. Available at: https://www.tandfonline.com/doi/full/10.1080/14681366.2020.1805493

Yrjö Engeström is Professor Emeritus and Director,
Centre for Research on Activity, Development and Learning (CRADLE),
University of Helsinki, Finland

Prologue

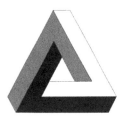

Exposed to death

Every life is a life exposed to death, or ultimately a 'bare life'. Such exposure to death, suggests Giorgio Agamben (1998: 88), "is the originary political element", for it is the ultimate expression of power – that of bare life's natural entropic course. There is no power greater than entropy – the gradual and inevitable decline into disorder that faces each of us as embodied thinkers, creating an existential dilemma.

Medicine is the primary cultural force that opposes entropy and death, and so is essentially political – as a power consciously and conscientiously exercised. Medicine joins the Welsh poet Dylan Thomas in exhorting us to "not go gentle into that good night,/ Old age should burn and rave at close of day;/ Rage, rage against the dying of the light". Medicine has adopted Thomas' plea as a modern oath and sentiment. No wonder that medicine has adopted martial metaphors ("the fight against disease") as it rages against the dying of the light on behalf of its patients.

Historically and culturally determined power structures within medicine and between its components (such as patients, educators, laboratory scientists, anatomists, managers, researchers and lawyers) have not been systematically researched and mapped, remaining largely a black box. While Daniel Dawes' (2020) *The Political Determinants of Health* engages with a limited landscape – that of American healthcare and politics – it nevertheless advertises a major, largely uncharted, contradiction between the ideal of global healthcare as patient-centred and interprofessional (suggesting horizontal power sharing and collaboration) and the reality. Division of labour within healthcare remains stubbornly hierarchical, with medicine occupying the tip of the hierarchy, while within medicine, there are historically determined hierarchical assumptions that place surgery above medicine, and hospital-based specialties above general or family practices.

Medical students are certainly treated as the base of the medical hierarchy in terms of status and realized power, and while patients may be treated courteously in most cases, they are largely excluded from meaningful involvement in medical decision-making, including shaping the purposes of medical culture. Further, where women now constitute 60% of entrants to medical schools globally, medicine's practices – particularly surgery, senior management roles and senior medical education positions – remain patriarchal, while in Europe in particular, black, Asian and minority ethnic (BAME) doctors remain under-represented, particularly at senior levels.

In other words, medicine is still juvenile in relation to the process of fully democratizing, despite advertising patient-centredness and inter-professionalism as its two great structural advances in recent times. Of course, democracy itself is a youthful work in progress (Keane 2009). Indeed, many perceived political democracies are radically in need of democratizing as right-wing populism has gained traction in the contemporary, neo-liberal world order. The world's biggest threat to health is social inequity (Navarro 2007; Marmot 2015), one of democracy's demons. And surely medicine should not still be advertising inequalities in its own household?

Equity and equality

A distinction must be made between equality and equity. Equality means treating everybody in the same way, but this assumes an initial level playing field. Equity means fairness and justice, or getting every person what they need to live a good life, and this will incur preferential treatment for the disadvantaged. The literature on social and health inequalities often confuses equity with equality or conflates them.

Global Health Europe defines inequity and inequality thus: "inequity refers to unfair, avoidable differences arising from poor governance, corruption or cultural exclusion while inequality simply refers to the uneven distribution of health or health resources as a result of genetic or other factors or the lack of resources". (http://www.globalhealtheurope.org/index.php/resources/glossary/values/17)

It is the job of healthcare education to challenge health-related structural inequity and inequality issues. Patient-centred practice does result in better health outcomes to improve equity (Bleakley 2014), while flattening hierarchies to increase collaboration within and between clinical teams results in better health outcomes, improved patient safety and greater worker satisfaction (Borrill et al. 2013).

Structural competence

Helena Hansen and Jonathan Metzl (2017: 279) describe "structural competency" as a "New Medicine for the U.S. Health Care System". The descriptor is ambiguous, perhaps purposefully so. Is the medicine, prescribed by politicians, to be taken by an ailing US healthcare system as a cure for a self-imposed stubbornness over the universal provision of affordable healthcare (Dawes 2020)? Or is the medicine one that the US healthcare system prescribes to the population, merely reproducing the long tradition of "the medicalization of everyday life", the promotion of a "pharmacracy" (Szasz 2007)? Further, the dosage of the "New Medicine" prescribed by Hansen and Metzl remains unspecified.

"Cultural competence" (or "competency") in undergraduate medical education is well established as a curriculum aim, particularly in North American and Canadian medical schools, defined as a cluster of values, knowledge and activities necessary to effectively provide care for, and interact with, patients from diverse ethnic and cultural backgrounds. Sunl Kripalani and colleagues (Kripalani et al. 2006: 1116) note that "Cultural competence programs have proliferated in US medical schools in response to increasing national diversity, as well as mandates from accrediting bodies". In 2006, however, when Kripalani and colleagues' paper was published, provision was patchy. Nearly two decades later, North American and Canadian medical education has become world leading in establishing cultural competence as core curriculum provision in medical education.

For some, however, cultural competence is necessary but not sufficient to turn medical students' attention away from "downstream" hospitalism, with its acute care focus, to "upstream" chronic care in the community, stressing prevention rather than cure. Cultural competence offers a restricted pedagogical horizon. Jonathan Metzl, a psychiatrist and sociology of medicine professor at Vanderbilt University, Nashville, has argued that cultural competence, or learning to be sensitive to ethnic differences, must be extended to learning to be sensitive to structural inequities such as poverty, diet and homelessness (Metzl and Hansen 2014).

In 2005, a pre-health major in medicine, health and society, drawing on social sciences, humanities and health sciences, was established at Vanderbilt (around 40% of the intake go on to study medicine) (Metzl and Petty 2017). This led to schemes for assessment of understanding and application of "structural health". In 2012–13, a curriculum overhaul led to an updating of material and expansion of ideas within the course, with students studying the politics of health and social activism.

Pedagogical innovations included a medical humanities component, where literary texts were studied for what they could teach about tensions between individual needs and social welfare provision, self-assessment and development of an evaluation instrument: the Structural Foundations of Health (SFH). Metzl and Petty (ibid.: 359), ahead of the Black Lives Matter uprising of Summer 2020 resulting from the police's murder of George Floyd in Minneapolis, conclude:

we aim to contribute to an evolving literature that suggests that teaching students about the social and structural aspects of race and medicine needs to begin sooner in the educational process, during the undergraduate years, when students can learn about structures and socioeconomic and historical contexts at the same time as they begin to learn about diseases and bodies.

Besides "race and medicine", of course, there is gender, poverty, stigma and other structural issues of which these authors are all too well aware.

Metzl's and colleagues' body of work around this topic names five "core competencies":

1. Recognizing the structures that shape clinical interactions.
2. Developing an extra-clinical language of structure.
3. Rearticulating "cultural" formulations in structural terms.
4. Observing and imagining structural interventions.
5. Developing structural humility.

All of this is to be welcomed, but such changes are advertised as "patient-centred" and "community-centred", so it is strange that a desire to turn medical and health education away from downstream acute care to chronic, structural social conditions upstream in communities should be dressed in such technical, rather than lay or (patient-friendly), language. Better, surely, to directly address the upstream population or communities the initiative is supposed to serve. Medicalized and sociology-tinged language will not strike a chord with a lay population. Perhaps the statements above can also be turned into questions suggesting multiple answers:

1. Why do doctors in clinics, primarily in hospitals, act and talk "clinically" rather than in everyday terms with patients in recognizing their primary social settings?
2. How might doctors talk with people (suspending the label of "patient") in terms of that person's common or everyday experience?
3. Rather than focusing on a person's ethnicity or first language, can the doctor re-focus on issues such as deprivation, stigma, poverty, housing, employment, access to food and medicines and whether or not they can afford healthcare?
4. How will a doctor help a person whose health is compromised by a lack of basic needs?
5. Will a doctor feel compassion and set aside judgement when meeting people in dire need of basics where this is compromised by health or lifestyle issues such as drug or alcohol dependency? And do a doctor's political persuasions affect this?

The language of "competencies", "skills" and "training" that infuses North American and Canadian medical education in particular is also both instrumental and reductive. And it is used habitually, without reflection. Community-oriented medical education, energized by the medical humanities, as I shall argue, should be an expansive, engaged learning saturated with unknowns and contradictions; this, rather than a list of competencies to be achieved in "tick-box" style. Such a "training" approach is deadening, where training, from the Latin *trahere*, means to "drag behind", as in the train of a wedding dress. (So also a railway train has a series of trailing carriages.) As teachers or facilitators, do we really want to drag our medical students behind us? Surely we want their learning to be expansive, adventurous, generous and challenging. Isn't this what they pay their tuition fees for? A better descriptor of expansive learning is "capability" (Nussbaum 2011), an as-yet undeveloped ability. This sees learning as a horizon project, one of unfolding potential.

In a pan-European context, Katja Lanting and colleagues (Lanting et al. 2019) assessed medical educators' preparedness to include cultural competence in their teaching of ethnically diverse cohorts of medical students. Of nearly 1,000 survey respondents across 11 European institutions, 40% felt they were unprepared for such teaching. A pan-European consortium for planning curricula to ensure lifelong cultural competence amongst medical doctors showed that while about half of medical schools surveyed were engaging with cultural competence, very few formally assessed students in this area of expertise (Sorensen et al. 2017: 28). Medical schools too were poorly resourced in this area, failing to provide tailored education for teachers. The authors concluded that "there are major deficiencies in the commitment and practice within the participating educational programs and there are clear potentials for major improvements regarding cultural competence in programmes". The cultural competency movement, addressing inequalities and inequities arising from issues such as gender, disability, race and ethnicity, has some way to go to develop programmes that have been established in areas such as ethics and professionalism. Indeed, issues of health inequities and inequalities grounded in culture are just as likely to be addressed through generic medical humanities provision as through tailored cultural competence provision (Kumagai and Lypson 2009; Kumagai and Naidu 2020). Most obviously, this would include well-established services such as medical translation for non-native speakers. Structural competency core, compulsory and assessed provision is some way off in most medical schools.

Political evolution

If we take the long view of archaeological anthropologists, there is a strong argument that the original condition of humankind – from emergence in Africa 300,000–200,000 years ago to the origins of art and cultural artefacts in Ice Age hunter-gatherers 15,000 years ago – was one of social collaboration (Flannery and Marcus 2012: x). Yet "By 2,500 B.C., virtually every form of inequality known to mankind had been created somewhere in the world". Ice Age hunter-gatherers, existing in family groups, must have had to collaborate with other family groups to hunt and prepare animals such as the woolly mammoth. Solidarity was not just based on task at hand and equitable division of labour, but also on myths, or a cosmology that gave a rationale for social structures. Drawing on evidence from extant hunter-gatherers that have evolved from social organizations based on family structures to a more complex cross-family clan structure (where clans are usually identified with a natural phenomenon such as a totem animal), Flannery and Marcus (ibid.: 65) note a common element: cultural lore described clans as descended as equals from originary cosmic forces or beings, as "The concept of the sacred which had once strengthened human society by encouraging selfless-ness and reducing status confrontation".

However, as such groups developed more complex social structures through a finer division of labour, this collaborative norm "would one day be manipulated to create a hereditary elite". Of contemporary societies, few match up to the "reducing status confrontation" rule exercised diligently in small hunter-gatherer groups. In 1968, a study of the !Kung on the Namibia/Botswana border in Africa showed a group of 12 men, 10 women and 13 children who largely foraged for food, displaying a social structure that "was as egalitarian as any ever studied" (ibid.: 31), where food was communally gathered and shared, with no argument over who was the "best" at the role (indeed there was a cultural counter-display of strenuous denial of any privilege); no one person ever claimed the kill in the hunt; and humour was regularly used to defuse potential conflict. It would be rare to find such efforts towards authentic "reducing status confrontation" within and between hospital-based multi-professional healthcare teams today, despite adver-tised subscription to democratized "*inter*-professional" activity.

Every culture has an origin myth, and this is drawn on as justification for social structures, either horizontal/egalitarian or vertical/hierarchical. The first two chapters of *The Book of Genesis* offer two origin myths – one promoting original democracy and one promoting original autocracy. The Western psyche is then grounded in contradictory origin myths. The first story is that of the Seven Days of Creation, set out as an unfolding hierarchy. The second story (actually com-posed before the first) tells of creation in the round, as the story of the Garden of Eden, with creation as a timeless set-piece into which Adam and Eve walk as innocents. Is this a metaphor for original democracy and equality?

The post–Ice Age shift to vertical power structures involved a change in reg-ister of origin myths, in which certain clans, genders or persons could assume authority over others through, for example, divine monarchies and hereditary elites. Division of labour became stratified vertically with accompanying levels of status. While resulting social inequalities in complex societies have become the norm, the sophistication of understanding of such social conditions and quality and strength of forms of resistance have also developed. Experiments in demo-cratic forms of politics have been tried since well before the famous Athenian assemblies in 5th-century BCE Greece (Keane 2009), but it is only in rela-tively recent historical times – through the English Civil War and overthrow of the monarchy in 1642–51, the American Revolution in 1765–83, the French Revolution in 1789–99 and the Haitian Slave Revolution in 1791–1804 – that democratic forms of government have been established.

By a modern, complex "democracy" I mean a "representative" democracy where, at a minimum: (i) all adult citizens can vote in a free and fair election for choosing or replacing a government; (ii) citizens, including children, can actively participate in civic life through assemblies; (iii) the media are free to investigate and report; (iv) laws are fair and apply equally to all citizens; (v) "democracy" itself in meaning and activity is constantly debated, modified and progressed; and (vi) human rights are protected. Human rights do not just equate with democracy but should be applied across the political spectrum. A majority of the world's countries are not democracies but autocracies, theocracies, plutocracies and meritocracies. Establishing democratic political structures obviously cannot be carried out in an autocratic manner but requires a social evolution that depends upon the psychological make-up of citizens to be able, first, to tolerate high levels of ambiguity; second, to compromise without feeling unduly cheated; and third, to engage in collaborative inquiry and debate into how best to communicate dialogically, while retaining high levels of reflexivity, self-awareness and insight.

These three conditions are the very capabilities that psychotherapists and health and social care professionals need in particular. If we are to reclaim any sense of our Ice Age ancestry, with capabilities to collaborate over the best use of resources, this must include how to afford equal opportunity for all – regardless of physical or mental states and within their horizons of capabilities. This is equality. But more, social life must also be equitable. We are not starting from a level playing field, and therefore everyone cannot be treated equally – some will need more help, or differing kinds of tailored help, than others to compensate for structural inequities. Medicine, with its pledge to treat all with equal attention and respect, must get its own house in order politically. Medical education is key to this project, and the medical humanities even more so, as we shall see.

The rise of Fascism in the 1930s threatened the progress of democracy, but this was quelled. After World War II, and then after the fall of the Berlin Wall, it looked as if democracy was picking up steam, challenging global injustices and the inexorable rise of free market neo-liberal capitalism, where "health" is treated as a commodity, healthcare is treated as a customer service and health inequities have become starker as the gap between rich and poor widens. But, since 2005, there has been a global decline in political rights and civil liberties in comparison with a widening of democracy.

A Freedom House report from 2018 shows global democracy in decline for a 12th consecutive year. In an age in which the climate crisis is our primary existential threat and is intimately linked with global health, and we have suffered a global pandemic from a novel coronavirus infection that has created worldwide mortality and morbidity and an accompanying major economic catastrophe, how will medicine and medical education respond? What will be the cure for the pandemic of social injustices?

Pernkopf's Atlas

Just as the Judaeo-Christian twin creation myths afford a contradiction, rarely discussed in everyday conversation, so throughout this book I set a series of questions prompted by contradictions. Following the pedagogical model of Cultural-Historical Activity Theory (CHAT) – originally devised by Lev Vygotsky (1896–1934), amongst others, after the 1917 Russian Revolution, and further developed in particular by the Finnish educational psychologist Yrjö Engeström (1987) and the American psychologist Michael Cole (1996) – I stress how learning is dependent upon contradiction as driver and motivator. I follow CHAT in seeing contradictions as resources rather than hindrances. As an illustrative example, let us consider a recent ethical and political contradiction faced by medical educators.

Among anatomical atlases, one in particular stands out for its accuracy in portraying nerve pathways and innervations. It was initially developed in the 1930s and is still in use today amongst surgeons specializing in delicate peripheral nerve surgery to relieve intense pain from damaged or trapped nerves. For some surgeons, it proves more useful as a guide than the most sophisticated images from scans. However, it was a Nazi surgeon, Eduard Pernkopf (1888–1955), who developed the atlas (planned for seven volumes, and developed over a period of 20 years working with four illustrators). Pernkopf, an Austrian, joined the Nazi party in 1933 while he was chair of the anatomy department at the University of Vienna's prestigious medical school. Later, he became dean for the medical faculty and then the university's president. The atlas was not finished until close to Pernkopf's death in 1955, and published in a two-volume edition in five languages, with an English-language version published in America in 1963.

By the 1980s, as part of an intense investigation into Nazi war crimes, the concentration camps and Nazi medical experiments prior to and during World War II, it emerged that Pernkopf's atlas was based on the dissection of cadavers of Austrians who had been tried and sentenced to death for anti-Nazi activities after the annexation. Artists who had worked with Pernkopf on the early drawings incorporated Nazi symbols such as swastikas and lightning bolts (SS insignia) into their signatures. Pernkopf himself spent three years in an allied prison camp after the war but, on release, continued to work on the atlas.

Elsevier, the Dutch publishers who had initially published the atlas in two volumes, stopped printing the book, and it was widely sidelined for clinical use on ethical grounds. However, copies still circulated and, despite the ethical concerns, are in use today. A 2017 ethical protocol committee had ruled that the atlas could still be used as long as full disclosure about its origins was conveyed to potential surgical patients or students. In an international survey of 182 nerve surgeons, 13% said they were using the atlas, 41% had used it previously and 41% were unaware of its existence, history and ethical status (Kershner 2020).

Nerve surgeons have a deep aesthetic sensibility for their work, engaging with delicate attachments, innervations and entanglements requiring an educated eye, fine eye–hand co-ordination and an admirable level of patience. This aesthetic side of medicine – in the case of Pernkopf's atlas a guide that is, reportedly, an exquisite map of the territory – is then intertwined with a problematic ethics and politics. But here, the ethics compromise the aesthetics as a political dilemma. But I have just illustrated how the contradiction inherent to the atlas affords a resource and not a liability. Medical students can now appreciate the atlas for the historical oddity it is while engaging with the ethical dilemma that it raises. Medicine and surgery are now extended from a functional platform to deeper ethical inquiry.

The structure of this book

This book addresses intersections between medicine, medical education, the medical humanities, politics, ethics and aesthetics. In an era in which medical education has become functional (such as competence-led) rather than expressive, such pedagogical conservatism dampens the possibilities of a more imaginative approach to pedagogy in which the vision of undergraduate medicine is expanded. Such an approach would value qualities to place appreciation of patients prior to the explanation of symptoms. And, importantly, such an approach would develop the question posed here as to how we might democratize medicine as an authentic service to the public.

Medicine has attempted to carry the contradiction that it must remain apolitical while it is blatantly an institution riddled with, and expressing, power issues. This is a generative contradiction, but its nature must be addressed before we can tap into its potential. For example, given the pressing issue of the climate crisis and lessons learned from the COVID-19 pandemic, we must surely reconceptualize undergraduate medicine and surgery curricula to turn away from the current emphasis on downstream hospital-based acute care to place more emphasis on upstream primary and community care. This is both an educational or curriculum development issue and a political one – fraught with power issues.

In the first half of the book – "Contradiction as Resource" – I look broadly at abstract issues before turning to concrete examples and activities in the second half of the book – "The Contradiction Cure". Saying this, I do have an aversion to separating out (and then opposing) "theory" and "practice". I prefer to think in terms of "praxis", or theory-in-action, where theories or hypotheses are not tested but rather evolve through stages of transformative questioning for possibility. Thus "the contradiction *cure*" is provisional, or 'under erasure' (c̶u̶r̶e̶), because in every cure is a potential side effect leading to a new symptom. The cure is a *pharmakon*, a healing poison. Thus, in part II, where I set out a blueprint for a medicine undergraduate curriculum as both political and aesthetic text, I imagine that this will not be to many educationalists' tastes, and parts of the blueprint remain untested and certainly under-developed – necessarily a work in progress. Paradoxically, then, the practical curriculum suggestions in Part II of the book are also conceptually demanding.

Throughout, I draw in particular upon Cultural-Historical Activity Theory (CHAT) (particularly the work of Yrjö Engeström); the curriculum reconceptualization movement (particularly the work of William Pinar); studies of biopower (particularly the work of Michel Foucault); the distribution of sensibility and emotional capital as a political issue (particularly the work of Jacques Rancière); and recent thinking on democracy (particularly the work of Michael Hardt and Antonio Negri).

In developing an argument for curriculum reconceptualization in medical education, I introduce the key role of the medical humanities in acting as a second stimulus in a double stimulation situation. This is a key idea and practice of the Russian psychologists Lev Vygotsky and Alexander Luria in particular, from the late 1920s and early 1930s. It is simple to grasp as an idea, but delicate in operation. Faced with a problem that seems intractable, Vygotsky found that children would find novel ways to move on from the problem or seek innovative approaches, if they were provided with a variety of parallel stimulus material to draw on, acting as "second stimulus" to the original problem. Adults use second stimuli in the same way, and often these appear serendipitously. In medical education, the arts and humanities have provided second stimuli that allow medical students to "think otherwise" about clinical issues. The medical humanities act as media for transformations of both agency and power, as we shall see.

If we return to the Ice Age hunter-gatherers described at the opening of this chapter, their development of cave paintings depicting animal forms, in particular, is often described as the origins of human art, beyond the aesthetics of stone and animal bone and horn tool making. It is viewed as a great leap of human consciousness in connecting sense perception, thinking and imagination to create a permanent language. But such images must have acted as double stimulation, modelling a core function of art and humanities. While hunters hunted, they also "thought otherwise" about the animals they hunted as sacred, offering up their lives for human survival. To ensure that the animal returns for the hunt next season, it must be revered and represented as a second stimulus and thanked for giving its life to maintain the life of the human community (Campbell 1988; Bleakley 2000).

The representation of the animal on the cave wall may be a "double" or a spirit appearing to the human as if manifesting from the depths of the rock. In the same way, the ubiquitous handprints of humans may not be a signature left by the artist, but rather the artist's own "ghost" hand coming back to meet him or her from the other side of the rock. This "doubling" too is a double stimulus causing an expansive leap in thinking and imagination. It is the shaman (the earliest "doctor") in the Palaeolithic hunting group who makes an imaginary ecstatic journey to an underworld in which s/he meets the spirit of the hunted animal and asks its forgiveness for being killed, or giving itself up for human life, to ensure its return next season. This hunt mythology provides a metaphor for all expansive learning, based on original contradiction and double stimulation.

As Michel Foucault (1976) famously argues in his historical reconstruction of the origins of modern diagnostic medicine from the late 18th century onwards, having "opened up a few corpses" in dissection, the doctor develops a medical gaze that "looks into" the body of the patient to locate the lesion (an area of abnormal tissue) that is the source of the disease whose expressive symptoms are all he has to go on (unless he is a dermatologist looking at the skin, or an opthalmologist looking at the eye as the most evolved part of the skin). This is akin to the shaman's journey, but now grounded in scientific certainty bolstered by the accompanying paraphernalia of laboratory tests. As the radiologist gazes at the images from X-rays and scans that allow direct access to the lesion, or the pathologist or laboratory scientist goes even deeper into flesh, investigating the qualities of blood samples, biopsies and tissue samples, is this not the contemporary equivalent of double stimulation and the shaman's journey to the underworld? Perhaps a closer parallel obtains in psychiatry, where the patient's language is divined and the lesion is heralded in the MRI brain scan, "speaking back" to patient and doctor.

References

Agamben G. 1998. *Homo Sacer: Sovereign Power and Bare Life*. Palo Alto, CA: Stanford University Press.

Bleakley A. 2000. *The Animalizing Imagination: Totemism, Textuality, and Ecocriticism*. PalgraveMacmillan.

Bleakley A. 2014. *Patient-Centred Medicine in Transition: The Heart of the Matter*. Dordrecht: Springer.

Borrill C, West MA, Shapiro D, Rees A. Team working and effectiveness in health care. *British Journal of Health Care Management*. 2013;6:364–71.

Campbell J. 1988 (2nd ed.) *The Way of the Animal Powers: Part 1 Historical Atlas of World Mythology*. Nashville TN: Vanderbilt University.

Cole M. Cultural psychology: a once and future discipline. *Nebraska Symposium on Motivation*. 1989;37:279–335.

Dawes DE. 2020. *The Political Determinants of Health*. Baltimore, MD: Johns Hopkins University Press.

Engeström Y. 1987. Learning by Expanding: An Activity-theoretical Approach to Developmental Research. Helsinki: Orienta-Konsultit Oy. Available at: http://lchc.ucsd.edu/mca/Paper/Engestrom/Learning-by-Expanding.pdf

Flannery K, Marcus J. 2012. *The Creation of Inequality: How Our Prehistoric Ancestors Set the Stage for Monarchy, Slavery, and Empire*. Cambridge, MA: Harvard University Press.

Foucault M. 1976. *The Birth of the Clinic: An Archaeology of Medical Perception*. London: Routledge.

Freedom House. 2018. Freedom in the World. Available at: https://freedomhouse.org/sites/default/files/2020-02/FH_FIW_Report_2018_Final.pdf

Hansen H, Metzl JM. New Medicine for the U.S. Health Care System: Training Physicians for Structural Interventions. *Academic Medicine*. 2017;92:279–81.

Keane J. 2009. *The Life and Death of Democracy*. London: Simon & Schuster.

Kershner I. 2020. In Israel, Modern Medicine Grapples With Ghosts of the Third Reich. *The New York Times*, May 14 2020. Available at: https://www.nytimes.com/2020/05/12/world/middleeast/nazi-medical-text-israel.html

Kripalani S, Bussey-Jones J, Katz MG, Genao I. A Prescription for Cultural Competence in Medical Education. *Journal of General Internal Medicine*. 2006;21:1116–20.

Kumagai AK, Lypson M. Beyond Cultural Competence: Critical Consciousness, Social Justice, and Multicultural Education. *Academic Medicine*. 2009;84:782–87.

Kumagai AK, Naidu T. On Time and Tea Bags: Chronos, Kairos, and Teaching for Humanistic Practice. *Academic Medicine*. 2020b; 95:512–17.

Lanting K, Dogra N, Hendrickx K, et al. 2019. Culturally Competent in Medical Education – European Medical Teachers' Self-Reported Preparedness and Training Needs to Teach Cultural Competence Topics and to Teach a Diverse Class. *MedEdPublish*. Available at: https://www.mededpublish.org/manuscripts/2188

Marmot M. 2015. *The Health Gap: The Challenge of an Unequal World*. London: Bloomsbury.

Metzl J, Hansen H. Structural competency: Theorizing a new medical engagement with stigma and inequality. *Social Science and Medicine*. 2014;103:126–33.

Metzl J, Petty J. Integrating and Assessing Structural Competency in an Innovative Prehealth Curriculum at Vanderbilt University. *Academic Medicine*. 2017;92:354–59.

Navarro V. 2007. *Neoliberalism, globalization, and inequalities: Consequences for health and quality of life*. London: Routledge.

Nussbaum MC. 2011. *Creating Capabilities: The Human Development Approach*. Cambridge, MA: Harvard University Press.

Sorensen J, Norredam M, Suurmond J, et al. Need for ensuring cultural competence in medical programmes of European universities. *BMC Medical Education*. 2019;19: 21.

Szasz T. 2007. *The Medicalization of Everyday Life. Selected Essays*. Syracuse NY: Syracuse University Press.

Part 1

Contradiction as resource

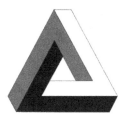

The Swedish artist Oscar Reutersvärd first created The Penrose triangle (above) - also known as the 'Penrose tribar' or 'the impossible triangle' - in 1934. The object can be depicted in a perspective drawing as an optical illusion, but cannot exist as a solid structure.

1 Politics

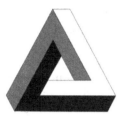

You are not welcome here, welcome!

At the acceleration of the coronavirus pandemic in America, with the death toll nearing 50,000 and rising (at the time of writing it is over 135,000 and rising), Dr Anthony Fauci, the primary medical and scientific advisor in the White House, said of his work: "You stay completely apolitical and non-ideological, and you stick to what you do. … I'm a scientist and I'm a physician. And that's it" (McCarthy 2019). Fauci, a distinguished public health expert, may have just been drawing a line between himself and the scientifically ignorant incumbent president of the United States, Donald Trump, a person who had overtly politicized the pandemic. Trump had supported conspiracy theories that China produced the virus in a laboratory, as well as right-wing protesters who took to the streets during lockdown, claiming that the government had curtailed their liberties.

In contrast, in the UK also at the height of the coronavirus crisis, Richard Horton, a doctor and longstanding editor of the prestigious medical journal *The Lancet*, vociferously challenged the UK government's response to the crisis as too little, too late. The government had dithered on mass testing and tracing, failed to acquire enough stock of personal protective equipment (PPE) for front-line healthcare workers, abandoned an early "acquisition of herd immunity" plan as both heartless and unworkable, and originally misreported numbers of deaths from COVID-19 by not including care home or domestic fatalities. In an interview with the *Financial Times*, Horton said, contra Fauci: "The idea you can strip out politics from medicine or health is historically ignorant. The medical establishment should be much more politicized, not less, in attacking issues like health inequalities and poor access to care" (Ahuja 2020).

Horton's claim can be backed up with any number of examples. Jacob King and Deniz Kaya (2016) – medical students from my own medical school, Plymouth Peninsula – have written a feisty critique of the lack of interest by doctors in party-political matters (noted first in a study by Grande and colleagues [Grande, Asch and Armstrong 2007] confirming voting apathy amongst doctors) that begins: "As a health professional working in a sterile environment one might easily find themselves feeling disparately removed from the slimy world of politics". This raises an interesting polemical standoff: sterile medicine versus slimy politics. But, actually, the authors note that one infects the other. Health professionals should not be passive observers of politics. The authors ask medical students and doctors to consider how they might influence healthcare through ballot-box politics.

Bram Wispelwey and Amaya Al-Orzza (2020) report a striking example of political influence upon health, one that should interest any medical student or doctor. We know that diabetes, along with respiratory and heart problems, is one of the pre-existing conditions making individuals vulnerable to serious development of COVID-19 infection. The authors note that Palestinian refugees on the West Bank have an incidence of 18% for diabetes and in Gaza 16%. This compares with 7.2% in Israel (Jaffe et al. 2017). These Palestinian refugees have poor diets, relying on cheap, highly calorific foods. There may be an ethnicity genetic predisposition whereby Arab populations show a higher incidence of diabetes than Jewish populations, but this is unlikely to be the principal cause (ibid.). A similar pattern can be seen amongst Indigenous Americans and African Americans, where the incidence of diabetes is twice as high as in the white, non-Hispanic population in North America.

Wispelwey and Al-Orzza (2020), in connecting the high incidence of diabetes in Palestinians, their political oppression and the subsequent impoverishment of lives, note that the "prevalence of the disease is linked to land dispossession, structural violence, colonial domination and oppression". Health and politics cannot be disentangled. As a consequence, the treatment of disease through medical intervention cannot be magically separated from conditions of inequity and inequality and their grounding and reinforcement in power structures. Downstream hospital medicine can no longer hide its gaze from upstream community health issues, where causes of ill health multiply under conditions of deprivation. Production of illness is the ghost industry that haunts the neo-liberal capitalist project. It compromises claims to democracy and shames the major proponents of our dominant modes of distribution of capital.

Such big issues trickle down to stain individuals' daily lives as forms of repression, often tangled up with identity politics as ills connected, for example, to ethnicity or gender. While a debate raged in the UK in the Spring of 2020 about the lack of availability of personal protective equipment (PPE) for frontline healthcare staff treating COVID-19 patients, this masked the fact that available PPE, such as masks, had been designed mainly for a larger male head template rather than for women, despite the fact that women make up 80% of the NHS workforce (https://digital.nhs.uk/data-and-information/publications/statistical/nhs-w

orkforce-statistics/march-2020). Absurdly, a survey showed that only one-third of women healthcare workers reported that their safety masks fitted properly, with more than a half of the rest reporting that ill-fitting masks hampered their work. But nothing was done to address this.

What relationship does, or should, medicine have with politics? This book widens that question to ask about the complex and often contradictory intersections between politics, aesthetics, medicine and medical education as these are mediated (and expanded) by the medical humanities (Figure 1.1). The book has no immediate close family as far as I am aware. Daniel Dawes' (2020) *The Political Determinants of Health* deals with relationships between politics and healthcare, but it is restricted to North America, focusing on the historical trials and tribulations of ObamaCare, and it does not engage at all with medical education or pressing issues such as health eco-literacy and the climate crisis.

There is significant literature in the fields of critical medical anthropology and sociology dealing with the relationships between healthcare and capitalist and socialist political systems, focused on health inequity and inequality, such as the work of Vicente Navarro (Navarro and Shi 2001, Navarro 2007, 2009), Howard Waitzkin (Waitzkin 1991; Waitzkin and Anderson 2020) and Hans Baer (Baer, Singer and Susser 2004). But this literature does not engage health pedagogies such as medical education, or the role of the medical humanities in educating medical students and doctors.

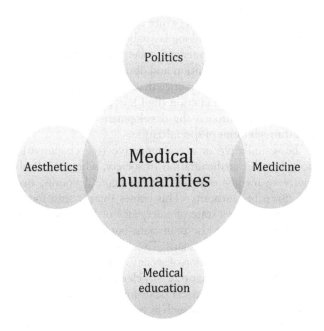

Figure 1.1 Intersections between politics, aesthetics, medicine and medical education with medical humanities as the mediator.

In this introductory section, I will define and delineate the areas this book addresses – medicine, medical education and politics – and begin to discuss their entanglements or intersections as a prelude to subsequent chapters. In chapter 2, I draw on aesthetics and medical humanities.

Medicine

Modern medicine is grounded in what Michel Foucault (1976) describes as the "birth of the clinic" (the modern hospital) in the late 18th century. Two practices in particular that delineated the birth of the profession of medicine conferred an identity construction and a code of practice: (i) learning anatomy through cadaver dissection, also providing a rite of passage into the profession; and (ii) doctors moving away from treating patients in their own homes, under the jurisdiction of the family, to treating patients in hospital (clinic) settings, thus gaining a "room of one's own" (to borrow from Virginia Woolf), having a uniform and developing a practice with an idiosyncratic language and code. The profession then closed ranks to cut off from public scrutiny and become an autonomous body, while patients were often objectified – treated as isolated symptoms or diseases rather than persons with symptoms embedded in a social context.

Medicine developed a "look" (Foucault's *le regard*), or a "gaze", in two senses. First, the doctor looked upon the patient as if looking into the dissected cadaver to see "into" the body for causes and effects of symptoms (lesions), isolating the person from his or her normal surrounds; and second, doctors came to gain a "look", or a self-presentation, through a uniform (white coats, stethoscopes) and a posture of confidence (Bleakley 2020b). Lifelong lay habits would be replaced by a set of "professional" habits. For example, medical students learned to control natural reactions of disgust through objectification and distancing so that medical students are educated for insensibility in a practice that calls out for deep sensibility – setting both a paradox and a contradiction (ibid.). In parallel, medicine adopted a quasi-militaristic structure through the development of a hierarchy based on experience gained through forms of specialization.

Medicine can broadly be assimilative or accommodative (see chapter 6). Assimilative medicine describes the medicalization of society, where medical interests shape social activity, or medicine is the Chronos figure devouring his own children in case they usurp his authority. This comes sharply into focus during epidemics and pandemics where a state of emergency or lockdown is in place, and the voices of authority are not the politicians but the medical and scientific community talking through the politicians. Thomas Szasz (2001, 2003, 2007), a psychiatrist, describes the medicalization of society as the emergence of a "pharmacracy" (see also Law 2006 and Montagne 2008). Here, society is dependent upon medical intervention such as pharmaceuticals for "everyday" anxiety and depression, beyond necessary interventions such as insulin for diabetics. But the society's psyche is shaped medically, thinking in terms of health and sickness even at the level of metaphor (a "healthy" economy), and framing life itself in terms of treatment regimes ("programmes"). Conversely, medicine can serve society or accommodate to it, acting as a critical friend. Here, medicine sits at a round table with social sciences, law, arts and humanities; is represented as popular culture in television "medi-soaps"; and invites collaboration with patients as experts in their own illnesses.

Medical education

Medical education – how medical students learn to become doctors (undergraduate), and the ongoing learning of doctors within a specialty (postgraduate and continuing) – is a species of pedagogy. Medical educators are not just clinicians; doctors in innovative medical schools have to learn basic and applied biomedical science, including anatomy, statistics, quantitative and qualitative research capabilities, communication and teamwork, education, psychotherapeutic skills, ethics, management, law, medical humanities and public engagement. Then there are the teachers who teach the teachers – those with pedagogical capabilities who educate, for example, anatomy teachers into good facilitative practices, and who design and evaluate curricula, to include assessment of learning. Medical education has the same academic apparatus as any discipline to include dedicated journals, conferences and academies.

From the late 18th century to the early 20th century, the medical "profession" was a craft guild with experts and apprentices who learned on the job. By the mid- to late-19th century, medicine was shaped more and more by science, such as Ignaz Semmelweis's discovery of the effects of hand sanitation from 1847, Louis Pasteur's late 1850s "germ theory" and Rudolf Virchow's late-19th-century work in pathology and public medicine showing how ill health and social deprivation are linked. How doctors were educated or trained, however, was unruly – haphazard and unregulated.

Modern medical education begins with Abraham Flexner's 1910 report on North American and Canadian medical schools and 1912 report on European medical schools. Flexner discovered that the majority of for-profit medical schools, run as businesses, were severely under-resourced and educationally naïve. As a result, many schools were closed rather than given resources to improve them, and these included schools that recruited women and African Americans (Hodges 2005). Perhaps as an unintended consequence, medical education was predominately white and male for over half a century after Flexner's report. Flexner also introduced a standard model of two years of laboratory-based dissection and science, followed by two or three years of largely hospital-based clinical experience. Downstream hospitalism became privileged over upstream primary and community care. Hospitalism, with its dress codes, ceremonies and intensivity or acute focus, was seen as sexier than community-based medicine and chronic care.

Since the 1960s, and influenced by the changes in social climate brought about by the Civil Rights and feminist movements, medical schools have slowly recruited women and black students. Women now constitute the majority of student intake globally – around 60%. Meanwhile, pedagogical methods have shifted from the transmission of knowledge and skills to interpretation models focused on learning by discovery and through experience and learning collaboratively. As medical culture changes – moving to more democratic structures such as patient-centredness and inter-professional teamwork – so traditions, such as learning anatomy through cadaver dissection and wearing white coats, have been challenged and changed (Bleakley 2020b). More radical pedagogies accept that the purpose of medical education is not simply to transmit known knowledge and skills (a "will-to-stability"), but also to develop climates in which innovation or the development of "possibility knowledge" can be fostered (Engeström 2018). This includes large-scale creative initiatives such as overhauling curricula, driven by emerging values including greater interest in public health and upstream issues – such as sources of health inequities and inequalities.

Meanwhile, medical education pedagogy remains in a fairly under-developed state globally, with some obvious sticking points when compared with pedagogical advances in other related disciplines such as clinical psychology, psychotherapy and counselling.

Medical education's pedagogical lack

1. There is a block in medical education about what "curriculum" can mean or be. There is an endless argument about content – what should and should not be "in" the curriculum. This mistakes syllabus for curriculum and takes our eye off the ball of meta-learning or learning to learn. Here, students do not learn "content" but learn how to access and critically think through issues pertinent to clinical work, whether grounded in science or the praxis of clinical work that has often been described as "science-using narrative work". This is a rather sweeping generalization, but medical education seems to have turned its back on the curriculum reconceptualization (Pinar 2006, 2011, 2012) movement that sees a curriculum as something to "think with", not something to be ingested and regurgitated. Medicine has what psychoanalysts would see as a fixation on "practical" or pragmatic activity, and brief flirtations with curriculum theory have ended badly, with medical educators irritated by the focus on theory rather than practice. They forget Kurt Lewin's aphorism that there is nothing so practical as a good theory. Later chapters in this book will grapple with these issues.
2. Work-based learning is central to medical education, but, with some outstanding exceptions, we do not do it well. For example, basics such as briefing and debriefing, to include scaffolding of new knowledge and skills, are often badly done or not done at all on work placements.
3. Given that collaborative learning is central to contemporary healthcare, it is strange how medical education has lagged in picking up on the value of socio-cultural and socio-material learning theories (Bleakley 2014). These approaches stress the important roles of mediating artefacts in learning (particularly important as we enter the age of artificial intelligence) and of the expansion of learning as innovation or the discovery of "possibility" through

collaboration. Part of the resistance to such approaches to learning, especially in North America, is that they eschew the individualism that is at the heart of the American way (Bellah et al. 2008); and, related to this objection, social learning theories have their origins in Soviet psychology that is both collectivist and dialectical-materialist. Further, such learning theories are grounded in the value of contradiction (see chapter 10) as engines of change. Conservative educators tend to feel uncomfortable with uncertainty and ambiguity, seeking resolutions.

4. If medical education were properly democratic, it would embrace rigorous, criteria-based self and peer assessment (Heron 1988; Orsmond 2004).

5. Medical schools are getting much better at this, but there is a history of poor emotional and psychological support for medical students, and this continues into junior doctoring and beyond (Peterkin and Bleakley 2017). Doctors are poor at looking after their own health, especially their mental health, and cultures of "gaining backbone", or expectations of resilience, still exist.

6. Where the evidence shows that tolerance of ambiguity is central to good medical practice, how will this be developed in a science-based culture that seeks resolutions? The medical humanities have been shown to provide a medium for the development of democratic habits, tolerance of ambiguity and humane approaches to others. It seems strange that the medical/ health humanities have not established themselves as core and compulsory elements of the curriculum, particularly as media, and "second stimulus", through which medicine can be "thought otherwise" or re-imagined.

Politics

Aristotle famously distinguishes between human and animal life by pointing to humanity's explicit need for regulation of social interaction through custom and law: "Man is by nature a political animal". This view is, properly, contested by cognitive ethologists who suggest that animal communities can be seen to engage socially through power structures that in turn structure communities (Abbate 2016). "Politics" comes from the ancient Greek *polis* or "city state". Fifth-century BCE Athens is often described as the first city-state to experiment with democratic votes through assembly (although only male citizens could vote, excluding women, slaves and exiles), although John Keane (2009) discusses widespread experiments with democracy prior to this across what is now the Middle East. The work of administering *polis* is *politeia* – the root of "police", where politics is about enforcement of law or custom and boundary making.

Kinds of power

Power, suggests Louis Althusser (2008), results in "ideological interpellation" – insertion into a social position that affords an identity, usually prescribed for us by dominant ideology. There is nothing that we think or do that is not subject to a value position that in turn shapes subjectivity. As values change, so subjectivities change (as a sense of self in the face of the Other), and as values are introjected, so persons follow predictable scripts or are inserted into cultures by playing out scripted roles. Interpellation into medicine once meant being apolitical or suspending political beliefs – but doctors are already socialized into wider political structures than their profession, such as a capitalist or a socialist system (compare a doctor who trained in Miami and is now in private practice as a successful aesthetic surgeon, with a doctor who trained in Cuba and now works for Doctors without Borders). Such professional interpellations can be complex and contradictory: a UK general practitioner works for the socialized NHS but runs the practice as a business.

The American social psychologists John French and Bertram Raven's (1959) typology of power was for many years the most influential modern text on the subject, eagerly studied by management in the post-World War II boom in corporate settings. In the 1958 chapter (published in two texts), five types were described:

1. Reward power (based on incentives such as tax cuts).
2. Coercive power (based on exercising bribes, penalties and threats)
3. Legitimate power (exercise of the law or custom)
4. Referent power (influence through identification, respect and trust, such as friendship)
5. Expert power (authority rests in expert knowledge or skills)

In 1965, French and Raven added a sixth component: (6) Informational power (the person may not exert power, but the information he or she holds does). The late 1950s and early 1960s produced a fetish object in psychology and organizational studies: "leadership" as a commodity. Having seen how absolute power can corrupt in the rise of Hitler and the Nazi party, North American psychologists were keen to square the values of personal liberty and entrepreneurship. Politics must be like a business. Medicine too must be based on a business model, with business-headed leaders. Doctors may have expert power, but that is not enough. Hospitals and healthcare systems must be run by people with management leadership capabilities, reward power giving way to referent power: respect for the boss.

We can add to French and Raven's typology: (7) power through deceit such as lying, cheating or dissimulating. Niccolò Machiavelli (1469–1527) preceded Hobbes and is perhaps history's most infamous political philosopher. In *The Prince*, Machiavelli famously advised that rulers gain more respect through fear than love or compassion, and thinking-on-your-feet realpolitik (practical responses and shifting values) always outlives political idealism. This remark by the British neurosurgeon and writer Henry Marsh is surely Machiavellian: we "have a very complicated relationship with patients … as soon as we have any interaction with patients, we start lying. We have to. There is nothing more frightening for a patient than an anxious or doubtful doctor" (in Adams 2017). Anybody who has experienced corridor talk – or rather gossip – in hospitals will know that such institutions paradoxically thrive on Machiavellian intrigue. Hospital managers soon learned that referent power, or charisma, was not enough to get by with in climates of cutthroat competition. Chief executives would quickly turn Machiavellian.

French and Raven's typology also assumes rational powers, so we can add a further category to the seven above: (8) irrational power through attraction and charisma, a kind of perverse referent power if the charisma is grounded in manipulation. Goodyear-Smith and Buetow (2001) have simplified French and Raven's typology, recognizing just three kinds of power:

(i)   muscle (force)
(ii) money (material)
(iii) mind (knowledge)

aligning more with Machiavellian realpolitik.

Sovereign power

Politics is the study of power, and power has three main faces: sovereign, capillary and absence of power, or powerlessness. Macro-politics, or sovereign power, describes power over others – by force or through the law, legitimate or illegitimate – as either a normal condition or as a "state of exception" (for example, during an emergency such as an epidemic, war or constitutional crisis). Theocracies and autocracies exert ultimate dictatorial power. Plutocracies shift the power base to the wealthy.

Democracies focus power in elected groups – governments, the police, councils and so forth – but can exert this in a sovereign way on the basis of being the elected party. This creates anomalies and anachronisms where the effects of a contemporary democracy can feel like living in a medieval kingship. Because of the multiplicity of parties, votes are divided and the governing party represents a minority of the voters, or, because of the nature of the electoral system, an American president or a British prime minister can be sworn in without receiving the majority of the public vote. Democracy in any case is best described as a project in the making, and, as the most complex of political forms, it has differing faces (Foreign Affairs May/June 2018).

John Keane (2009) distinguishes between three kinds of democracy: assembly, representative and monitory. The ancient world modelled public assembly democracy, where in certain cities all male citizens could gather, listen to or participate in the debate, and vote by a show of hands. Such public assemblies originated in the Middle East around 2500 BCE and spread throughout classical Greece and Rome, also engaging the Islamic world until around 950. Keane notes that rural assemblies in Iceland and the Faroe Islands in particular replaced such city-based assemblies. Iceland's field-based common assembly lasted from 930 to 1800. As noted, Athenian assemblies of the 5th century BCE were not the earliest, and also not necessarily the best, model of such assemblies, where women, slaves and foreigners were excluded.

A second historical phase of democracy occurred from around the 10th century as a representative democracy, the model we are most familiar with today. Assembly democracies are popular at a grassroots level to address local issues and may be invited nationally through occasional referenda, but the government of a large population requires elected representation in a national assembly or parliament. Such democracies are nevertheless fragile. As Keane (ibid.: xvii) notes, by the 12th century, forms of parliamentary assemblies were common across the Atlantic region – Europe and the east coast of the Americas, but "It ended on a sorry note, with the near destruction worldwide of democratic institutions and ways of life by the storms of mechanized war, dictatorship and totalitarian rule that racked the first half of the twentieth century". There was a fear on the part of the ruling classes that government by the multitude would lead to anarchy. While necessarily bureaucracy-heavy, the English Civil War revolution in the mid-17th century, the French and American revolutions in the late 18th century, and the Haitian slave uprising against French colonial rule in 1791–1804 showed that representative democracy was a functional and fairer alternative to monarchies or colonial oppression. There would always be major contradictions to such models – particularly women not being given the vote, and the continuation of slavery in America until the Civil War aftermath and subsequent outcomes of civil rights legislation.

Keane suggests that we are entering an era of what he calls "monitory" democracy, where global organizations such as the United Nations and the World Health Organization can monitor and help shape a new world order. This is a surveillance democracy, where the rules of democracy themselves are democratized, despised by right-wing libertarians. Keane is right about this emerging global era, fractious and fragile as it is, but what he misses is that such a monitory democracy functions largely through capillary power rather than sovereign power, as discussed below. Sovereign power is the work of an explicit authority traditionally bent on submission, so that power is oppressive and repressive. Capillary power is a generative or productive force running through all activity that can be ordered, such as an introjected moral conscience or a will for good, as a "habit of the heart" (Bellah et al. 2008). Monitory democracy will not be imposed from above but will grow from below, as social conscience, and its engines are social media that can network the populus. This is relational power, a contemporary formulation evident in the work of Michael Hardt and Antonio Negri (2000, 2006, 2009, 2017), who envisage an emergent "multitude" and "common wealth" as a reaction against class-based neoliberal capitalism, or rampant free-market economics, that they see as inevitably collapsing in the face of the climate crisis and the balance in the world order shifting from American dominance to the influence of China.

Democracies may mask plutocracies, in which power follows wealth, and so an outwardly democratic structure actually serves to benefit those who are already privileged through holding wealth or capital resources such as access to fossil fuel, property or land. Democracies can resort to authoritative rule without the normal processes of representative votes during a state of emergency (such as the COVID-19 pandemic, or in times of civil unrest, with policed "lockdowns"). Mature, or "technical", democracies advertise relational power – informed collaborative or collective decision-making through compromise, exercised particularly through "micro-democracies" as "hybrid forums" – local, town hall and community debates that feed into larger parliamentary structures (Callon, Lascoumes and Barthe 2011).

Michel Callon and colleagues (ibid.) make a distinction between delegative, deliberative and dialogic democracies. In a delegative process, advertised in particular through the way that governments have drawn on scientific advice during the coronavirus pandemic to guide policy, experts pass on their judgements to politicians who act on them as they see fit and then announce policy to the public. The public learns one thing through formal presentations from government, and another through the media's investigative journalists, who may have accessed leaked material that shows the reality of the situation. For example, scientific advice may be discarded, distorted or manipulated (data can be presented in such a way that it flatters the government even when it is actually bad news). In a deliberative process, the public can hear experts' views in small forums that allow for debate. A consensus is aimed at. The job of politicians is then to frame activity and legislation around the advice they receive from such hybrid forums.

Hybrid forums developed from consensus conferences were initiated in the USA but pursued in Denmark in particular as Citizens' Conferences. Their success depends upon the selection of participants who receive education in how to conduct a hybrid forum based on dialogue with experts. The outcomes of forums may not be consensus. These structures, suggests Callon and colleagues (ibid.: x), are not necessarily about "agreement" but rather learning and expanding dialogical activity, where "democracy will not be increased by seeking agreements at any cost. Politics is the art of dealing with disagreements, conflicts, and oppositions; why not bring them out, encourage them, and multiply them, for that is how unforeseen paths are opened up and possibilities increased". This intensively contradictory situation affords dialogic democracy: a democratization of democracy itself.

Such hybrid forums can act as nodes of resistance to centralized government. Callon and colleagues, as noted, importantly describe their work not in terms of end points or clean and clear conclusions, but rather to multiply uncertainties. The work of hybrid forums is summarized below.

The work of hybrid forums

1. To challenge the view that the knowledge of specialists cannot be grasped by laypersons, by inviting specialists to engage with the lay public, as "public engagement" work. This may be arts-based: in galleries, performance spaces and so forth.

2. To encourage secluded research (for example in laboratories) to "come out" and engage a lay audience in public spaces. This can extend to, for example, autopsies (such as Gunther von Hagens' notorious televised autopsy) (https://www.youtube.com/playlist?list=PLV6F-vYLHBFar7mIb5hLtm3-7 g-N5XLhD). There are already established art movements that draw on

laboratory-based scientific work to make this accessible to the public (http s://cordis.europa.eu/project/id/266682).

3. To provide consensus conferences and other hybrid forums representative of delegative democracy and transform these into dialogic democracy.

4. To develop new pedagogies to inform, explore and explain the work of hybrid forums where collective and collaborative learning generates new objects of inquiry and experiments with new social configurations. For example, medicine curricula are designed with scientific, clinical and pedagogical experts sitting alongside "expert patients" (persons who are experts in their own illnesses) and laypersons, given an equal voice.

In the same vein as hybrid forums, Pierre Rosanvallon (2018) describes a "democracy beyond elections", pointing to the contradiction that our regimes are democratic, but we fail to govern democratically. There has been a shift globally, for example, to presidential styles of government even where parliamentary democracies exist. Rosanvallon suggests that elected central governments must maintain touch with the populus as a "permanent democracy" through large-scale exercises in consultation. In other words, the populus must discipline its elected executives. This can lead to technocracy and burnout on the part of the populus through extended referenda. Some medical schools, such as my own (Peninsula UK), have experimented with forms of "permanent democracy" through the executive's relationship to a student parliament acting as a counterweight to critical decision-making. Certainly at the curriculum planning level, it is common for students to sit on decision-making groups.

Such intensive dialogic spaces provide a model for future medical education. Hybrid forums for example can readily be set up within medical schools and inter-professional health faculties to involve the lay public in the role of "patient voice" and to include hybrid experts such as actor patients familiar with simulation learning for clinical and communication skills. However, they do require expert facilitation, where the intensity of dialogue inevitably raises emotional issues, some of which may remain unresolved and may be brought to the forum "charged". In chapter 14, I suggest that all medical students should learn co-counselling as a way to better engage in dialogical democracy, and this could apply to any hybrid forum participants. Given the public unrest during the coronavirus pandemic in relationship to many politicians' handling of advice received from scientific experts, Callon and colleagues' (2011: 9) cautionary note is apposite: "Science and technology cannot be managed by the political institutions currently available to us … they must be enriched, expanded, extended, and improved so as to bring about … technical democracy".

In democracies too, it is all too easy for authority structures or hierarchies to emerge or fail to transform, overriding democratic habits – such as default-position, or habitual, hierarchical teams in surgical contexts. A typical tactic of more authority-led surgeons who do not exercise a dialogical imagination, but prefer monologue (telling, cajoling, challenging rather than asking or debating), is to set up a mini state of emergency in the operating theatre by invoking, typically, a siege mentality, such as "siege by management" or "bureaucracy" (for example, clinical guidelines that challenge established habits – "this is the way we do things around here"). The surgeon sets up a climate in which all must rally around his (rarely "her") directives (Bleakley 2014).

During the coronavirus pandemic, governments too took the opportunity to declare a state of emergency. This gave them powers to take independent decisions without due process of debate and vote. For example, the UK government typically took decisions *for* the National Health Service (NHS) to implement, rather than *with* the NHS (for example through forums).

Capillary power

The poet Wallace Stevens makes a distinction between two kinds of energy: "force" and "presence". "Force" is power acting on things to change them. "Presence" is power inherent in things as a living expression of potential. In *The History of Sexuality: An Introduction*, Michel Foucault (1980: 136) turns the notion of power as a controlling authority (Stevens' "force") on its head to describe a subtler form of power (Stevens' "presence"): "a power bent on generating forces, making them grow, and ordering them, rather than one dedicated to impeding them, making them submit, or destroying them". While Foucault describes this "capillary" power as one that generates "force", his descriptions are closer to Stevens' notion of "presence" – an inherent capability for productive formation and change that runs through any system.

As "capillary", the power reaches into every aspect of life; and more, into every fibre of the body – as potential, as well as regulation and modulation (biopower at the individual level). In chapter 7, I look at capillary power in more depth, as this morphs (in Foucault's scheme) to "biopolitics" and "governmentality" – various strategies that come to shape and control persons at the level of the public body, as positive transformations in the way that we are governed. This includes the development of formal provision of public health. I discuss these later in terms of a strategy of resistance to authoritative sovereign power.

Capillary power can be treated as a metaphor, a poetic device that helps us to imagine a web of forces like a mycorrhizal spread (Engeström 2008), a hidden, symbiotic permeating presence ready to energize or organize an activity. Power here is an impetus to collaborative leaps of the imagination feeding into an activity that is inconceivable at the personal level but achievable when we are "connected" (Oliver 2020). Such a web also operates in the world implicitly to grease social exchanges, as "manners" and "social responsibility" – importantly through bodily presence and intimacy. Without this, there would be no acting on conscience for social responsibility that the psychologist Alfred Adler called "fellow feeling", "community feeling" and "social interest" (*gemeinschaftsgefühl*) (see Papanek 1963 for an account of how "social interest" underpins and shapes social justice activism). Further, there would be no "self help" in looking after one's own health (something, so the research literature (Bleakley 2020b) tells us that doctors are notoriously poor at – a medical conundrum and contradiction).

We need a poetic imagination to capture the beauty of Foucault's notion of capillary power at the bodily level. The American poet Ralph Waldo Emerson said: "The poet turns the world to glass" (*The Poet* 12–13), or makes the invisible visible. His successor, Walt Whitman, celebrated the body with the same vision as Foucault, a poetic form of medical gaze: "The thin red jellies within you or within me, the bones and/ the marrow in the bones/ the exquisite realization of health" – not just an anatomical listing or "naming of parts" but also a celebration of Wallace Stevens' "presence" over "force".

In his later lectures on power, Foucault (2008), as noted above, coined the terms "biopolitics" and "governmentality" to describe an embodied biopower at the level of the population as well as the individual. Governmentality refers to a host of historically and culturally inflected ways in which the body of the populace is controlled or controls itself. A recent example has been the ready adoption of the habits of "lockdown" and "social distancing" during the coronavirus pandemic. Capillary power morphing into governmentality as a "presence" rather than a "force" (legislative rule) exhibits literally in the ways that the body is regulated by introjected values that make up a social-sensory fabric: we willingly exercise and eat well at one end of the scale, or we refuse to look after our bodies through poor diet and lack of exercise at the other end. From a health biopower perspective, the first habit is conformist and welcome as it ultimately places less strain on healthcare, while the laissez-faire attitude of letting the body go is a form of resistance to an introjected governmentality as a pattern of health rules. Simultaneously introjected and distributed, biopower as governmentality is then a way of governing a population body without explicit (sovereign power) government, while maintaining the possibility of resistance that any liberal democracy will tolerate or encourage. Introjected biopower and public governmentality often conflict in the field of health. For example, recreational drug taking continues for personal pleasure in the face of legislative control of such drugs as a health safeguard.

Capillary power as governmentality is then a micro-political power that runs through a system, often unnoticed or unaccounted for. Its most common form is again "naturalized" power operating on the body and between bodies. This can be experienced, again, as surveillance of the body in other-control or self-control (personal hygiene, public hygiene, diets, exercise regimes). Where sovereign power has a number of regimes of truth – verifiable fact through scientific experiment, observation, opinion or religious belief – capillary power is usually productive, rather than controlling, where its primary telos is the formation of identity. Capillary power works primarily to produce subjectivities. We will meet many examples of such power effects in discussing how medical students (as proto-professionals) learn to take on the identities of "doctor" and "professional".

Powerlessness

Beyond sovereign and capillary power (power exerted) is powerlessness. While Aristotle suggested that what distinguishes humans from other animals is our political will, thus separating nature from culture, we might think that the most natural political force of nature is life morphing into death. As the Preface notes, death is the most natural of powers as the universal exercise of entropy, while it is medicine's sworn cultural role to thwart nature's death drive. This is a power struggle, a political venture, whether it is critical interventions in downstream hospitalism or "at source" prevention in deep upstream primary and community care.

Beyond facing death, powerlessness is the absence of personal power in conditions of carrying a stigma, exile, isolation, lockdown, ecological disaster, refugee status from war, political and religious conflict, homelessness and extreme poverty, imprisonment, isolation and loneliness, mobility challenges, mental illness such as psychotic episodes and the body under anaesthetic and in coma. Stripped of power and a point of identification, and often in transit, such a person may struggle to form an identity. Powerlessness can also be experienced by subjection to an authority that restricts personal choices, such as women under strict Islamic law or excommunicated individuals.

Powerlessness and states of emergency are particularly pertinent to learning medicine and surgery, as often high-risk endeavours. Patients who become seriously acutely ill can lose all sense of power as they put themselves in the hands of professional healthcare. This is a kind of political exile in which capillary power can dry up and the sovereign power of medicine is the mirror into which such patients look, sometimes in a state of terror or at least high anticipation. Medical students in this circumstance can then reconceptualize patient-centredness as a power structure where the patient paradoxically has no power and must be empowered, at a minimum, for dignity. Early years medical students are, by definition, powerless as they lack status through clinical experience. The primary form of power they do possess is emotional integrity, but this capital too, as explored particularly in chapter 9, is appropriated as part of the fabric of the sensible, or the aesthetic fabric of the medical culture. Here, seniors decide how emotional capital might be re-distributed through pedagogic interactions with students focused on "professionalism" or historically conditioned approved patterns of behaviour with patients and students.

The UK General Medical Council's "Outcomes for Graduates" (GMC 2018a) offers a blueprint for undergraduate medical education, stating the professional capabilities and values for newly qualified doctors. Medical students and newly qualified doctors should be able to "Recognise the potential impact of their attitudes, values, beliefs, perceptions and personal biases (which may be unconscious) on individuals and groups and identify personal strategies to address this". This is an example of how institutionalized medicine appropriates the emotional capital of medical students under the guise of emancipating them and their patients and colleagues. Students, as voting citizens capable of intimate relationships, and who we consider are old enough to be sent to war, must be reminded that their self-presentation to others has an effect. Is this not patronizing? Are they supposed to strip themselves back to value-free persons (robots) prior to being re-educated, or indeed, re-programmed?

Students can resist the stripping of emotional capital in various ways: through formal sovereign power institutional forums such as students' parliaments, formal feedback, mentorial sessions and research into areas such as professional lapses by seniors, and through capillary forms of resistance such as inauthentic play acting as supplication, and "sly civility" or tactics of sarcasm disguised as compliance. Resistance is intrinsic to power. It is central to power plays and has many faces. I devote three separate chapters to the topic (chapters 7, 8 and 9).

Identity politics

Following from Foucault's analysis of the making of subjectivities as an exercise of power, and Giorgio Agamben's (1993, 1998) "Homo Sacer" – the person who is set adrift from civil society or stigmatized, such as, again, the immigrant without rights; those displaced by famine, conflict or natural disaster; the homeless; the person without healthcare cover; the severely disabled; those kept in a coma; the lonely; the sectioned; the abused living in a permanent state of fear; and those with severe memory loss – "politics" and "identity" have now fused. Identity politics, as the list above shows, has two faces. One is a face of pride, reclamation, statement and affiliation (such as gender identities and fluidities in the LGBTQ movement); the other a face of shame or despair, such as the homeless, the disfigured and persons displaced by conflict or natural disaster, given "refugee" status that affords both stigma and identity. In light of the "Black Lives Matter" consciousness-raising and social activism movement, we now recognize clearly that structural racism has produced populations of the "configured" acting as scapegoats for not only explicit white supremacy but also implicit and cumulative micro-aggressions by a white majority. This, as we shall see, has consequences for the health of the black and ethnic minority communities.

Identity politics flowered in the late 1960s to parallel party politics. Here, gender, sexual, racial, ethnic, religious, disability, social and cultural groups offer the bases for identity constructions. It is in this arena, through a focus on social justice issues within the medical/health humanities, that medical education has primarily engaged openly and expressively with politics. This has grown partly out of medical ethics' interests in issues such as gender bias in pharmaceutical trials (bias towards male participants even where women turn out to be the major consumers of a drug). For example, women are twice as likely as men to be prescribed antidepressants, and one in eight women worldwide takes antidepressants, yet pregnant women are excluded from clinical trials, with drug companies arguing that they do not want to expose the foetus to potential harm (van der Graaf et al. 2018).

In the arena of identity politics, "disability" in particular has become a central issue, with a new politics of protest emerging over the negative connotations or stigma of "disability". And thanks to the work of advocates such as Therese "Tess" Jones at the University of Colorado, disability studies are prominent in contemporary medical/health humanities. In an interview with Cynthia Pasquale (2019), Tess Jones says that some people "think of medical humanities as frivolous or simply enrichment, but over the years, I've witnessed a strong political and social advocacy in which the arts are critical".

As examples of self-advocacy, "deafness" has been redefined by radical "ability" proponents as another kind of human capability, rather than restrictive, with its own culture and language of signs. The "dis-" in "disability" has been roundly challenged. So-called gypsies have re-oriented around the term "Romany travellers" (distinct from "Travellers", who identify with a nomadic lifestyle but do not identify with traditional Romany culture) to challenge stigma. But identity politics also has a sinister side that can be seen with the rise of neo-fascist white nationalist groups, extreme evangelicals and belligerent terrorist cells. In medicine, particularly through the rise of social media, people have come to identify through their illnesses, particularly with rare physical conditions and widely with mental health support groups, where "patients" lose this identity tag by becoming experts in their own conditions, often forming support groups through social media networking.

Identity politics can be traced to the Suffragette movement of the early 20th century and the Pacifist movement during the two world wars, but it was given a high profile by the Civil Rights and "first wave" feminist movements of the 1960s and 1970s. Identity politics are also advertised by anti-colonialist resistance movements such as Mahatma Ghandi's non-violent protests against British colonization of India over more than 30 years, from 1919 to 1948, and the psychiatrist Franz Fanon's support of the protest in the Algerian resistance movement against French occupation from 1954 to his death in 1961. Again, a resurgence of Black Lives Matter has recently injected new passions into identity politics inviting activism.

The private, the public and what is held in common

Asked what comes to mind if medicine is mentioned in the same breath as politics and you might say "the difference between private and public medicine". This would equate with medicine as a business for profit (private) and medicine as a public service supported by taxation and donation (public). Both of these are forms of capitalism, one "hard" (private medicine as businesses set up for profit), and the other "soft" (a government providing public healthcare through the investment of capital gained through taxation). The former is capitalist medicine, the latter socialist – or state capitalist – medicine. The idea of the latter – as advertised in, for example, the UK's National Health Service (NHS) – is that a society in principle does not compete for healthcare services, with an understanding that healthcare provision is a collaborative effort in which some people will benefit more than others. The benefit of the latter is the provision of a safety net for all as accident is just as likely to lead to medical intervention as sickness. The much-admired NHS, as noted above, is in fact constituted by 75% public ownership through the state and 25% privatized.

Globally, we are so entrenched in neo-liberal capitalism as the only viable economic model, advertised through the "growth" of economies, that we find it difficult to envisage other models. We also, strangely, equate capitalism with democracy (free choice as free-market or open competition). In principle, however, there is an alternative to individual venture capitalism for profit and socialism or state capitalism supported by taxation that is reinvested in the market economy. Indeed, while we embrace democracies of various kinds, there is a fundamental block to our development of better democracy (eradicating poverty and fundamental inequity and inequality) where we have top-down imposition of democracy because we are always choosing between two alternative forms of capitalism: competitive free-market neo-liberalism and state capitalism as the acceptable face of socialism.

The alternative, described in the work of Michael Hardt and Antonio Negri (2000, 2006, 2009, 2017), is a bottom-up society in which the "multitude" or populus have genuine and widespread access to political life based on common wealth and not just on economic wealth. The idea of an authentic "patient-centred" and "inter-professional" medicine would be a model of the multitude drawing on common wealth. Despite claims that "patient-centredness" is now every day in healthcare (Bleakley 2014), this remains a radical "horizon" model for medicine, where embracing multitude and common wealth has not yet been achieved. We have yet to realize a "patient-directed" medicine, although models for this exist, such as "informed" patient groups with unique conditions who form support networks online and remain in touch with the latest research in their field of disease or disability, as mentioned above.

By "common wealth" I mean that which we hold in common as beyond private ownership and manipulation that affords the quality of life: (i) aspects of the natural world in which we all participate such as breathing air, swimming in fresh or sea waters and watching and listening to animal life (all of which have been shown to have effects on health and quality of life); (ii) a social life free from oppression or coercion, following democratic principles of collaboration, debate and compromise; and (iii) ownership of our bodies and their dispositions in human relationships, particularly our affective or emotional lives, without subjugation or abuse. Capitalism, necessarily divisive and exploitative, should have no claim on such common wealth.

In this chapter, we have seen how medicine, medical education and politics are entangled to form complex webs of associations. In the following chapter, I introduce aesthetics and ethics into this complex, referring in particular to the varied roles of the medical humanities in medical education. As we embrace the engagements of politics and medicine in medical education, we find ourselves facing a number of key contradictions. The medical humanities can act as a second stimulus to allow us to think differently about such contradictions, although we are still in for a bumpy ride.

If the worlds we are entering through the subject matter of this book are non-linear, or complex, systems, then politics, aesthetics, ethics and medical education are phase-space attractors – models towards which such systems may evolve but in ways that evade linear modelling. The medical humanities may be thought of as a strange attractor. Here, deep transformations can occur where two points on the attractor are close together and multiply intensities of change. I am think-ing of the two faces of the medical humanities as in an embrace and kiss: first, the arts and humanities applied to medicine to increase its power; and second, the study of the culture of medicine through the inter-disciplinary arts and humani-ties such as the history of medicine, where medicine is appreciated more deeply, while its educational or pedagogical aspects are treated as secondary or even ignored (Bleakley 2020a).

Bibliography

Abbate CE. "Higher" and "Lower" Political Animals: A Critical Analysis of Aristotle's Account of the Political Animal. *Journal of Animal Ethics*. 2016;6:54–66.

Adams T. Henry Marsh: The Mind–Matter Problem is Not a Problem for me, Mind is Matter. NEUROSCIENCE: *The Observer*, 16 July 2017. Available at: https://www.the guardian.com/science/2017/jul/16/henry-marsh-mind-matter-not-a-problem-inte rview-neurosurgeon-admissions

Agamben G. 1993. *The Coming Community*. Minneapolis, MI: University of Minnesota Press.

Agamben G. 1998. *Homo Sacer: Sovereign Power and Bare Life*. Palo Alto, CA: Stanford University Press.

Ahuja A. Richard Horton: "It's the Biggest Science Policy Failure in a Generation": Lunch with the FT Richard Horton. *Financial Times*, 25/26 April, 2020: 3. Available at: https://www.ft.com/content/8e54c36a-8311-11ea-b872-8db45d5f6714

Allthusser L. 2008. *On Ideology*. London: Verso.

Baer HA, Singer M, Susser I. 2004 *Medical Anthropology and the World System*, 2nd ed. Westport, CT: Praeger.

Bellah RN, Madsen R, Sullivan WM, et al. 2008. *Habits of the Heart: Individualism and Commitment in American Life*. Berkeley, CA: University of California Press.

Bleakley A. 2014. *Patient-centred Medicine in Transition: The Heart of the Matter*. Dordrecht: Springer.

Bleakley A. 2020a. Don't Breathe a Word: A Psychoanalysis of Medicine's Inflations. In: A Bleakley (ed.) *Routledge Handbook of the Medical Humanities*. Abingdon: Routledge, 129–35.

Bleakley A. 2020b. *Educating Doctors' Senses Through The Medical Humanities: "How Do I Look?"* Abingdon: Routledge.

Callon M, Lascoumes P, Barthe Y. 2011. *Acting in an Uncertain World: An Essay of Technical Democracy*. Cambridge, MA: MIT Press.

Dawes DE. 2020. *The Political Determinants of Health*. Baltimore, MD: Johns Hopkins University Press.

Engeström Y. 2008. *From Teams to Knots: Activity-Theoretical Studies of Collaboration at Work*. Cambridge: Cambridge University Press.

Engeström Y. 2018. *Expertise in Transition: Expansive Learning in Medical Work*. Cambridge: Cambridge University Press.

Foreign Affairs. *Is Democracy Dying?: A Global Report*. Vol. 97, May/June 2018.

Foucault M. 1976. *The Birth of the Clinic: An Archaeology of Medical Perception*. London: Routledge.

Foucault M. 1980. *The History of Sexuality: Vol I. An Introduction*. New York: Vintage Books.

Foucault M. 2008. *The Birth of Biopolitics: Lectures at the Collège de France 1978–1979*. London: Palgrave Macmillan.

French J, Raven B. 1959. The Bases of Social Power. In: D Cartwright (ed.) *Studies in Social Power*. Ann Arbor, MI: Institute for Social Research, 150–67.

General Medical Council (GMC). 2018a. Outcomes for Graduates. Available at: https://www.gmc-uk.org/-/media/documents/dc11326-outcomes-for-graduates-2018_pdf-7504 0796.pdf

Goodyear-Smith F, Buetow S. Power Issues in the Doctor–Patient Relationship. *Health Care Analysis*. 2001;9:449–62.

Grande D, Asch DA, Armstrong K. Do Doctors Vote? *Journal of General Internal Medicine*. 2007;22:585–89.

Hardt M, Negri A. 2000. *Empire*. Cambridge, MA: Harvard University Press.

Hardt M, Negri A. 2006. *Multitude.: War and Democracy in the Age of Empire*. London: Penguin.

Hardt M, Negri A. 2009. *Commonwealth*. Cambridge, MA: Harvard University Press.

Hardt M, Negri A. 2017. *Assembly*. Oxford: Oxford University Press.

Heron, J. 1988. Assessment Revisited. In: D Boud. (ed.) *Developing Student Autonomy in Learning*. London: Kogan Page, 77–90.

Hodges B. The Many and Conflicting Histories of Medical Education in Canada and the USA: An Introduction to the Paradigm Wars. *Medical Education*. 2005;39:613–21.

Jaffe A, Giveon S, Wulffhart L, et al. Adult Arabs Have Higher Risk for Diabetes Mellitus than Jews in Israel. 8 May 2017. Available at: https://doi.org/10.1371/journal.pone.017 6661; https://journals.plos.org/plosone/article?id=10.1371/journal.pone.0176661

Keane J. 2009. *The Life and Death of Democracy*. London: Simon & Schuster.

King J, Kaya D. Clinicians Should Understand How They Can Use the Ballot Box to Advance Their Patients' Health Interests. *Medical Humanities Blog, Politics and Medicine*, December 2016. Available at: https://blogs.bmj.com/medical-humanities /2016/12/09/politics-and-medicine/

Law J. 2006. *Big Pharma: How the World's Drug Companies Control Illness*. London: Constable.

McCarthy J. 3 Ways People in Poverty Suffer the Most From Pollution. *Global Citizen*, 17 May 2019. Available at: https://www.globalcitizen.org/en/content/how-pollution-affects-the-poor/

Montagne M. Review: Thomas Szasz. The Medicalization of Everyday Life. Selected Essays. *American Journal of Pharmacy Education*. 2008;72:123.

Navarro V. 2007. *Neoliberalism, Globalization, and Inequalities: Consequences for Health and Quality of Life*. London: Routledge.

Navarro V. What We Mean by Social Determinants of Health. *International Journal of Health Services*. 2009;39:423–41.

Navarro V, Shi L. The Political Context of Social Inequalities and Health. *International Journal of Health Services*. 2001;31:1–21.

Oliver T. 2020. *The Self Delusion: The Surprising Science of How We Are Connected and Why That Matters*. London: Weidenfeld & Nicolson.

Orsmond P. 2004. Self- and Peer-Assessment: Guidance on Practice in the Biosciences. Leeds: Centre for Bioscience: Higher Education Academy. Available at: https://www.ucl.ac.uk/teaching-learning/sites/teaching-learning/files/self_and_peer_assessment. pdf

Papanek E. 1963. Social Interest, A Purposeful Motive for Constructive or Destructive Behavior. Available at: https://www.adlerpedia.org/concepts/15

Pasquale C. 2019. Five Questions for Tess Jones: Painting a Picture of the Role of Humanities in Medicine. University of Colorado CU Connections. Available at: https ://connections.cu.edu/spotlights/five-questions-tess-jones

Peterkin A, Bleakley A. 2017. *Staying Human During the Foundation Programme and Beyond: How to Thrive after Medical School.* Baton Rouge, FL: CRC Press.

Pinar WF. 2006. *The Synoptic Text Today and Other Essays: Curriculum Development after the Reconceptualization.* New York: Peter Lang.

Pinar WF. 2011. *The Character of Curriculum Studies: Bildung, Currere, and the Recurring Question of the Subject.* New York: Palgrave Macmillan.

Pinar WF. 2012. *What Is Curriculum Theory?* 2nd ed. London: Routledge.

Rosanvallon P. 2018. *Good Government: Democracy Beyond Elections.* Cambridge, MA: Harvard University Press.

Szasz T. Beware of Pharmacracy. *Independent Institute*, 21 August 2001. Available at: https ://www.independent.org/news/article.asp?id=276

Szasz T. 2003. *Pharmacracy: Medicine and Politics in America.* New York: Syracuse University Press.

Szasz T. 2007. *The Medicalization of Everyday Life. Selected Essays.* Syracuse, NY: Syracuse University Press.

Van der Graaf R, van der Zande ISE, den Ruijter HM, et al. Fair Inclusion of Pregnant Women in Clinical Trials: An Integrated Scientific and Ethical Approach. *Trials.* 2018;19:78.

Waitzkin H. 1991. *The Politics of Medical Encounters.* New Haven, CT: Yale University Press.

Waitzkin H, Anderson M. 2020. *Social Medicine and the Coming Transformation.* Abingdon: Routledge.

Wispelwey B, Al-Orzza A. Underlying Conditions. *London Review of Books*, 18 April 2020. Available at: https://www.lrb.co.uk/blog/2020/april/underlying-conditions

2   Aesthetics

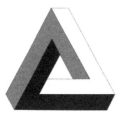

Distribution of the sensible

While medical education in general has failed to address links between aesthetics and politics, within the field of the medical/health humanities there is a growing interest in addressing health inequities and inequalities through two aesthetic channels: a "pedagogy of the oppressed" as proposed by Paulo Freire (2017), and a "theatre of the oppressed" as proposed by Augusto Boal (1991), who was directly influenced by Freire. Such frameworks have been applied globally to medical and healthcare education to help students to develop an appreciation of health inequalities (Ramaswamy and Ramaswamy 2020). One body of work that has not as yet had an impact upon medical education or the medical humanities is that of Jacques Rancière (1991, 1995, 2006a, 2006b, 2010, 2011, 2013), whose life's work has been to create dialogue between politics and aesthetics.

Where capital is utilized to produce profit, such profit is typically unfairly redistributed in a free market capitalist economy. It is not just physical or intellectual labour that is exploited, but also "emotional labour", a term coined by Arlie Hochschild (1983). In any work context, feelings have to be regulated and managed appropriately and this, in for example the "front end" service industries, is a central part of the job. Famously, in *Being and Nothingness*, Jean-Paul Sartre (2003) describes an over-eager waiter who adopts a façade in order to please customers and then to be tipped. Sartre describes this as acting in "bad faith" or engaging in self-deception by deceiving others. Sartre distinguishes between authenticity (the waiter who does not play act) and bad faith.

But Erving Goffman's (1990) dramaturgical model of social interaction would say that so-called "authenticity" is itself simply an example of "managing impressions". In medical education we call this learning "professionalism". For Goffman, there is no dividing line between good and bad faith; rather there are polished and clumsy, artful and pedestrian ways of managing impressions or presenting a "self", both "frontstage" (public) and "backstage" (private). Such a view, however, hollows out any ethical dimension to interactions and raises the question of "who writes the scripts?" For Jacques Rancière (2013), those in whom power is invested write the scripts of social exchange, so that an aesthetic of the multitude is displaced by a minority aesthetic of the elite.

Medical students must learn how to manage feelings and present an appropriate professional front or demeanour in often intensive and pressing circumstances. Emotional labour, from the beginning of their education, is channelled and formed according to "professional" expectations. Such capital is no longer owned by the students but becomes the property of the institutions of the medical school and the clinic. It is redistributed according to historically determined patterns of expected professional behaviour. Such emotional or affective capital is intimately linked with sense-based dispositions and actions (perceiving, feeling, making value judgements, developing tastes) that Rancière (2006b, 2010) calls "the fabric of the sensible". Such a personal perceptual scheme, and associated social code of manners, is subject to a power structure, or "policed". Breaches of professionalism are considered to be serious in the socialization of trainee doctors, so much so that medical students themselves can come to police the behaviour of their seniors if they spot breaches of professionalism (see Chapter 7). These may be reported back to core medical school faculty who in turn can police the pedagogical behaviour of clinical teachers. These interactions then form a fabric of the sensible through highly structured and coded patterns of distribution of emotional capital, as acts of governance and counter-resistance (Gill et al. 2015; Monrouxe et al. 2014; Shaw et al. 2018). Such interactions involve both politics and aesthetics – or power and sensibility.

Rancière (2013, ix) describes aesthetics broadly as "ways of perceiving and being affected", where again boundaries or transgressions are "policed". Tyson Lewis (2012: 1) describes the cultural "system of divisions and boundaries … that define what is visible and audible within a particular aesthetico-political regime". Lewis would include here all the senses, or their interactions, to form a fabric of the senses as "an organizational system of co-ordinates that establishes a distribution of the sensible" (ibid.: 3). The novelist China Miéville (2018) describes the education of sensibility as "reconfigurations of experience" in accordance with the habits of a dominant social group.

In *The Politics of Aesthetics*, Rancière (2006b: 50) notes that the relations between power and sensibility are not grounded in some transcendental abstract principles, but are immanent and fluid, or subject to historical conditions: "The visibility of a form of expression as an artistic form depends on a historically constituted regime of perception and intelligibility". Medical students (who have signed up for a vocational programme) effectively work for, or are employees of, medical schools in conjunction (usually) with university hospitals and primary care facilities. They are educated in time to adapt largely to hospital performance spaces: clinics, operating theatres, admissions units, intensive or critical care units, accident and emergency units, both generalist and specialty-based wards, and inter-disciplinary team meetings.

They know relatively little of how the patients they meet also "circulate" through a medical system: as blood or tissue samples, through pathology laboratory spaces; as discharged patients through physiotherapy or support services; as admissions through ambulance and paramedic services; or as patients discharged into the community and cared for by social services, community services and formal and informal carers. More, they know little of object-oriented ontologies that treat these circulating objects (such as human tissue or patients' notes) without objectifying them, while having equal ontological status within a system of practice (Mol 2002; Harman 2018). They come to know a little about palliative care and nursing homes, and more about family or general practice. Their physical, intellectual and emotional labour is then fairly focused clinically.

As they progress in their careers to medicine or surgery, and then to specialties (including general practice), what Tyson Lewis (2012) calls "acclimation pedagogy" – focused on work-based learning – intensifies. This is a pedagogy that does not primarily open up an inquiring mind and teach critical thinking. Rather, it is one that narrows down learning to specifics that are tightly policed or subject to a strong ethical and professional frame, following a pattern of induction and socialization. Performance spaces (Bleakley 2016) such as operating theatres, morgues, laboratories, wards, critical care units, dermatology clinics, maternity units, lecture theatres and so forth cultivate ways of emoting and being that are tightly controlled by conventions and traditions, where emotional capital is held by an authority and a fabric of sensibility is formed so that you sense according to how you should and not necessarily how you wish, as a circulation of tradition.

Modes of perception and regimes of emotion tailored historically for specialties are performance scripts demanding close reading, leading to an identity construction. But of course change and progress must happen and this is not just knowledge- or technique-based. Styles and approaches change too, and for such innovations to happen, the fabric of the sensible must be rent, and sensibility capital must be redistributed. Forms of counter-resistance (see Chapters 7–9) seed such innovations. Medical culture shifts from the default position of a "will-to-stability" to seek "possibility knowledge" through forms of political resistance.

This can happen in a large-scale shift of values, such as democratization of medicine through patient-centredness and inter-professional practices – both engineered and promoted by medical education. Lewis (2012) describes how "the aesthetic principle of democracy" by its very nature breaches acclimation pedagogy. Here "Empire" morphs into "Multitude", then "Common Wealth", and finally "Assembly" as processes of democratization intensify and are refined (Hardt and Negri 2000, 2006, 2009, 2017). This follows Hegel's evolution of "spirit" through dialectic, as the passage from individualism to collectivity; and Marx's evolution of social equity as common ownership of the means of production of goods, services, ideas and emotional capital. This is echoed in collaborative, democratic pedagogical practices such as small group learning with student-led components.

Ten kinds of aesthetic work

The sum of the intersections between medicine, medical education, politics and aesthetics can be framed as the work of the "medical humanities" (Bleakley 2015, 2019; Bleakley, Marshall and Brömer 2006). Aesthetics in medicine – and not "aesthetic medicine and surgery" as corrective, or as embellishment and enhancement – is a minefield and rarely discussed in medical education. With some notable exceptions (Macneill 2014; O'Neill 2015; Bleakley 2017), even the field of the medical humanities resists in-depth discussion of aesthetics. While medical ethics – the issue of moral principles guiding practices and choices – is established in medical education, aesthetics is not yet afforded a similar status. Yet ethics and aesthetics are inextricably mixed, where what is valued is a mix of a job done thoughtfully and sensitively (ethics) and well, or of quality (aesthetics). Aesthetics has lost its tether and become inflated where it is seen to refer to "high art" rather than the *quality* and *form* of activity based in close noticing or cultivation of the senses, as sensibility (Bleakley 2020b).

The root of the word "aesthetic" is the ancient Greek *aisthesis* – "sense impression", meaning experience gained directly through perception and sensation without cognitive interpretation or interference. As a formal modern study, "aesthetics" began with the German philosopher Alexander Baumgarten's particular use of the word in 1735 to describe refined responses to high art or the appreciation of beauty. But this approach goes beyond the root meaning of the word, that, as noted, is to engage the senses fully – precisely what doctors do in conducting an examination and making a diagnosis, for example. While aesthetics is now used to describe qualities and form, this can range across a spectrum of emotional and sensory responses to embrace disgust as well as pleasure. Thus, in medical education, the aesthetic realm can include dealing with disgust in first clinical encounters with wounds and death, as well as the sensory pleasures of watching someone return to health. Aesthetics in particular describes the education of the senses to make finer discriminatory clinical judgements, for example through auscultation, percussion and palpation, as well as close observation and smell (Bleakley 2020b).

In medical education, aesthetics is a lost or unknown territory. This is understandable where scientific medicine has displaced interest in form and appearance for dominance of function. Appreciation of form has then been an-aesthetized or dulled rather than aestheticized. Good anatomy and applied science teachers cannot have lost their wonder at the display of the natural world, yet this aesthetic response will usually be lost where explanation precedes appreciation, rather than the other way around. I would recommend that those teachers embed themselves in the work of the biologist Adolf Portmann (for example 1967) – who argues for appreciation preceding explanation in biology – to restore a sense of wonder to their interests. Typically, Portmann resists the reduction of form to function, such as the territorial explanation for birdsong. Much of birdsong, suggests Portmann, is for the sake of it – expression of beauty rather than fence building that smells too much, in any case, of human capitalist interests projected onto the animal world.

Below, I consider ten kinds of aesthetic that can, and should, engage medical education. Each of these is entangled with politics or power, and ethics or value choices.

1. Appreciation of science

The science informing medical practice is explanatory, but science should not be reduced to function alone. Science should be appreciated for its beauty, and natural wonders for their expression. Natural science precedes and embraces experimental and laboratory science. There are, however, ethical issues to consider – pathologized tissue may look beautiful under the microscope, especially when stained, but this tissue is from a person's body and being, and that person may be suffering. Electron microscopy images are generally stunning, but this is not how we normally see the world.

2. Modification of the senses

Medical students undergo a radical re-orientation of the senses, dictated by the authority of medical education, to which they must willingly submit to eventually attain a medical identity. A whole slice of sensibility concerned with disgust and revulsion must be re-educated to accept what will be a daily part of an assault on the senses – illness, wounding, bodily harm and death. The primary aesthetic education is then an an-aesthetizing or dulling of the ordinary. In parallel, however, is an education of an extraordinary sensibility and sensitivity to suffering and hurt – and a celebration of return to health through treatment – as these are presented in symptom patterns for close diagnostic noticing.

3. Democracy

Engaging democracy is an art, and is evolving. In the face of historical traditions of hierarchies within medicine broadly and within specialties, particularly in surgery, medical students are encouraged to develop democracies of patient-centredness and inter-professionalism. There is a strong evidence base that flattening hierarchies in healthcare creates conditions for improved patient outcomes, safety and worker satisfaction. The blunt tactics of authority-led or arrogant behaviour are devoid of art. Democratic debate, collaboration and work of consensus require artful reflection and adjustment.

4. Clinical judgement

Students and junior doctors develop formed diagnostic capabilities as they progress. Balancing normative scientific evidence (guidelines) and personal judgement about the individual patient is an art – the forming of "mindlines" (Wieringa and Greenhalgh 2015; Gabbay and le May 2016), or clinical judgement based largely on experience rather than on evidence-based clinical guidelines.

5. Cultural style
Style is a cohesive set of qualities, such as the Minimalism that characterizes the clinical space and the reporting styles of doctors – brief and to the point.

6. Personal style or taste
This is what characterizes the individual clinician, to include innovations, adaptability and improvisation. Value judgements are appropriate to context (ethical and sensitive). While taste is often reduced to relativism ("personal taste"), there is a common factor. Taste is essential to medical diagnostics, where a blunt or dulled range of senses makes for a poor diagnostic radar.

7. Beauty
Words such as "form", "elegance" and "beauty" do not readily roll off the tongues of hard-pressed and hard-bitten doctors. "Beauty" has its root in the Latin *bellus*, meaning "fine" or "refined". Medicine is a fine art and a refined application of science and humanities. Nobody wants a medicine that is clumsy, dull or ugly.

8. Cognition and creativity
Medical education above all aims to engage a creative imagination that moves beyond conservatism and a will-to-stability in learning to nurture innovation and possibility knowledge.

9. Resistance
Acts of resistance to perceived injustices, sleights or abuse of power and authority (dissensus rather than consensus) can power creative change or modification, or turn the ordinary into the extraordinary. The arts and humanities are identified by their powers of dissensus, to make us "think otherwise". Individuals may cultivate sophisticated forms of resistance to perceived injustices and authorities such as "sly civility", a mocking of authority disguised as conformity.

10. Appearance
Self-presentation affords a trustworthy impression for patients and colleagues. Doctors want to appear professional and confident, but not arrogant. Management of impressions is an art and medicine can be readily understood as theatre, with tight scripts and specific roles. In fact, soap opera representations of medicine ("medi-soaps") are one way that the public can be informed about medical culture while retaining value as entertainment. Once a vocation but now a job, doctors manage appearances in a broader variety of ways than in previous generations, and this is inflected particularly by the disappearance of major props such as the white coat and stethoscope. Thinking about art that deals with surfaces can help the understanding of the significance of appearances (inauthentic or insincere self-presentation, as in Jean-Paul Sartre's fawning waiter embodied in *Being and Nothingness* as the choice of inauthentic Nothingness over authentic Being). A whole school of art – Pop Art – has taken the surface culture of everyday life such as advertising and kitsch as a formal

statement of what is to be valued, and has questioned cherished notions in art such as "authenticity". Andy Warhol produced cheap prints of everyday items that could be made in multiples, where the "original" is lost. Before Warhol, Walter Benjamin had foreseen the "age of mechanical reproduction", bemoaning the potential loss of the unique article. Warhol parodied this view by making single collectibles of mechanically reproducible items that now, ironically, sell as unique art objects for millions of dollars. The most successful of contemporary artists, Jeff Koons, has made one-off versions of kitsch objects. A three-feet-tall stainless steel sculpture reminiscent of a silver balloon animal is currently the most expensive piece sold by a living artist, fetching $91.1 million at auction. This kind of aesthetic again is of little use to doctors, who need to look beyond surface symptoms to the deeper causes of illness. However, medical students are told to heed "Sutton's Law". Willie Sutton was a notorious American bank robber who, when asked why he robbed banks, supposedly answered: "because that's where the money is". Sutton's Law refers to not ignoring the obvious. But "appearance" in medicine is not an aesthetic quality that should interest medical educators. We need to go beyond appearance to authenticity. All the above are necessarily micro-political acts of what Michel Foucault (1988) calls "aesthetic self-forming". Just as a practice is formed aesthetically, or has contour, grace and beauty, so an identity is formed – not just informed "doctor", or "surgeon", but "professional" and "trustworthy person".

Educators might ask of the ten faces of aesthetics:

1. "Are these components important or of interest?"
2. If they are of interest, then, "how do I address these?"
3. Further, "does this require modification of curriculum content or process (reviewing the ways that students learn current content)?"

In response to (3) above, a process curricular approach (see Chapters 11–13) would embrace all ten aesthetic dimensions as ways that current curriculum content can be inflected rather than replaced. All ten aspects of aesthetics also embrace issues of power, primarily because the ways that the senses are used are not simply biological or natural, but are also affected and shaped by culture, changing historically. What is noxious and disgusting in one culture may be pleasurable or soothing in another, and sensory responses differ in the same culture through history. This applies to body odours, the smells of animals and the tastes of foods.

But sensibility too is cultural capital (see Figures 2.1– 2.3). When a medical student has to unlearn a response of disgust to bodily fluids, for example, senior members of the profession, as teachers, mentors and role models, drain off the emotional capital involved and retain this. Again, the distribution of emotional capital is frustrated where it is retained in the lore of the elders and conservation of bad habits, and the emotional responses of neophytes are seen as illegitimate or do not constitute legitimate capital. While symptoms of unprofessionalism include objectification of patients and overt cynicism, they also embrace lack

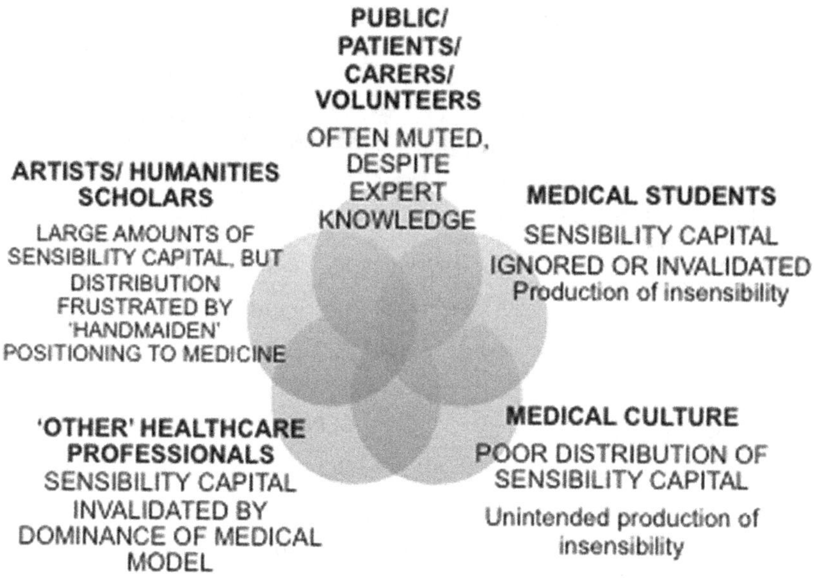

**PUBLIC/
PATIENTS/
CARERS/
VOLUNTEERS**

OFTEN MUTED,
DESPITE
EXPERT
KNOWLEDGE

**ARTISTS/ HUMANITIES
SCHOLARS**

LARGE AMOUNTS OF
SENSIBILITY CAPITAL, BUT
DISTRIBUTION
FRUSTRATED BY
'HANDMAIDEN'
POSITIONING TO MEDICINE

MEDICAL STUDENTS

SENSIBILITY CAPITAL
IGNORED OR INVALIDATED
Production of insensibility

**'OTHER' HEALTHCARE
PROFESSIONALS**
SENSIBILITY CAPITAL
INVALIDATED BY
DOMINANCE OF MEDICAL
MODEL

MEDICAL CULTURE

POOR DISTRIBUTION OF
SENSIBILITY CAPITAL

Unintended production of
insensibility

Figure 2.1 Mapping the distribution of sensibility capital (1).

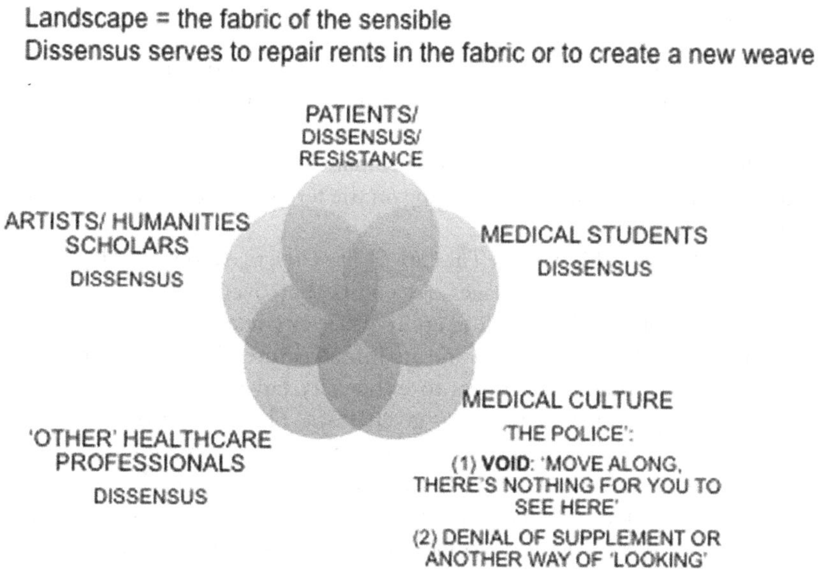

Landscape = the fabric of the sensible
Dissensus serves to repair rents in the fabric or to create a new weave

PATIENTS/
DISSENSUS/
RESISTANCE

ARTISTS/ HUMANITIES
SCHOLARS

DISSENSUS

MEDICAL STUDENTS

DISSENSUS

MEDICAL CULTURE

'THE POLICE':

(1) **VOID**: 'MOVE ALONG,
THERE'S NOTHING FOR YOU TO
SEE HERE'

(2) DENIAL OF SUPPLEMENT OR
ANOTHER WAY OF 'LOOKING'

'OTHER' HEALTHCARE
PROFESSIONALS

DISSENSUS

Figure 2.2 Mapping the distribution of sensibility capital (2).

RESPONSE AT PENINSULA MEDICAL SCHOOL

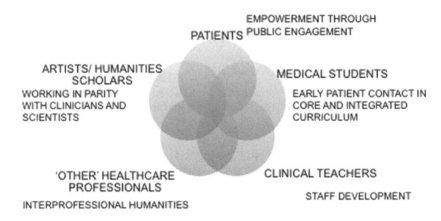

EMPOWERMENT THROUGH
PATIENTS PUBLIC ENGAGEMENT

ARTISTS/ HUMANITIES
SCHOLARS
WORKING IN PARITY
WITH CLINICIANS AND
SCIENTISTS

MEDICAL STUDENTS
EARLY PATIENT CONTACT IN
CORE AND INTEGRATED
CURRICULUM

'OTHER' HEALTHCARE
PROFESSIONALS
INTERPROFESSIONAL HUMANITIES

CLINICAL TEACHERS
STAFF DEVELOPMENT

Figure 2.3 Mapping the distribution of sensibility capital (3).

of emotional insulation and over-involvement with patients: both ends of the spectrum (under- and over-involvement) demonstrate insensibility.

Acclimation pedagogies

Returning to the (mal)distribution of sensibility capital, introduced in the first part of this chapter, acclimation (American usage) or acclimatization (British usage) is the process and result of becoming accustomed to a new climate or to new conditions. Lewis (2012) describes "acclimation pedagogy" as the formalized learning of an identity or new way of being on the terms of an externally imposed authority.

In China Miéville's 2009 novel *The City & The City*, two cities sit side-by-side with differing cultures and languages. At points they overlap ("crosshatching" and living "grosstopically"). Growing up in either city requires learning how to "unsee" members of the other city and its infrastructure. This is an acclimatization process. Prospective travellers to either city have to undergo intensive acclimation pedagogy before they are given visas. Should a citizen of either city consciously or inadvertently "see" the other city and its inhabitants, this is called "breaching" and the person is immediately arrested by the Breach police and given re-education in perception, in how to sense appropriately and selectively. Persistent breaching leads to more severe punishment. The novel offers a metaphor for the shaping of the senses by culture and history. Aesthetics, the manipulation of the sensible fabric of the world and responses to qualities, is a historically and culturally inflected phenomenon.

There is nothing necessarily sinister about this – we are subject to learning new sensibility practices through external authority all the time. Lockdown and social distancing in a climate of emergency are recent global examples. Vigilance in the face of "terrorist threat" is another example. All professional socializations, or regimes of formal rule-bound activity such as sports, require acclimation.

The point is to be reflexive about patterns and possibilities. Where does an acclimation pedagogy become an oppressive socialization, frustrate innovation or slowly erode patience and resilience through micro-aggressions?

Socialization into medicine requires divesting oneself of key lay emotional capital (ways of being) and intellectual capital (ways of thinking and problem solving) in order to engage with the professional culture that is oriented to emotional insulation (potentially numbing empathy) and practical action (potentially numbing conceptual acuity). It is a process of unlearning one set of habits in order to learn a new set. An important work of political resistance occurs as medical students retain personal signifiers in the face of medical socialization. Millennials and Generation Z medical students and junior doctors may come to constitute the force of resistance that radically changes the nature of medical education post-coronavirus pandemic. The inevitable social change post-pandemic must surely alert medical education to the central importance of health eco-literacy and radical upstream medicine where the climate emergency can be seen as a pandemic in slow motion (see Chapter 4).

Emotional (or affective) capital, produced from emotional labour (Hochschild 1983; Brook 2013), is extremely important in medical education. Such capital is central to how communication is exercised, and communication is key to patient care and safety. In recent years, we have accrued research evidence that the majority of medical errors or iatrogenic mistakes are products of poor communication not between doctors and patients, but between doctors and other healthcare professionals in "liquid" clinical team settings – fast-paced clinical encounters with little room for error. This is particularly acute in surgical settings, both within and across teams (Bleakley 2013).

Such a draining off of affective capital has consequences – medical students feel dried out and dehumanized, just as patients might. In light of this, medicine has developed professional codes and engineered climates of democracy – patient-centredness and inter-professional teamwork. Students expect seniors to model professional behaviour as sensitivity to patients. In most cases, seniors do this well. When they do not, students can and do organize modes of political resistance to recover emotional capital that has been lodged in the apex of the hierarchy. For example, contra acclimation, students do not necessarily "unsee" professional lapses by seniors and are ready to report perceived unprofessional behaviour and, in the worse cases, to whistleblow (see Chapter 7).

Intellectual knowing and practical doing are held together by affective glue, by feelings and sentiments. The easiest way to test this is to look at symptoms of breakdown or burnout (Peterkin and Bleakley 2017). Knowledge and practices are valued for their qualities, and it is the value complex that holds a practice together. If the practice is devalued, then the practitioner loses interest. Around any set of practices, a web of values forms that holds the practices, and these are represented in medical aphorisms ("patient-centredness", "do no harm", "treat the person not the disease") (Levine and Bleakley 2012). This affective glue represents a set of interests that are "formed" or "shaped" and that form an identity in turn. This shaping gives qualities to a practice such as elegance, sensitivity, assuredness and so forth. The quality of a practice is its aesthetic dimension, readily known by how it engages the senses. Where senses are tuned, there is vibrancy and readiness, or an aesthetic presence. Where senses are dulled, there is a bluntness or dullness, and practice is an-aesthetized.

Any set of practices underpinned by knowledge and values, such as medicine and medical pedagogies, can be seen to form a fabric, a connectedness. These fabrics are also known by their locations: the hospital ward, clinic and operating theatre; the primary care clinic; the hospice. Often this fabric of the sensible is heavily specialized, such as a paediatric audiology clinic with video playback facilities for observing how parents interact with a deaf child. The fabric embraces practitioners and family members engaging in affect-laden work around a child to seek possibility knowledge as parents learn new ways of communicating and the child gains confidence.

The medical humanities

In the past two decades in particular, the medical humanities (also referred to as "health humanities" to embrace all healthcare) have become an important component in undergraduate medicine and surgery curricula globally (Bleakley 2015). There is also a growing interest in medical/health humanities in postgraduate or continuing medical education (Peterkin and Skorzewska 2018), dental education (Zahra and Dunton 2017) and wider health professions (such as nursing) education (McFarlane 2018), where again the "health humanities" (Crawford et al. 2015) descriptor is more appropriate. The medical humanities originally developed within the post-WWII arts for health movement through arts therapies, focused not on the education of doctors or health professionals but on the recovery from ill health of patients, often as an adjunct to psychiatric care (Bleakley 2015).

The use of techniques such as voice projection from drama education were brought in to some postgraduate and continuing education programmes for doctors, and this might be complemented by study of film and television portrayals of doctors, but the introduction of the medical humanities into undergraduate medical education grew first from the establishment of medical ethics into curricula. Here, instead of functionally imbibing knowledge and skills and then doing, medical students were asked to reflect on the consequences of their actions, and to think also about the historical and cultural contexts of their chosen profession and the values that shape their actions. They would thus gain a critical metaperspective on medicine and become reflective practitioners (Bleakley 1999). Subjects such as the history of medicine widened students' perspectives from the confines of basic and applied science, but were usually only studied by the few as electives. As students and faculty often played instruments, music might be introduced as a break from medical studies, treated in the same way as sports – as recreation.

But subjects such as life drawing, complementing surface and living anatomy, were seen to have pragmatic educational value, and were readily absorbed into the curriculum. As arguments were made for educating students in communication, so psychology and drama amplified core curriculum studies. Actor patients were used in clinical and communication skills training, and students learned from them about performance, scripts, impression management, role-playing and identity construction. This psychological input was also found to be useful in better understanding the cognitive processes of clinical diagnostics.

Careful thought about the way that patient care happened on the ground revealed a strong component of narrative or story, with interest in switching from the doctor's interpretation to the patient's telling. Patients told stories in consultations, and doctors had to make sense of these in dialogue with patients. A "narrative-based" medicine came into being (Hunter 1991; Chambers 1999; Charon 2006; Milota, van Thiel and van Delden 2019; Schleifer and Vannatta 2013). Doctors used specialist language while patients used lay language, and bridges had to be built for common understanding. A study of the metaphors used in medicine helped with this (Bleakley 2017). Doctors could capture the complexity of clinical episodes through poetry, and also wanted to write about the experience of practising medicine, so that the medical auto-ethnography became a popular genre (for example Kalanithi 2019).

As deeper reflection on the social, gender and ethnic stratification of medicine revealed institutional fault-lines, so medical education took more interest in social justice issues. Medical humanities interests started to swell and split into three camps, often competing for scarce research resources: one – based in the community – identifying with the older streams of arts therapies with service users at the centre; a second – based in universities – focusing on the inter-disciplinary study of medical culture with application to medical education as a secondary consideration; and a third – based in medical schools and clinics – focusing on how the arts, humanities and social sciences could enrich medical education to produce "rounded" doctors who were questioning, caring and creative. Three recent synoptic texts document state-of-the-art thinking and activity in each of these areas: (i) community-based arts therapies (Crawford et al. 2015); (ii) inter-disciplinary critical study of medical cultures (Whitehead and Woods 2016); and (iii) arts and humanities informing applied medical education (Bleakley 2020a).

Central to this third approach is finding ways in which doctors' senses can be educated for improving diagnostic acumen (Bleakley 2020b); their sensitivities educated for closer listening, narrative intelligence, emotional sensitivity and more democratic dialogue with patients and colleagues; and their sense of justice energized to work against health inequities and inequalities and for patient advocacy. A fourth synoptic text in particular addresses these social justice and advocacy issues (Jones, Wear and Freidman 2014). In the latter, politics joined ethics and aesthetics to energize the scientific imagination at the heart of medicine.

Medical students needed to be reminded that science is intrinsically aesthetic and that the body, bearing complexity and beauty and inviting wonder, cannot be reduced to a linear engineering problem.

So, contemporary medical students studying anatomy might also learn from medical history that Andreas Vesalius in the 16th century, the father of the anatomical text, also seeded the modern discourse that the body can be viewed as a machine, objectified and stripped of the mind, feelings and social context. They might learn from the psychologist and cultural commentator Michel Foucault (1976) that the objectifying clinical gaze in Western medicine was established through the sudden proliferation of cadaver dissection at the end of the 18th century – a gaze that would not develop in Chinese medicine as human cadaver dissection was taboo until the 20th century. Medical students would have their gazes turned inward to the effects of pathology in the body – lesions – and how these would be managed in the hospital setting, and away from the sources of diseases in the environment and in society, so medical education gained a bias, away from population health and civic issues, spurning politics, for example. Students of all skin colours might (and should) wonder why the dermatology texts they study, and the hi-tech manikins they use in simulation settings to learn clinical skills such as intubation, show white, and not black or brown, skins. Surely Black Lives Matter in medical education too?

To return to medical humanities in medical education, clearly, as multiple topics and subjects come into view to provide multiple possibilities, they cannot simply be crammed into the curriculum as content. New ways of thinking about curriculum as process have to be adopted. A pedagogical imagination must be exercised where the purpose of the curriculum is re-imagined. No longer cramming facts and learning techniques as an individual, medical students must now learn how to learn; how to learn collaboratively; and how to navigate work-based learning by thinking on one's feet, tolerating uncertainty, asking for help and guidance, reflecting and innovating. This does not have to be complicated – shifting the register of medicine from instrumental description to aesthetic appreciation can involve a simple analogy such as taking the beat of the heart ("lub-dup/ lub-dup/ lub-dup/ lub-dup/ lub-dup") as the basis for Shakespearean iambic pentameter: "But soft/ what light/ through yon/ der win/ dow breaks?"

Evaluation studies show that medical humanities in the medicine curriculum play an important role in shaping doctors as meta-learners, or good at learning how to learn, how to tolerate ambiguity, and how to collaborate (Bleakley 2015, 2019, 2020a). These are essentially the capabilities needed for effective participation in a democracy. As noted, issues of social justice have recently become a major focus for the medical or health humanities, debating the parameters of "humane" medical practice. Given that the aim of the humanities is to explore and expand what it is to be human, and that the arts do not merely embellish but also critically interrogate this, it is no wonder that the medical humanities provide a point of engagement with social justice issues in medical education.

A good example, mentioned earlier, is the widely employed "Theatre of the Oppressed" (Boal 1991). In Brazil in the 1970s, Augusto Boal developed a set of theatrical forms based on the ideas of the liberatory educationalist Paulo Freire, to give voices to oppressed peoples. Boal aestheticized Freire's political project by using theatrical frameworks through which protest and resistance could be rehearsed as critical interrogation of oppressive social and political forms. Addressing themes of "difference" and "identity" as these relate to poverty, inequality, disability, inequity, gender and ethnic discrimination, isolation, oppression and activism, Boal's theatre invites performers and audience to collectively rehearse responses to such themes with a view to turning inquiry into liberatory or emancipatory activity. The caveat is that the new "emancipator" does not repeat the old habits of the oppressor to become neo-colonial.

The workhorse of the medical humanities

In subsequent chapters, I argue that aesthetics and politics in medical education can be brought into fruitful dialogue through mobilizing key pedagogies, particularly Cultural-Historical Activity Theory (CHAT) and curriculum reconceptualization; and through adopting the medical humanities as core and integrated provision through which medical education is mediated. As noted in the Preface, the medical humanities afford a second stimulus in double stimulation learning, to widen horizons of possibility. Where the formal curriculum is the first stimulus in learning medicine, a more adventurous and innovative learning is promised through enrichment by the medical humanities as the second stimulus creating a "thinking otherwise" about the topic.

For some, the medical humanities (or health humanities) have a beguiling charm as a distraction from the blood and guts of clinical medicine, bringing some sophistication also to the blunt instrumentalism of applied biomedical science. Patients are portraits and stories, their symptoms poetry, while everyday clinical procedures afford notable drama. These are the pearls of the medical humanities beyond the sweat and tears of everyday medical work that does not engage a creative imagination or pursuit of possibility knowledge. But this is to idealize the medical humanities. There is common grit that makes these pearls. This is the medical humanities as collective workhorse – bringing the fullness of humanity to medicine in the form of democracy at work within medical education. Central to this is (often bruising) politics – the machinations of power. Medical humanities produce tangible effects (Mangione et al. 2018) because blood, sweat and tears are involved. Often caricatured as play, the medical humanities demand work.

Politics is often cast as the intrusive shadow of medicine and medical pedagogy that can turn artistry into sinister Machiavellian power plays. This is akin to what William Blake called the "infernal machine" or "Chiaro Oscuro," the "hellish" brown shadows beloved by Venetian and Flemish painters that Blake saw as a mean-spirited treacle coating denying potential light and joyous celebration. Politics in medicine – most immediately in policy and healthcare management – need not be sticky brown shadows. Indeed, it is time to bring politics out of the shadows and celebrate power in medicine and medical pedagogies as potentially liberatory; and certainly as terrains for artful resistance to heavy-handed and unimaginative pedagogies, particularly in curriculum development, where medical education has shown a strange resistance to contemporary innovations.

More, where it situates such innovative thinking in the field of medical humanities, this constitutes a "thinking-politics-with-curriculum-in-mind" as a poetic device. Here, politics and aesthetics meet such that power is not conceived as blunt, material and instrumental (acting as an an-aesthetic) but rather as an aesthetic gesture that shapes democratic habits as things of beauty and elegance, awakening the senses. The curriculum is then not dull and dulling, but sharp, pointed, challenging and enervating. It is an approach to curriculum that should enlighten and needle at the same time. Such a curriculum literally makes sense, raising levels of sensibility to create medical students who are alive to what patients want – or medical students that have their antennae up.

I will critically address curriculum stagnation and conservatism to set out a blueprint for radical change to embrace issues of politics or power as these meet aesthetic concerns. The medical/health humanities have been shown to educate the sensibilities and sensitivities of medical students as a platform for improving clinical diagnostic capabilities and shaping doctors who listen to their patients and respond caringly. But this work, to which I have made a contribution (for example Bleakley 2015, 2019, 2020a), is limited by its previous refusal to engage with politics or power structures. Despite a global interest in incorporating medical humanities in medicine and surgery curricula, there is a danger of producing dilettante pearl fishers rather than artisanal grit shifters, the former perhaps interested more in the delicate intricacies of narrative theory or obscure historical fact rather than the everyday incessant noises of power plays and resistances that characterize both the joys and tensions of clinical work.

Crudely, I want to encourage a shift in gaze of the medical humanities from art gallery to contemporary eco-factory, and of medical education generally from downstream hospitalism, or hospital-based work experience, to upstream primary care and "deep upstream" community care focused on the long-term implications of an ecological crisis as an exploitation of common wealth by cynical private interests. Again, such exploitation supports and deepens health inequities and inequalities.

From concept to activity

Hegel's Master : Slave formula says there is no master without the slave. In other words, the slave affords the master's *raison d'être*. This gives the slave a paradoxical power. Without customers there are no shopkeepers. Without the populus or multitude there are no politicians. And without medical students there are no medical educators. Medical students have power because they provide the medium through which medical educators can continually transform and develop their pedagogies. Jacques Rancière's (1991) *The Ignorant Schoolmaster* posits a pedagogical thought experiment: what if the teacher knew the same as, or even less than, the pupils? How would "teaching" and learning progress once "teaching" is made redundant? The point is to bring our focus back to the resources that are provided by learners and the potential for adapting content-heavy curricula into "learning to learn" processes. "Teaching" then becomes "facilitation of learning", as explored in Chapter 14. More radical approaches to such a pedagogy develop collaborative inquiry as the primary mode of learning (what do we need to know and how can we best learn this?) and criteria-based self and peer assessment as the most democratic ways of judging whether or not learning has taken place, and if expertise is being acquired.

This book follows the logic of CHAT, perhaps the most informative of social learning theories for medical education, in moving from concept to activity. CHAT brings together the two strands of the politics and aesthetics of pedagogy by (i) constantly referring learning back to the learner's needs within a democratic collectivist learning experience (the politics); and (ii) through the arts of graceful double stimulation and scaffolding of learning (the aesthetics). Frederick van Amstel (http://fredvanamstel.com/blog/double-stimulation-experiments) describes double stimulation in the context of design education: "The first stimulus is a contradictory situation and the second stimulus is an ambiguous instrument that may be used to overcome contradictions". "Overcome" may not be the best descriptor here. "Develop" or "nourish" may be better.

The ideas in this book are neither "other worldly" nor utopian, but rather grounded in the realities of clinical work. We must ask what are the most appropriate learning experiences for a medical student that turn mere events into experiences. What processes turn the surface into depths? CHAT provides a tried and tested framework for addressing this question. In the context of medical treatment, the patient is the object of the activity system, and the shared outcome is improving both patient care and safety. There is a further primary outcome and this is worker satisfaction, "measured" not economically but aesthetically, as quality of work embracing artistry and expression. The shared outcome is then quality of patient benefit from healthcare intervention plus quality of work satisfaction for practitioners. In line with "third wave" Activity Theory's interest in the shared objects of differing but adjacent activity systems, a third activity – in the context of this book, that of medical education – has as its primary object the "rounded" doctor who is educated clinically but also emotionally, socially and politically. This is the doctor as democratic worker. A double stimulation is at work here – that of the fundamental acquisition of clinical capabilities to diagnose and treat symptoms, in turn deepened by a cultural and historical education as an artful doctor who treats persons in the contexts of their communities. The point of a contemporary medical education in times of global ecological crisis is to shift the medical gaze from symptom to cause, and from hospital treatment to community prevention, primarily through addressing health inequities and inequalities. This is a medico-political task.

Within these activity systems, communities (such as healthcare workers) interact with multiple objects or artefacts that mediate learning, such as computers, patients' notes, pharmaceuticals and a range of technologies. Every community has a set of rules and a series of roles forming a complex division of labour.

This gets tasks done more efficiently, but can also creatively investigate new ways of learning by members of communities of practice collaborating democratically.

Every person (subject) implicated in the activity system is "creating" themselves, or developing identities and subjectivities in the light of the complex dynamic working of the whole system. Every system, as noted above, interacts with other systems (such as sets of care teams working around a single patient's needs). Every part of the system is potentially in a relation of contradiction or ambiguity with every other part, and it is the constant movement of such dialectic within a democratic, dialogical framework that makes the system dynamic and expansive, refusing collapse or crystallization but moving into new territories. The basic activity system can be mapped as in Figure 2.4.

In Figure 2.5, we see tensions between kinds of learning within and across activity systems:

What if the object of the activity is now politics or power? So, the overall object is still looking after the welfare of the patient, but within this, sets of power structures – often contradictory – are at work. Division of labour and consequent roles, and the exercise of rules such as protocols and clinical guidelines, necessarily enact a variety of power plays. In medicine, hierarchies form around expertise, but these are usually focused on technical expertise, and so issues such as communication capabilities, democratic habits (dialogue rather than monologue, close listening rather than habitual talking) and emotional intelligence are overshadowed. Function precedes and occludes form, rather than functions being shaped by forms. The aesthetics of political exchanges are squeezed out or forced under, only to return in distorted forms, as ugly politics – Machiavellian, and cut-throat neo-liberal.

As conversations, contradictions and dialogues go on between elements of an activity system, so tolerating the consequent ambiguities and uncertainties, and

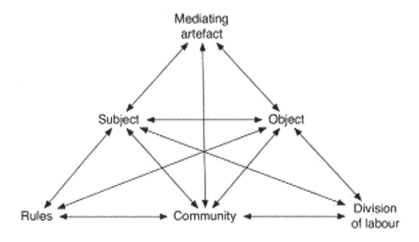

Figure 2.4 Basic Activity System – the primary object in medicine is the patient.

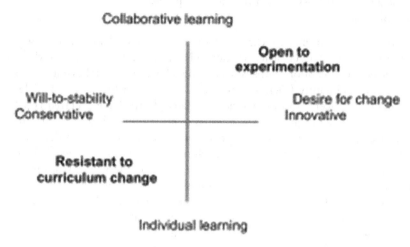

Collaborative learning

Open to experimentation

Will-to-stability
Conservative

Desire for change
Innovative

Resistant to
curriculum change

Individual learning

Figure 2.5 Kinds of learning.

then transforming the contradictions into opportunities (where events become experiences), requires transformative expertise that is an aesthetic capability or an art. This artful shaping of opportunity out of potential collapse or crystallization of a system is what the aesthetics (and ethics) of politics demands, where the exercise of creative imagination again turns mundane events into meaningful experiences. Democracy, necessarily an unfinished business or a "horizon" project (a democracy-to-come and a democratizing-of-democracy) is a work of art, a shaping of politics against the odds for the benefit of all. The art of democratic shaping of the project of medical education – through thinking with curriculum as a political text and use of the medical humanities as media for productive change or possibility knowledge – offers a potential transformation of the modern medical gaze.

As long as competences are met at graduation, to make sure that medical students are able to make the transition to junior doctoring, medical schools globally have latitude to innovate in the curriculum. Yet, there is reluctance to do so, and this is often a legacy of a longstanding tension between conservative clinician educators and scientists and non-clinical pedagogical experts. The latter, fired up by new approaches to educational theory and practice, often seek radical curriculum change during times of global social unrest that impact upon healthcare. Now is one of those times. An unprecedented alignment of ecological catastrophe and global political shift to the right that embraces climate change denial has brought into focus the need for a radical shift in how we educate doctors for the future. This has been acutely focused by the global coronavirus pandemic that has revealed, in many countries, a fatal disjunction between the worlds of politics and medicine, and a raw exposure of the effects of health inequities and inequalities.

From downstream hospitalism to "deep" upstream community care

Where the coronavirus insult focus rests with acute hospital-based critical care, availability of ventilators, critical care staff and beds, this is because here is where the perceived focal point of deaths is happening. However, this takes our eye off deaths in the community (such as care homes), where, in England and Wales for example, well over a third of Covid-19 related deaths have occurred (BMJ 2020). Medical students globally are oriented to hospital-based early training to gain experience in acute care, yet the great burden of healthcare is in the community linked to management of multiple, chronic illnesses in older age. Where hospitals treat downstream patients at the point of acute intervention, upstream primary and social care is the ground for multiple causes of illness, both in physical and mental health (and it is time that we stopped separating these territories). The following Chapters 3 and 4 expand this. First, what is the historical relationship between politics, medicine and medical education; and second, what is, and what could be, the relationship between the climate emergency and medical education?

Bibliography

Bleakley A. From Reflective Practice to Holistic Reflexivity. *Studies in Higher Education*. 1999;24:315–30.

Bleakley A. Working in "Teams" in an Era of "Liquid" Healthcare: What Is the Use of Theory? *Journal of Interprofessional Care*. 2013;27:18–26.

Bleakley A. 2015. *The Medical Humanities and Medical Education: How the Medical Humanities Can Shape Better Doctors*. Abingdon: Routledge.

Bleakley A. Bargaining with Hypnos: Sleep Deprivation in Junior Doctors as Durational Misperformance. *Performance Research*. 2016; 21: 49–52.

Bleakley A. 2017. *Thinking With Metaphors in Medicine: The State of the Art*. Abingdon: Routledge.

Bleakley A. Invoking the Medical Humanities to Develop a #MedicineWeCanTrust. *Academic Medicine*. 2019; 10: 1422–24.

Bleakley A. (ed). 2020a. *Routledge Handbook of the Medical Humanities*. Abingdon: Routledge.

Bleakley A. 2020b. *Educating Doctors Senses Through The Medical Humanities: "How Do I Look?"* Abingdon: Routledge.

Bleakley A, Marshall R, Brömer R. Toward an Aesthetic Medicine: Developing a Core Medical Humanities Undergraduate Curriculum. *Journal of Medical Humanities*. 2006;27:197–213.

Boal A. 1991. *Theatre of the Oppressed*, 2nd ed. London: Pluto Press.

British Medical Journal (BMJ). Covid-19: Deaths in the Community Approach 20 000 in the UK. *BMJ*. 2020;369:m2449.

Brook P. Emotional Labour and the Living Personality at Work: Labour Power, Materialist Subjectivity and the Dialogical Self. *Culture and Organization*. 2013;19:332–52.

Chambers T. 1999. *The Fiction of Bioethics: Cases as Literary Texts*. London: Routledge.

Charon R. 2006. *Narrative Medicine: Honoring the Stories of Illness*. Oxford: Oxford University Press.

Crawford P, Brown B, Baker C, et al. 2015. *Health Humanities*. Basingstoke: Palgrave Macmillan.

Foucault M. 1976. *The Birth of the Clinic: An Archaeology of Medical Perception*. London: Routledge.

Foucault M. 1988. *Technologies of the Self*. Amherst, MA: University of Massachusetts Press.

Freire P. 2017. *Pedagogy of the Oppressed*. Harmondsworth: Penguin.

Gabbay J, le May A. Mindlines: Making Sense of Evidence in Practice. *British Journal of General Practice*. 2016;66:402–03.

Gill A, Nelson EA, Mian A, et al. Responding to Moderate Breaches in Professionalism: An Intervention for Medical Students. *Medical Teacher*. 2015;37:136–39.

Hardt M, Negri A. 2000. *Empire*. Cambridge, MA: Harvard University Press.

Hardt M, Negri A. 2006. *Multitude.: War and Democracy in the Age of Empire*. London: Penguin.

Hardt M, Negri A. 2009. *Commonwealth*. Cambridge, MA: Harvard University Press.

Hardt M, Negri A. 2017. *Assembly*. Oxford: Oxford University Press.

Harman G. 2018. *Object-Oriented Ontology: A New Theory of Everything*. London: Pelican.

Hochschild AR. 1983. *The Managed Heart: Commercialization of Human Feeling*. Berkeley, CA: University of California Press.

Hunter KM. 1991. *Doctors' Stories: The Narrative Structure of Medical Knowledge*. Princeton, NJ: Princeton University Press.

Jones T, Wear D, Freidman L (eds.) 2014. *Health Humanities Reader*. New Jersey: Rutgers University Press.

Kalanithi P. 2019. *When Breath Becomes Air*. London: Bodley Head.

Levine D, Bleakley A. Maximising Medicine Through Aphorisms. *Medical Education*. 2012;46:153–62.

Lewis T. 2012. *The Aesthetics of Education: Theatre, Curiosity, and Politics in the Work of Jacques Rancière and Paulo Freire*. London: Bloomsbury.

Macneill P (ed.) 2014. *Ethics and the Arts*. Dordrecht: Springer.

Mangione S, Chakraborti C, Staltari G, et al. Medical Students' Exposure to the Humanities Correlates with Positive Personal Qualities and Reduced Burnout: A Multi-Institutional U.S. Survey. *Journal of General Internal Medicine*. 2018; 33: 628–34.

McFarlane A. 2018. *Nursing Humanities. April 17, 2018*. Available at: https://blogs.bmj.co m/medical-humanities/2018/04/17/nursing-humanities/

Miéville C. 2018. *The City & The City*. London: Picador Classic.

Milota MM, van Thiel GJM, van Delden JJM. Narrative Medicine as a Medical Education Tool: A Systematic Review. *Medical Teacher*. 2019;41:802–10.

Mol A-M. 2002. *The Body Multiple: Ontology in Medical Practice*. Durham, NC: Duke University Press.

Monrouxe L, Rees C, Dennis I, et al. Professionalism Dilemmas, Moral Distress and the Healthcare Student: Insights from Two Online UK-wide Questionnaire Studies. *BMJ Open*. 2014;5(5). Available at: http://dx.doi.org/10.1136/bmjopen-2014-007518

O'Neill D. *Surprised by Beauty*. 19 June 2015. Available at: https://stg-blogs.bmj.com/bmj/ 2015/06/19/desmond-oneill-surprised-by-beauty/

Peterkin A, Bleakley A. 2017. *Staying Human During the Foundation Programme and Beyond: How to Thrive After Medical School*. Baton Rouge, FL: CRC Press.

Peterkin A, Skorzewska A. 2018. *Health Humanities in Postgraduate Medical Education*. Oxford: Oxford University Press.

Portmann A. 1967. *Animal Forms and Patterns: A Study of the Appearance of Animals*. New York: Schocken Books.

Ramaswamy R, Ramaswamy R. 2020. Desire imagination Action: Theatre of the Oppressed in Medical Education. In: A Bleakley (ed.) *Routledge Handbook of Medical Humanities*. Abingdon: Routledge, 250–56.

Rancière J. 1991. *The Ignorant Schoolmaster: Five Lessons in Intellectual Emancipation Paperback*. Stanford, CA: Stanford University Press.

Rancière J. 1995. *On the Shores of Politics*. London: Verso.

Rancière J. 2006a. *Hatred of Democracy*. London: Verso.

Rancière, J. 2006b. *The Politics of Aesthetics*. New York: Continuum.

Rancière J. 2010. *Dissensus: On Politics and Aesthetics*. London: Continuum.

Rancière J. 2011. *The Emancipated Spectator*. London: Verso.

Rancière J. 2013. *Aisthesis: Scenes From the Aesthetic Regime of Art*. London: Verso.

Sartre J-P. 2003. *Being and Nothingness: An Essay on Phenomenological Ontology*. Abingdon: Routledge.

Schleifer R, Vannatta JB. 2013. *The Chief Concern of Medicine: The Integration of the Medical Humanities and Narrative Knowledge into Medical Practices*. Ann Arbor, MI: University of Michigan Press.

Shaw MK, Rees CE, Andersen NB, et al. Professionalism Lapses and Hierarchies: A Qualitative Analysis of Medical Students' Narrated Acts of Resistance. *Social Science & Medicine*. 2018;219:45–53.

Whitehead A, Woods A (eds.) 2016. *The Edinburgh Companion to the Critical Medical Humanities*. Edinburgh: Edinburgh University Press.

Wieringa S, Greenhalgh T. 10 Years of Mindlines: A Systematic Review and Commentary. *Implementation Science*. 2015;10:45.

Zahra FS, Dunton K. Learning to Look from Different Perspectives – What Can Dental Undergraduates Learn from an Arts and Humanities-Based Teaching Approach? *British Dental Journal*. 2017; 222:147–50.

3   Common wealth

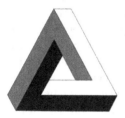

Medicine is naturally political

Geographical areas in America with the highest incidence of reported and treated physical pain are also those that most strongly supported Donald Trump at the 2016 USA presidential election and have gone on to form the rump of Trump's populist base. In these areas too are high incidences of addiction and deaths from the strongest of painkillers – prescription opioids such as OxyContin (Case and Deaton 2020). Alcohol abuse and suicide rates are also high, and the sufferers are mainly white, male and working class, often unemployed or in low wage, part-time or temporary "gig economy" jobs. Their distinguishing characteristic is lack of a university-level education. The anxiety of this group is huge, leading to such high suicide rates, and part of this anxiety rests with America's notoriously unfair healthcare system. Without a public health system, individuals who can afford health insurance find that it soaks up 18% of their annual income, and this figure is rising – in 1960, it was just 5%. An estimated 8.5% of Americans do not have health insurance (ibid.). Ironic, then, that this very group voted for a president who has tried to rip up ObamaCare.

For over a century up to the 1990s, life expectancy had increased year on year for Americans. And then something tipped. Relatively poor white, working-class Americans were at risk of dying at an earlier age than their parents and were living with more health problems. Two Princeton economists, Anne Case and Angus Deaton, worked out why, calling the toxic causative afflictions "deaths of despair" (ibid.). These communities, living in impoverished areas that had high unemployment in the wake of the loss of manufacturing or extraction, were wracked with despair; many people were offered prescription opioids by their family doctors, turned to alcohol abuse or committed suicide. As deaths from heart disease in the USA declined between 1990 and 2020, death from drug abuse and overdose, alcohol-related illness and suicide increased to outnumber cardiac illness–related deaths.

You would think that medical students and their educators would be falling over themselves to get their teeth into this upstream social issue affecting health. But medical schools are by and large myopic – focused on the thin, leading edge of the wedge that is downstream hospital-based acute care. Isn't this why students, especially the men, came into medicine? Isn't it here in sexier medicine that the fireworks happen? Sarah Barber et al. (2018: 160), in a study of medical students' preferences for future work, describe the "low perceived value of community-based working".

Certainly the complexity and technological wizardry are mainly concentrated in hospitals, and this is why they consume far larger budgets than primary care and community care combined. Of course, some students globally opt to study for social care or public health at the undergraduate level, but this is not a medical degree; some medicine graduates will study for a Master's degree in public health or community medicine or may study for a module in community medicine in their undergraduate programme. But by and large, undergraduate medicine fails to embrace community interests. This territory will only come fully into view if you train in general or family practice, care of the elderly or community psychiatry.

As much as 75% of medical issues globally are public health concerns or are socially determined – such as tainted water; lack of food and shelter; displacement as a consequence of war, political, ethnic or religious strife; and consequences of environmental disasters. Yet medical students spend very little time studying public health and policy issues. Recent research (Vaidaya et al. 2019) shows that in UK medical schools (31 were surveyed), students spend an average of 85 weeks on clinical placements over the whole course, of which around 63 weeks on average are spent in hospital medicine specialties and surgery placements, while 8 weeks are spent in general practice. Public or community health and care attracts little attention (only six UK medical schools provide public health placements).

But some centres for medical education are passionate about not only community health, but also how the medical humanities, with their interests in social justice issues, can feed into a community-oriented medical education. An international conference was planned for March 2020 at Vanderbilt University, Nashville, Tennessee, entitled "The Politics of Health" (Vanderbilt 2019). The conference was postponed due to the COVID-19 pandemic. The pre-conference advertising assumes the value of the social sciences and humanities in medical education, asking in what ways these contemporary inflections of medicine embrace issues of health equity, inclusion and justice. How does real-life medicine intersect with its virtual versions, such as television medical soap operas, in the portrayal of political issues? How should doctors respond to divisive political interventions in healthcare such as the anti-abortion, anti-vaxx and pro-gun lobbies? In what sense is there a "poetics of politics" that relates to health? What is a desired political future that best engages health interventions? How do we address both health inequities and inequalities?

The medical humanities offer medical students in particular media through which they can grapple with these issues of health inequality and inequity. Such work also brings medicine into contact with the social sciences beyond functional or instrumental engagements such as learning communication skills and the cognitive psychology of clinical decision-making. As medical education addresses politics, there is a danger that this is reduced to functional accounts of population health, the economics of medicine or instrumental policy issues, at which point students may be warned off entanglement with politics, where policy is traditionally seen as the job of politicians and managers, and doctors are too busy dealing with the clinical issues of patients to get tangled up in politics. As the American doctor and activist Alexander Leaf noted with a large dollop of irony, doctors get too caught up in "the cold dope" of traditional diagnosis and therapeutics to be bothered with issues of health and politics (Dunk and Jones 2020). Day-to-day clinical pressures become all consuming.

But this narrow focus on the functional-clinical not only places politics on the back burner but also strips out what gives the clinical encounter body and presence for both patients and health workers – ethics and aesthetics. Ethics brings value decisions to the forefront, so important to social justice and advocacy issues in medicine. Further, medical interventions can be handled clumsily, devoid of form and sensibility. This invites aesthetics to the table. Where this book is about politics in medicine and medical education, as we have already seen, ethics and aesthetics are necessarily bound into the discussion (Figure 3.1).

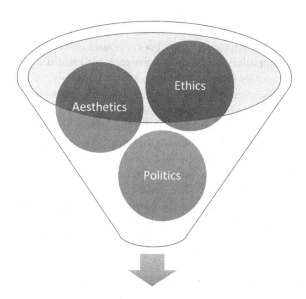

Medical education as a political text

Figure 3.1 The anatomy of the book.

Singing the "body electric"

As more of the world's natural resources such as oil and mineral deposits – in principle "common wealth", or owned by the multitude – have been appropriated as the capital by big business, and where most land is privately owned, common wealth has shrunk considerably, and health inequities and inequalities have expanded. While ground we tread, the air we breathe and seas and lakes we swim in can be considered as common wealth, such spaces have been appropriated by private enterprise – housing, industry, extraction such as mining, industrial agriculture, commercial planes and boats, transport in general, the leisure industries – and generally exhausted of raw materials, or left polluted. Of course we are complicit, as customers, in this colonization of our common wealth, but we would not wish upon ourselves the pollution and consequent health hazards that this brings, such as respiratory disorders from bad air. Again, the distribution of such ailments is undemocratic – the poor suffer more than the wealthy because their housing is concentrated in the most polluted areas where traffic congestion is worse.

Air pollution contributes to nearly nine million premature deaths annually, but these deaths are not distributed equally. People living in low-income countries suffer the most, where heavily polluting industries are outsourced and environmental regulations are lax. Sub-Saharan Africa has an incidence of death from air pollution that is 23 times higher than that of New Zealand, for example (McCarthy 2019). In America, black and Hispanic populations are more likely to live near to fossil fuel–dependent industrial sites that cause heavy air pollution, and these populations consequently have a higher incidence of respiratory disorders (Tessum et al. 2019). Studies in the UK show that in urban areas, richer households produce more air pollution, while poorer households have the highest level of exposure to such pollution and then suffer greater ill-health consequences. As Barnes and colleagues (Barnes, Chatterton and Longhurst 2019: unpaginated) conclude: "The research provides a stark argument for treating air pollution in the UK as a social justice issue as much as an environmental one".

The human body might be seen as the last bastion of common wealth – surely we own our hearts, lungs and genitalia – but of course this is not the case. We are subject to cultural expectations of how bodies should be and act: how they should be gendered, what thoughts we should have about our own and others' bodies and appearances, how bodies should perform and what constitutes both somatic and psychological health and illness. Our bodies are distributed. More importantly, we are subject to health issues from pollution or cross-species infections as our bodies are co-existent with other life forms as part of a global market. Despite the novel coronavirus pandemic, wet markets trading in "exotic" animals continue to flourish in South-East Asia.

The body is subject to both intimate and global powers, its health controlled by forces beyond its assumed identity, such as ambient pollution, and the poor and vulnerable body suffers most. Our collective existence is distributed across a fabric of sensory membranes. More, this global distribution of the sensible, controlled by big corporations and implicated in illegal animal trading, extends also to the mind – where our extended cognitions are part of the world-wide-web, as digitalized information. But this fabric of the sensible, and its associated pathologies, is subject to structural health inequities and inequalities. COVID-19 was hailed as a "great leveller", indiscriminate in its power to infect. But this turns out to be untrue – in the UK, for example, the virus has hit black, Asian and minority ethnic (BAME) groups the hardest. Black persons are four times as likely to die from infection and Bangladeshi and Pakistani persons nearly twice as likely as the white population, where BAME groups suffer the highest levels of social inequity and inequality, resulting in a high incidence of illnesses such as cardiovascular disease and diabetes. A similar pattern has been found in the USA (Bailey and West 2020).

To better understand the relationship between the personal body, the body of democracy and common wealth (or what is ideally held in common as a shared capital, such as the body and the body of the sea) prior to extensive contamination through pollution and bombardment through the age of information, I will return to the 19th century to consider what we can learn from the American poet Walt Whitman (1819–1892) as a champion of a people's medicine. Although a layperson with no qualification in medicine, Whitman gained experience as a volunteer nurse during the American Civil War, where he witnessed death, wounding and disfigurement, helping to treat hospitalized and recovering soldiers. Whitman offers an antidote to the contemporary insults to body and mind listed above, and a lesson in how medicine may be democratized, shifting from medicine assimilating society ("medicalization") to medicine accommodating to society's and individuals' needs (discussed in Chapter 6).

As already noted, the American writer and philosopher Ralph Waldo Emerson (1803–1882), a major influence on Whitman, had said: "The poet turns the world to glass", or makes the invisible visible. Whitman sees into the body to find: "The thin red jellies within you or within me, the bones and/ the marrow in the bones/ the exquisite realization of health" (from "I Sing the Body Electric"). Again, this is akin to the modern medical gaze as described by Michel Foucault – a "looking into" the body for the lesion, as if examining the dissected and anatomized corpse, that becomes a diagnostic "seeing", echoed in anatomy texts. This is the fabric of sensibility that has bound modern medicine for well over two centuries. Whitman offers an aesthetic form of political resistance to the dominant functionalism of the anatomical text and gaze. As a poet, he democratizes the body, refusing to privilege ideals, or kinds of bodies, but rather celebrating ordinary function – "My respiration and inspiration, the beating of my heart, the/ passing of blood and air through my lungs,/ ..." – as extraordinary, a "body electric" (ibid. *Leaves of Grass*: 51).

As a volunteer wound-dresser or auxiliary nurse in Unionist field hospitals during the American Civil War, Whitman had no need of learning anatomy through cadaver dissection or anatomy texts. He saw many badly wounded soldiers, both recovering and expiring: "in one of the hospitals I find Thomas Haley, Company M, 4th New York cavalry – a regular Irish boy ... shot through the lungs – inevitably dying" (Whitman 1961). Trained as a journalist, Whitman had a keen eye for detail, and this was amplified by being a close observer of the natural world. His 1882 book *Specimen Days* switches seamlessly between heart-rending descriptions of wounded soldiers and loving engagement with country lanes, ponds and grasses. Already exposed to the suffering body, Whitman's gaze is not the penetrating medical look, but a long, sinuous meandering glance that is reflected in his experimentation with long sentence prose poems.

His gaze on the body is literary: a double stimulus, the first a naïve, appreciative and exploratory glance; the second a reflective re-cognition through the loping sentences of prose poetry. The humanities take the contradiction of the body (it shines as it inevitably dies) to the second level of inquiry that celebrates the existential dilemma of the knowledge of ageing and death. Medical educators agree that medical students must meet the dead body early in their studies, either through cadaver dissection, attending an autopsy or encountering death in the hospital or community. But the second stimulus is vital: how will the death be sensitively and creatively acknowledged and then explored? The arts and humanities collectively afford primary media for such exploration.

Whitman then models an alternative medical gaze to that described by Foucault. Foucault describes a gaze of power and authority that sets the trainee doctor apart from the layperson where the ownership of organs and functions is temporarily assigned to the diagnostic and treatment regimes of medicine, stripping the patient of bodily capital. Whitman's "body electric", in contrast, is a shared current and pulse, a common wealth, identifying with wider nature as common property. This vision is aesthetic as well as democratic or political. It addresses beauty in common access to experience.

Where Foucault's medical gaze becomes dispersed to technologies such as high-end imaging (CT, MRI, CAT scans), Whitman's project is to use poetry and prose as a second stimulus in educating for citizens to grasp the right to know their own bodies. Poetry is the layperson's scanner, relying on metaphor as well as a literal description. The scan can be impressionistic rather than specific, educating a sensibility for a "body without organs", to borrow Gilles Deleuze and Félix Guattari's descriptor, which acknowledges a body refusing objectification and boundary, but one that is free-floating and "de-territorialized" (resisting colonizing, such as through medicalization). This is considered in more detail below.

Whitman's (1892/1961) late period *Specimen Days* is an interleaving of nature notes, written largely while he was recovering from a stroke in 1874–1875, and memoirs of his time working voluntarily as a wound-dresser or auxiliary nurse during the American Civil War largely in Washington DC. With sickness (the memory of wounded soldiers and his own partial paralysis) as a background, Whitman (1961: 114) describes "Nature's aroma" as a balm and "cooling breeze" to "some fevered mouth". He was horrified by the results of battle. Helping out in a field hospital at Falmouth, near Fredericksburg, Virginia, Whitman (ibid: 42) describes a scene "Outdoors, at the foot of a tree, within ten yards of the front of the house" (used as the hospital) "I notice a heap of amputated feet, legs, arms, hands, etc., a full load for a one horse cart".

At the close of the Civil War, Whitman (ibid.: 37) notes that the victory for democracy is "the peaceful and harmonious disbanding of the armies in the summer of 1865". For Whitman, authentic democracy follows the same trajectory as the emergence of the Hegelian Mind or Spirit – it is the natural, emergent, collaborative form of political organization, currently imperfect, readily distorted, a "horizon" historical project, more readily described as an ideal than achieved. Democracy is an unfolding state of inevitable human collaboration to better humanity. It then has an aesthetic curve to its process, a natural unfolding shape. Thus (ibid.: 268) "Democracy most of all affiliates with the open air, is sunny and hardy and sane only with Nature – just as much as Art is". Democracy will not flourish, claims Whitman, if it is cooped up in buildings, subject to instrumentalism and starved of aesthetics. Politics must engage beauty and form, and their models are self-evident in Nature. But the democratic gaze begins in recognizing the beauty of every part of the body as contributing equally to the whole, resisting a functional reading.

A person's "expression … appears not only in his face/ it is in his limbs and joints also, it is curiously in the joints of his hips and wrists/ it is in his walk". Such generosity towards the body is demanded even after illness. After Whitman suffered a stroke, he moved to Camden, New Jersey, where his health declined, and he died at 72. His funeral was a public event, embracing his own vision of the beauty of the ordinary multitude, where "There is something in staying close to men and women and/ looking on them, and in the contact and odor of them".

Whitman's lay medical vision, contra Foucault, is again echoed in the contemporary idea of Gilles Deleuze and Félix Guattari (2013) of the "body without organs". A territorializing or colonizing impulse overlays a conquered space with classifications: grids, mapping, co-ordinates, naming. This is an exercise of power, a means of control. It is reflected in the traditional "organ-based" and "systems-based" curricula of medical schools, as if persons could be understood bit-by-bit, inviting objectification and de-personalizing (Mannino and Pregler 2018). In contrast, a de-territorializing or nomadic impulse has no desire to colonize. The anatomized body (with organs) is the body colonized by medicine – for good reasons, as it must be understood before it is treated. But such colonization has a darker side – medicine exerts authority or sovereign power, and this can readily become distorted, as patronizing practices, for example, and ultimately as the Chronos Father that is "medicalization", eating his children as they are born lest they usurp his authority.

This anatomical "divide and rule" model for the human body has served medicine well. Deleuze and Guattari – echoing Whitman – would "sing the body electric" as the undivided and unconquered body – free from a directive and controlling gaze, but rather subject to an appreciative, poetic (and erotic – putatively banned in medicine) glance. This is the body of common wealth, democratized and shared in patient-centred and patient-directed medicine. Whitman's medicine is not *looking into* the body, but *looking after* the body.

Plague

My son, a geographer and athlete who makes films about surfing in wild locations around the world (and how surf eco-tourism projects can be developed to help local communities), returned in early March 2020 from filming in Algeria just as the first COVID-19 cases were registered in the UK. An image that stuck in his mind was a bookstall in the airport at Algiers that was stacked high with copies of Albert Camus's (1948) novel *The Plague*. The story is set in a fictional town, Oran, on the Algerian coast. It tells of how an animal-borne virus runs uncontrollably through the population of the town, killing half of its inhabitants. Even as the bodies heap up, people say that "this is not happening to us" and "plagues are medieval not modern"; further, as one of Camus' characters says: "everyone knows it has vanished from the West". In Camus' existentialist novel, in close proximity to death and the complete absence of safety, the lives of these people are drained of meaning. As hope recedes, so the world is turned from home to hospital and hospice.

The key character in the novel, Dr Rieux, works tirelessly to help the dying in Oran. Commended for his heroic work, the doctor says he is no hero, and that the only way to address the plague is "with decency". "What is decency?" somebody asks of Rieux, to which he replies: "doing my job". After a year or so, the plague ebbs away and the city returns to some sense of normality.

COVID-19 (novel coronavirus), Ebola, Sars, bird flu, HIV-AIDS – we are increasingly subject to epidemics and pandemics involving a crossing of pathogens from animal species to humans. Research on the genome sequence data of COVID-19 shows that it was not engineered in a laboratory – as conspiracy theories have suggested – but originated through natural processes. It may be that the virus entered the human population as a non-pathogenic entity and then evolved or mutated into the pathogen. A more likely scenario, however, is that COVID-19 (a SARS-Cov2 spike protein pathogen) most resembles related viruses found in bats and pangolins.

Direct bat–human transmission is unlikely. It is more likely that a human ate an animal that had been bitten by a bat. Or, a pangolin was eaten, or a human bitten by a civet or ferret that had in turn been infected by a pangolin. We may never know the exact chain of events, but there is a principle at play – we are increasingly exposed to animal life in a way that is unique in human evolution, and the reasons for this include our extensive industrial-like forays into previously untouched natural environments, for example through intrusive logging, mining and clearing for cattle ranching; this is exacerbated by extensive unregulated global trading in "exotic" animals promising large profits.

As the COVID-19 pandemic gripped, countries were desperate for critical care hospital beds, ventilators, masks and other equipment and trained staff to look after very ill patients. Nobody wished to see any deaths from this virus, but the numbers of people who become critically ill in relation to those who may be infected remained relatively small. Meanwhile, upstream medicine has to be more "home cooked" and user-friendly, often based on advice rather than treatment – "self-isolate", "look after yourself", "if you get symptoms rest and self-medicate", "see us if things get really bad". The tone is less hysterical than that of acute or critical care. Yet, if upstream primary care and community medicine, mixed in as it is with patients' "folk wisdom", were to be more successful, the numbers in hospitals would be less pressing. So, there is one vital lesson here: prevention rather than last ditch cure – or "trace, test, and treat". New Zealand, Australia and South Korea modelled it well.

Add to this the fact that a high proportion of deaths from COVID-19 occurred in community care homes. In relation to the theme of this book, there is a lesson here for medical education. Again, downstream hospitalist clinical activity has long held the gaze of medicine and has been the focus for undergraduate medical education at the expense of upstream community education. As noted previously, the vast majority of a UK medical student's clinical placement time is spent in hospital medicine specialties and surgery placements, rather than in general practice and public or community health. In the USA, there are dedicated public health schools (they do not offer medical degrees), and medicine graduates can study for a Master's degree in Public Health in many countries. But here, I am concerned with the relative lack of public health input in medicine and surgery undergraduate courses. A 2019 USA survey (Knight 2019) reports that American medical students are less likely to choose to become primary care doctors:

> Despite hospital systems and health officials calling out the need for more primary care doctors, graduates of US medical schools are becoming less likely to choose to specialize in one of those fields. A record-high number of primary care positions was offered in the 2019 National Resident Matching Program – known to doctors as "the Match." It determines where a medical student will study in their chosen specialty after graduation. But this year, the percentage of primary care positions filled by fourth-year medical students was the lowest on record.

There are historical reasons for this resistance to community medicine. In the context of European medicine, again, Michel Foucault (1976) has traced these reasons in *The Birth of the Clinic*. In a nutshell, the rise of hospital-based clinical treatment gave doctors a "room of their own" (to borrow from Virginia Woolf) away from the traditional visit to patients' own homes. This created a unique location for identity construction as a physician with a set of rituals, a uniform and a specialist knowledge and language. More, the hospital became a site for medical schools and clinical research, while anatomy laboratories aligned with mortuaries to provide teaching areas for anatomy through dissection. Medicine's face turned from the community to the hospital. Patients who once received doctors into their homes on the family's terms were now placed in the role of customers at hospital sites, where they had no role as stakeholders, although they had the right to expect hospitality. More, the hospital at first offered doctors a firewall from direct political interference, while politics stuck closely to the body of primary and community care.

Eventually, hospitalism too became subject to direct political influence, and the medical profession lost autonomy as it also was challenged to become more transparent in its practices. As noted, medical education has retained the two-tier system: a highly favoured hospital-based education and a significantly less-favoured primary and community-based education. As a result, medical education has kept away from politics and partially shunned the importance of issues such as health inequities and inequalities and prevention rather than cure. But now we have a third set of factors at work that I call "deep upstream". Medical education rarely casts its gaze in this direction – it is too busy with hospitalist concerns. But the "deep upstream" is fast becoming the major health challenge of our times. It embraces the health implications of the climate disaster, including global warming and environmental degradation, to which I turn in the following chapter; and the global trade in live animals through wildlife markets. To return to viral epidemics and pandemics, as noted here, new thinking suggests that the destruction of biodiversity may create conditions for the rise of new diseases. Emerging science of "planetary health" (Leaf 1989a, 1989b; Salas, Malina and Solomon 2019) moves us further upstream than classical population health medicine and its interests in health inequalities. Now, we must face the new wave of raw encounters between humans and pathogens from animals disturbed as their habitats are ravaged.

Where Michael Marmot (2015) asks, in the first line of *The Health Gap*: "Why treat people and send them back to the conditions that make them sick?" we should see a shift in the medical education gaze from downstream hospitalism to upstream community health as natural. A second shift to "planetary health" and "deep upstream" would make many anatomists and biomedical scientists uneasy, fearing they would lose curriculum space to fuzzy social scientists, anthropologists and do-gooder ecologists. Yet this shift can be made, and this book suggests how. This turn of the medical gaze embraces what socially conscious doctors have long demanded – active engagement with health inequities and inequalities as a priority and not an afterthought. This is a political engagement, the responsibility of citizens in a democracy.

We must embrace the fact that the medical gaze has already shifted from doctor-centred to patient-centred and patient-directed dialogue. Diagnosis was always by definition patient-centred – you do not get the diagnosis unless you observe and listen to the patient on his or her terms, where symptoms are in patients and not in textbooks, and where diagnoses are often in the patient's narrative of the illness. But treatment regimes have never been democratic, traditionally embracing hierarchical teams and doctor-centred practices. Dialogue with patients and authentic inter-professional engagement should follow the example already set upstream by primary and community practices, but this does not abandon core scientific biomedicine. Rather it embraces biomedical methods but filters these through a new literacy: critical health eco-literacy, defined and discussed in the following chapter.

Such health eco-literacy, as we shall see, describes a shifting landscape of politics as this engages medicine. A first wave of population medicine, introduced by

Rudolf Virchow in Germany in the mid- to late-19th century, embraced a socialist agenda in the challenge to structural health inequities and inequalities. It was explicitly about resistance to Government politics and policy in broad daylight – a battle about the exercise of sovereign power. Michel Foucault, looking at historical examples of regimes of "care of the self", noted that since late Greek and early Roman times, another form of politics besides sovereign control operated.

This was "biopower", introduced in Chapter 1 and developed in Chapter 7. It operates on and through the body, displaying in how people look after their appearance, hygiene and self-presentation to form an identity. A set of rules shapes the ways that self-care, such as hygiene regimes, operates within cultural and social groups that reach into the fine structures of behaviour (hence this kind of power is also called "capillary power"). Within these webs of self-imposed regimes, "governmentality" emerges that is both about external authority imposing rules, as public health, and internalized patterns of self-care. A contemporary example of the latter would be fitness classes, going to the gym, meditation, mindfulness and so forth.

None of these are externally imposed, but they are nevertheless highly regulated or rule-bound within each discipline. Sovereign power and capillary power can meet. "Wash your hands", "don't touch your face", "wear your mask in public", "don't shake hands", "socially distance", "self-isolate" are sovereign power imperatives in the coronavirus crisis that were quickly internalized as conscience or capillary biopower. Sovereign power remains as sanctions or fines for transgressions.

One of the greatest breakthroughs in hospital care and subsequently in public health was the hygiene regime of hand washing that becomes habitual or internalized, a healthcare worker's "conscience". In 1846, Ignaz Semmelweis, a doctor from Hungary working in Vienna, noticed a difference between the health of women giving birth in a midwife-run maternity ward to those in a medical student- and doctor-run ward. The latter had a much higher death rate from fevers. Noticing that medical students and doctors often came onto the wards after performing autopsies, he hypothesized that they had picked up what he called "cadaverous particles" and carried these into the maternity wards, subsequently infecting women. The end product of this story is hospital hygiene, saving many potential deaths.

Now, a "deep biopower" has emerged that has potentially sinister sovereign power implications. While hand washing is an "over the skin" form of surveillance leading to capillary power habits, a new "under the skin" form of surveillance is emerging in which governments can – and will in some cases – survey citizens as a sovereign power arrangement through health technology mobile phone apps and biometric bracelets that record and monitor temperature, blood pressure and proximity to others. Contact tracing legitimizes such surveillance.

The medical gaze (and with it the gaze of medical education, how medical students learn to become doctors) must shift from "opening up a few corpses", as Foucault described the modern medical education gaze of the late 18th and early 19th century that inaugurated a scientific, anatomy-based diagnostic medicine, to issues of health inequities and inequalities, and then to the "deep upstream" of damage to the health of the planet itself. The "lesion" here is in global health inequities and inequalities and the increasingly polluted and exploited body of the planet, including its oceans, lakes and waterways.

This shift of gaze embraces political issues and responds to them through activism. Indeed, conscious and thoughtful medical practice and medical education can both be thought of as kinds of resistance and activism, but these need a wider reach to embrace democratic habits for the health of the environment. How we can do this is to reconceptualize the undergraduate medicine curriculum and begin to think with this curriculum. How will we translate, for example, what we can learn from Walt Whitman about celebrating the democracy of the body, from inventive social activism responding to needs for PPE during the COVID-19 pandemic, or from "deep upstream" health inequality issues to shape a responsive medicine undergraduate curriculum? As this book unfolds, we will turn our gaze to such pressing pedagogical issues. Meanwhile, we turn from personal health and public health to the health of the planetary body of Earth itself, where humans are both its viral contaminators and its dependent guests – a strange contradiction. The planet provides hospitality and hostility in equal measures, but must we continue, in the Anthropocene Age, to only return the insult, as if the complex history of humanity were to conclude with hot air?

Bibliography

Bailey S, West M. 2020. *Ethnic Minority Deaths and COVID-19: What Are We to Do?* King's Fund. Available at: https://www.kingsfund.org.uk/blog/2020/04/ethnic-minority-deaths- COVID-19

Barber S, Brettell R, Perera-Salazar R., et al. UK Medical Students' Attitudes Towards Their Future Careers and General Practice: A Cross-Sectional Survey and Qualitative Analysis of an Oxford Cohort. *BMC Medical Education.* 2018;18:160.

Barnes JH, Chatterton TJ, Longhurst JWS. Emissions vs Exposure: Increasing Injustice from Road Traffic-Related Air Pollution in the United Kingdom. *Transportation Research Part D: Transport and Environment.* 2019;73:56–66. Available at: https://www.sciencedirect.com/science/article/pii/S1361920919300392#!

Camus A. 1948. *The Plague.* London: Hamish Hamilton.

Case A, Deaton A. 2020. *Deaths of Despair and the Future of Capitalism.* Princeton, NJ: Princeton University Press.

Deleuze G, Guattari F. 2013. *A Thousand Plateaus.* London: Continuum.

Dunk JH, Jones DS. Sounding the Alarm on Climate Change, 1989 and 2019. *New England Journal of Medicine.* 2020;382:205–07.

Foucault M. 1976. *The Birth of the Clinic: An Archaeology of Medical Perception.* London: Routledge.

Knight V. American Medical Students Less Likely to Choose to Become Primary Care Doctors. *Medical Xpress,* 24 July 2019. Available at: https://medicalxpress.com/news/2019-07-american-medical-students-primary-doctors.html

Leaf A. Potential Health Effects of Global Climatic and Environmental Changes. *New England Journal of Medicine.* 1989a;321:1577–83.

Leaf A. Health in the Greenhouse. *Lancet.* 1989b;1:819–20.

Mannino N, Pregler J. 2018. *Benefits of an Organ-Based Block Curriculum*. Available at: https://medschool.ucla.edu/body.cfm?id=1158&action=detail&ref=27

Marmot M. 2015. *The Health Gap: The Challenge of an Unequal World*. London: Bloomsbury.

McCarthy J. 3 Ways People in Poverty Suffer the Most From Pollution. *Global Citizen*, 17 May 2019. Available at: https://www.globalcitizen.org/en/content/how-pollution-affects-the-poor/

Salas RN, Malina D, Solomon CG. Prioritizing Health in a Changing Climate. *New England Journal of Medicine*. 2019;381:773–74.

Tessum CW, Apte JS, Goodkind AL, et al. Inequity in Consumption of Goods and Services Adds to Racial–Ethnic Disparities in Air Pollution Exposure. *PNAS*. 2019;116:6001–06.

Vaidaya HJ, Emery AW, Alexander EC, et al. Clinical Specialty Training in UK Undergraduate Medical Schools: A Retrospective Observational Study. *BMJ Open*. 2019;9:7.

Whitman W. 1961. *Specimen Days*. New York, NY: Signet Classics.

Vanderbilt 2019. International Health Humanities Consortium. *The Politics of Health Conference*. Available at: https://www.vanderbilt.edu/mhs/2019/06/2020hhc-2/

4 Climate emergency

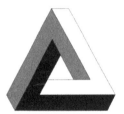

The climate emergency and medicine

Medicine's most pressing global issue (and political problem) is the climate emergency: global warming, increasing pollution and loss of biodiversity (WHO 1998). I will use this as a frame to illustrate how medicine, medical education, politics and aesthetics are intertwined in complex ways. They form what William Pinar (2006, 2011, 2012), the father of the "curriculum reconceptualization" movement in postmodern pedagogy, has called "complicated conversations" to describe a variety of expressions of curricula. I prefer "complex conversations". "Complicated" implies a linear problem that can be solved, where "complex" describes interacting dynamic systems that are appreciated and understood but remain beyond "solution-ism" (van der Niet and Bleakley 2020). My focus is on the undergraduate curriculum, where medical students begin their journeys to gain legitimate identities as doctors. My ever-present filter in thinking through these curriculum issues is a range of approaches common to the medical humanities.

The perils of global warming, pollution and loss of biodiversity – now commonly referred to as a "Climate Emergency" – are well documented (Vollmann 2018; Wallace-Wells 2019). Such perils have been widely discussed, particularly since the 1992 Earth Summit in Rio de Janeiro and its groundbreaking pre-conference meeting at Porto Alegre (Baird Callicott and da Rocha 1996), which led to a declaration of how university education could respond by encouraging "ecological literacy" (Orr 1992) across courses. This has now developed into a full-blown "ecopedagogy movement" as a variety of critical pedagogy, articulated particularly well by Richard Kahn (Kahn 2010).

Thirty years ago, there seemed to be "No Immediate Danger" of environmental impact from inexorable economic "growth" – to poach the title of William T. Vollmann's (2018) masterwork on "carbon ideologies". Vollmann's neologism "carbon ideologies", the subtitle to his book, plainly links carbon emissions and industrial-economic power structures bent on maximizing profit. This complex has come to cause our major public health threat, and those who will suffer most are the poorest and most vulnerable people who actually contribute least to carbon emissions.

Breaking the promises of neo-liberal capitalism, as economies "develop", the metaphorical rising tide does not in fact bring all boats with it (Picketty 2014). Rather, the very rich get much richer, as the poor sink and do not profit at all. Global neo-liberalism has brought a widening in income inequality with a knock-on effect on health disparities. Literal rising tides promise to be the downfall even of the rich, as our current trajectory of carbon emissions will increase global temperature by at least 3°C threatening to flood cities worldwide, including Miami and New York. A global survey conducted by the Royal Society of Tropical Medicine and Hygiene across 79 countries (Marzouk and Choi 2019) reported that the climate crisis was seen as the most important of global health concerns, where 92% of respondents believed that governments and health bodies were lagging in their response to the crisis. Madelon Finkel (2019: 265) describes how "planetary health" impacts on "poverty, nutrition, gender equity, water and sanitation, energy, economic growth, industrialization, inequality, urbanization, human consumption and production, climate change, ocean health, land use, peace, and justice".

Again, the most vulnerable social groups will also be those most severely affected by climate change outcomes, linked also with increasing levels of pollution. Large areas of the globe will be too hot to inhabit, and rising sea levels, as noted here, are already driving out low-lying communities, causing mass migrations. The "climate migrant" will be an increasingly common phenomenon, bringing new pressures on healthcare services. Air pollution in cities, already a major cause of death, will intensify. Increased sea levels and temperatures will lead to an increase in water-borne infectious illnesses such as cholera and toxin-related illnesses such as shellfish poisoning. Threats from extreme weather conditions such as forest fires, tornadoes and hurricanes will become more frequent and will have a major impact on biodiversity. There is no need to go on cataloguing disasters. These narratives are well known, reported daily in the media. Importantly, the existential threat of the climate crisis is a source of poor mental health – anxiety, depression and suicide ideation (Ciancon, Betrò and Janiri 2020) – most obviously for those who are already immediately threatened, such as delta farmers who once relied on the annual rise of rivers but now find that the tidal rise is overwhelmingly high and their livelihoods and homes are at risk or already destroyed.

But this, for many, is old news, and the tardiness of governments to respond is not just frustrating but shocking. Over two decades ago, a World Health Organization (WHO 1998) report linked climate change and health issues. *The*

Lancet (1989) medical journal ran an editorial "Health in the Greenhouse", warning that an environmental disaster would outreach the threat of nuclear war (Leaf 1989b). The evidence from science had already stacked up. Now it was time for global political action to address changes in the way that energy was being produced and consumed. In the same year as *The Lancet* editorial, the *New England Journal of Medicine* ran an article by Alexander Leaf entitled "Potential Health Effects of Global Climatic and Environmental Changes" (Leaf 1989a). Leaf was a chemist who later trained as a doctor, and he was also an activist, in particular an anti-nuclear demonstrator (Leaf 1986), who believed that the growing ecological crisis demanded political intervention.

By 2018, *The Lancet's* Countdown Report on the climate emergency and health repeated that "climate change is the biggest global health threat of the 21st century". As Finkel (2019) notes, around a quarter of our current global health burden can be directly or indirectly attributed to the effects of "environmental risks", such as air pollution, that could be modulated through cultural change of lifestyles or patterns of consumption (see Table 4.1). And this health burden will increase sharply.

Renee Salas and colleagues (Salas, Malina and Solomon 2019) led a call by the *New England Journal of Medicine* (NEJM) to prioritize the climate emergency as a primary risk to health (https://www.nejm.org/climate-crisis). They list increasing numbers of allergies due to increasing pollen, asthma increase due to deterioration in air quality, and increase in vectorborne diseases as a consequence of an expansion of the range of insect vectors. Ironically, again, those who will suffer most are those who have least contributed to carbon emissions. Salas and colleagues also note that health systems themselves have large carbon footprints and are thus simultaneously part of the problem and the solution. Caren Solomon and Regina LaRocque (2019), also in the NEJM, remind readers that the USA health care system accounts for a tenth of the country's carbon emissions and that if it were a country in its own right, this system would rank as the seventh globally in terms of volume of emissions.

The NEJM further notes a new kind of voice in medical research and reporting: not simply passively describing, but actively encouraging response, or direct action – in other words, politicizing. James Dunk and David Jones (2019, 2020) describe how Alexander Leaf sounded alarm bells about climate change three decades ago when few were listening. More, they also note that Leaf was not simply

Table 4.1 Climate change risks

Kinds of risk	Illustrative example
Immediate and direct	Air quality, heatwaves, extreme weather
Indirect	Infectious disease distribution, fish stocks, water quality
Deferred and diffuse	Existential concerns and impact on mental health
Associated with conflict and refugee flow	Civil conflict, exposure to risks in temporary camps, loss of citizenship, discrimination affecting the quality of life

a theorist but, as noted above, an activist. As a Harvard professor, in 1961 Leaf co-founded Physicians for Social Responsibility and joined the International Physicians for the Prevention of Nuclear War (IPPNW). He urged doctors to extend their vision and activities beyond the clinic. His memoir noted that "there are social and man-made hazards with possibly disastrous consequences to human health" ignored by medical education (Leaf 1996). Doctors must then stand "in the vanguard".

As Dunk and Jones note, by the early 1980s, Physicians for Social Responsibility "had established a significant public presence and won substantial political clout". Leaf bemoaned the lack of engagement amongst his colleagues and medical students with policy, as noted earlier, and was disappointed to find that many students preferred to learn just "the cold dope" — traditional diagnosis and therapeutics. At this moment in time, in the wake of Leaf's inspiration, for Dunk and Jones (2020: 207), "It may no longer be appropriate for physicians to remain apolitical", where "activists have turned from research to advocacy to civil disobedience. They promise to sound the alarm on climate change and human health ever more forcefully until our societies are transformed".

The climate emergency and medical education

Already at the cliff's edge, medical schools are waking up to the fact that the health implications of the climate emergency should be central to any undergraduate medicine curriculum. It is not a luxury but an imperative. The American "Physicians for Social Responsibility" website for August 2019 reported that "medical schools (are) now moving to teach future doctors to address climate change". "Moving" is a troubling word here, where rapid curriculum development is necessary. It would be preferable to see medical schools actively doing, rather than planning to do. Further, pedagogically, should we be "teaching" medical students about the climate emergency, or rather drawing on their interest and motives to *facilitate* independent and collaborative learning? What medical students need, again, is *health eco-literacy*: not an inventory of facts about how climate change is impacting upon health, but rather a language and conceptual apparatus, or way of understanding that allows critical appreciation and leads to choosing the most appropriate tools for engagement. Students need to learn a sustainable practice deriving from the values of health eco-literacy.

As noted in previous chapters, where medical education still tends to favour the production of downstream hospitalists engaging in acute and critical interventions, health issues are largely situated upstream, in communities and concentrated in multiple chronic issues in the elderly population. Structural social injustices have a direct impact upon life expectancy – for example, politically led economic austerity over the past decade in the UK has led to an unprecedented lowering of life expectancy for those living in the most deprived areas (Health Foundation 2019). Medical students need to engage with this at first hand, not just in primary care clinics but also in food banks, shelters, drug and alcohol rehabilitation units and housing units.

While there is an urgent need to address knowledge of the health impact of climate change for medical students, a prior question is: "are medical schools open to curriculum change as a pedagogical principle"? A 2017–18 survey of 147 North American medical schools carried out by the Association of American Medical Colleges (AAMC 2018) reported that 35% planned to make future curriculum changes, and 31% already had such changes in process. Some medical schools have moved quickly, such as the University of California – San Francisco, to weave "climate health" into the medicine curriculum. But, given the urgency of need presented by the global climate crisis, are these numbers enough? There is momentum; however, Beth Howard (2019) notes a number of important initiatives across North American medical schools, including an elective "Climate Medicine" at the University of Colorado School of Medicine. But, again, why an elective and why not core and compulsory provision?

The American Medical Association (AMA 2019) suggests "incorporating the health implications of climate change into the spectrum of medical education, including topics such as population displacement, heat waves and drought, flooding, infectious and vector-borne diseases, and potable water supplies". But we should note that these are material health issues and do not include crucial psychological, social or cultural dimensions. As our primary global existential threat (replacing the threat of nuclear war that the Cold War brought and the fall of the Berlin Wall dissipated), climate change's impact as noted here is psychological as well as somatic – bringing widespread anomie or dread.

Perhaps in the near future, climate change denial will be categorized in the *Diagnostic and Statistical Manual of Mental Disorders* (DSM). "Denial" after all is one of the key Freudian ego defence mechanisms and a common neurosis that can become uncommonly large amongst politicians in particular as the ego grows and "alternative facts" are mobilized. It is shocking to see that, in 2019, a commentator can suggest that "Climate change curriculum in med school is a waste of time and money" (Schieber 2019). In an article first published in the *Epoch Times* (an alarmist right-wing paper) and republished in the *Heartland Institute* newsletter, AnneMarie Schieber (ibid.), a journalist, warns of "progressive politics that are seeping into the medical school curriculum at an alarming rate".

Further: "Medical schools should be focused on the how of treating disease, *not being indoctrinated with politically tinged subjects such as climate change*" (my emphasis). More: "When medical schools engorge their curriculums with the political fare, it comes at the expense of something else. … There is no room today in our daunting health care system to be wasting time and money teaching doctors about climate change". It is ironic that a blatantly politically motivated paper commenting on medical issues would suggest that medicine and politics should not mix. The *Guardian* newspaper has exposed the Heartland Institute, a global warming–denying right-wing think tank, as "financed by fossil fuel and coal companies" (Kirschgaessner and Holden 2020).

Schieber's notion that medical schools might "engorge" their curricula shows faulty thinking about what a curriculum is, failing to differentiate between content (syllabus) and process (curriculum thinking). Undergraduate study could never encompass the huge informational content of contemporary medicine in any case, so students must learn how to learn, or to gain knowledge independently and collaboratively. A typical problem-based learning (PBL) session for early years medical students does not encompass the teaching of set content, but is a facilitated process in which students find out collaboratively what basics or essentials needs to be known, and what could, or should, be done for a particular illustrative patient or healthcare issue.

Rather than "engorging" the curriculum, a smart educational approach is, again, to facilitate the learning of literacies, in this case eco-literacy, or more specifically, health eco-literacy (Maxwell and Blashki 2016). The "medical text" (the patient and his or her social context) can then be read ecologically. This means not only a literal reading of the relationships between ecology and health, but also consideration of metaphor, such as a reconceptualization of the way that, for example, cancers are talked about – no longer in unhelpful militaristic metaphorical language ("fighting disease", "the war on cancer") that can exhaust already exhausted patients (Bleakley 2017), but in terms of ecological metaphors such as "resources", "balance" and "conservation of energy". This is a checks-and-balances approach rather than an aggressive battle. We should note that when the novel coronavirus pandemic hit, reporting reverted to industrial-strength use of martial metaphors – a knee-jerk, rather than a considered, response.

Eco-literacy is not just learning facts about challenges from climate change. Rather, it is acquiring a language that allows for understanding of, and critical discussion about, environmental issues, such as through complexity and chaos models – both of which should already be established in medical education as paradigms by which "health" and "disease" are understood, but which are still gaining a foothold as essential knowledge paradigms in the field. This "meta" approach has been described as building "adaptive expertise" through medical education (Bell et al. 2012). Again, such an approach is not content-led but process-led, in the tradition of problem-based learning, one that might be better described as patient- and population-based learning (see Chapters 11–13). Just as clinical diagnostic reasoning is learned through exposure to patients in tandem with discussions with experts, so eco-literacy is a diagnostic and treatment method best learned through inter-disciplinary contact with, for example, geographers, earth scientists and oceanographers.

As with much content and process in the medicine curriculum, medical students can learn to extend functional medicine to medicine as artistry, embracing both humane and imaginative approaches such as narrative approaches to improve understanding of patients' stories. The medical humanities in medical education can stimulate this shift from learning what is already known to learning for innovation and change. Problem-based learning "cases" (usually individual "paper" patients) can be extended to extreme weather case studies and their impact on public health, such as Hurricane Katrina and the 2009 extreme wildfires in California and bushfires in Australia. Cases will then embrace communities. Resources can be extended beyond scientific issues to involve double stimulation, using as the second stimulus, for example, auto-ethnography insider accounts, photographic documentation and literary accounts or "ecofictions" such as Tom Piazza's (2009) *City of Refuge* and Jenny Offill's (2020) *Weather*.

Importantly, medical students should become reflexive about the carbon footprints of the medical systems in which they work, learning how they can help to reduce those footprints. For example, as noted earlier, the USA health system is the seventh-largest producer of carbon emissions globally (Rappleye 2017), contributing to increasing air pollution and causing, for example, the very pulmonary problems that doctors end up treating. The National Health Service (NHS) is responsible for 5.4% of the UK's greenhouse gas emissions, with over 20 million tonnes of CO_2 emissions annually, costing over £50 million on carbon permits (Bawden 2019). A leading organization for ecologically responsible healthcare, *Health Care Without Harm*, reports that the global carbon footprint for the healthcare industry worldwide accounts for 4.4% of net CO_2 emissions (https://noharm.org). If it were a country, global healthcare would be the fifth largest emitter on the planet.

There are, however, model healthcare organizations that have taken steps to reduce their carbon footprints. Newcastle NHS Trust in the UK installed combined heat and power plants in its hospitals in the late 1990s, where all electricity used comes from 100% renewable sources. New staff, patient and visitor electric bus services have been commissioned, and catering and estates vehicles are electric. Since 2011, the combined Trust has sent zero waste to landfill and recycles more than 40% of non-clinical waste (where the average in the NHS is 23%). Details matter – the hospital cafes and restaurants all provide compostable cutlery and plates.

Pockets of concerned medical students and doctors worldwide have prompted urgent action on the climate emergency in both medical education and publicly as professionals who are first and foremost concerned citizens. The University of Hawaii's John A. Burns School of Medicine has created a Division of Ecology and Health to research and develop innovative, community-based projects at the interface of ecological and health sciences that can be incorporated into the medicine curriculum. This educates medical students to extend biopsychosocial models to embrace "ecohealth" perspectives. This in turn invites inter-disciplinary learning and trans-disciplinary problem solving that can be carefully woven into the existing curriculum by imaginatively reconceptualizing process rather than adding new content.

A group within the Canadian Federation of Medical Students has called for more education on climate change to be implemented by 2020 (Mercer 2019) in the face of global lag. The International Federation of Medical Students' Association is urging medical schools to integrate climate topics into the curriculum urgently in the wake of its survey of schools across 118 countries, which showed that less than 16% engage with climate emergency issues as part of their curricula (Earls 2019). In the USA, by 2019, 187 schools and programmes had joined a coalition set up in 2017 by Columbia University's Mailman School of Public Health to network curriculum ideas about climate change education, where The Global Consortium on Climate and Health Education has set up a resource bank including links to slides, videos and online courses, as well as

curriculum   ideas   (https://www.mailman.columbia.edu/research/global-conso
rtium-climate-and-health-education).

Meanwhile, the American Medical Association (AMA) has urged teaching on climate change to all physicians and medical students. Individuals such
as Caroline Wellbery, a family physician, medical educator and professor at
Georgetown University Medical Center, Washington DC, has for some time
been a leading figure in calling for medical schools to urgently incorporate
health eco-literacy in medicine curricula, noting that this is a "transboundary"
issue requiring imaginative collaborative pedagogical responses (Wellbery et al.
2018). Where translational medicine has linked bench science research to clinical practice and population health, we must now add environment and ecology
as a fourth factor.

Recognizing that, as noted here, the health and care systems in England alone
are responsible for more than 5% of its total carbon footprint, the UK NHS has
launched a "Greener NHS" campaign to tackle health issues arising from the
climate emergency. This initiative will attend first to home-grown carbon emissions, with the reduction of air pollution as a key concern. This is estimated to
cut new asthma cases by a third. The NHS plans to become the world's first major
health service to get to net-zero emissions and is working in tandem with "Lancet
Countdown", an independent international expert group researching and advertising the links between health and the climate emergency. Health services can
reduce emissions and pollution through using renewable energy sources; building energy-efficient hospitals; using electric vehicles; sparing patients unnecessary trips to hospitals through better use of technologies such as telemedicine;
changing pharmaceutical packaging and habits of pharmaceutical consumption
through schemes such as the "green" and "blue" gyms (encouraging exercise,
lifestyle changes and environmental awareness); updating medical devices; and
changing patterns of use of polluting anaesthetics.

A parallel process to these "greener" health service schemes must be consciousness-raising about appropriate activism and protest. Clinicians and medical
school staff should be able to engage in open discussions with their employers
about the right to peaceful protest in joining non-violent action groups such
as Extinction Rebellion (https://www.doctorsforxr.com/health-hub). Doctors are
citizens first and foremost, and, given their commitment to cure and care, are
surely morally implicated in ecological issues that bear on health.

Behind the climate issue is a spectre haunting medical education

Medical education must remain nimble and responsive to changing social conditions and emergent issues such as the climate crisis. The modern period of medicine since the late 18th century embraces a golden era of hospital medicine and
hospital-based acute care. Yet the contemporary face of healthcare across many
nations is one centred on an ageing population with multiple chronic morbidities
that are largely managed in the community, drawing on a large cohort of unpaid
carers (usually family members).

Again, medicine has focused on the downstream fallout from upstream health determinants such as poverty and environmental degradation, and medical education has echoed this. Hospital care has the biggest concentration of resources such as technologies, testing and research, but primary and social care in the community constitutes most of healthcare. The coronavirus pandemic brought these issues into sharp focus where a significant number of deaths occurred in the community in care homes, and crowded institutions such as prisons and refuges have proved to be particularly vulnerable to the spread of the virus. Crowded shantytowns such as Brazil's favelas have, predictably, also been particularly vulnerable.

Scientists and public health journalists continue to do their job of studying and advertising climate change trends, but the climate emergency has now become a political issue. A cabal of major political figures (and their supporters) remains as climate change deniers or sceptics, seemingly in the grip of the oil, gas and coal conglomerates. At the time of writing, the countries with the biggest carbon footprints are China (28% global emissions and the biggest coal producer), USA (15% and third-biggest coal producer), India (8% and second-biggest coal producer), and the Russian Federation (5% and sixth biggest coal producer). Each has at the time of writing a leader who is not committed to a radical change in energy policy and each is, in turn, a plutocracy – run by and for the wealthiest.

Add to this that the biggest carbon sink, the Amazon forest, is being decimated for political gain by Brazil's currently autocratic government, while Australia, the world's fourth-biggest coal producer and the largest net exporter of coal, has recently been subject to the worst bushfires ever experienced and has a government which has buried its collective head in the sand over the climate emergency while its backyard burns by committing to opening extensive new coal mines. The climate emergency can only be addressed by radical shifts in politics, but the political will must be evident.

Medicine's relationship to the climate emergency – where, as already noted, health services are major contributors to carbon emissions worldwide – is necessarily mediated through policy and politics. Before health eco-literacy, medicine must make its political entanglements clear and gain political literacy. Politicians take as their right and responsibility governance of health services, yet doctors – while engaging with policy – have characteristically steered clear of mixing party politics and medicine, or have been unable to square their political affiliations with their duties to provide equitable healthcare and engage with patient advocacy. In order for future doctors to gain political literacy, the medicine undergraduate curriculum must engage with politics; or, the curriculum must be treated as a political text. The climate emergency is medicine's springboard into the world of politics.

In the following chapter, I show that there is a spectre haunting climate change that we can call a "political will". At the time of writing, the major polluting nations of the world and the major coal and oil producers and exporters are led by governments who are in climate denial, and by standard (and stale) neo-liberal models that refuse to accept that "economic growth" based on carbon ideologies in the current climate emergency are unsustainable. This blinkered vision is a health hazard affecting us all.

Bibliography

American Medical Association (AMA). 2019. *Global Climate Change and Human Health H-135.938*. Available at: https://policysearch.ama-assn.org/policyfinder/detail/climat e%20change?uri=%2FAMADoc%2FHOD.xml-0-309.xml

American "Physicians for Social Responsibility". 2019. *Medical Schools Now Moving To Teach Future Doctors To Address Climate Change*. Available at: https://www.psr.org/ blog/2019/08/09/medical-schools-now-moving-to-teach-future-doctors-to-address-cl imate-change/

Association of American Medical Colleges (AAMC). 2018. *Curriculum Change in US Medical Schools*. Available at: https://www.aamc.org/data-reports/curriculum-reports/in teractive-data/curriculum-change-us-medical-schools

Baird Callicott J, da Rocha FJR. 1996. *Earth Summit Ethics: Towards a Reconstructive Postmodern Philosophy of Environmental Education*. New York: State University of New York Press.

Bawden A. 2019. The NHS Produces 5.4% of the UK's Greenhouse Gases. How Can Hospitals Cut Their Emissions? *The Guardian*, 18 September 2019. Available at: https ://www.theguardian.com/society/2019/sep/18/hospitals-planet-health-anaesthetic-g ases-electric-ambulances-dialysis-nhs-carbon-footprint

Bell E, Horton G, Blashki G, Seidel BM. Climate Change: Could It Help Develop "Adaptive Expertise"? *Advances in Health Sciences Education*. 2012;17:211–24.

Bleakley A. 2017. *Thinking With Metaphors in Medicine: The State of the Art*. Abingdon: Routledge.

Cianconi P, Betrò S, Janiri L. The Impact of Climate Change on Mental Health: A Systematic Descriptive Review. *Frontiers in Psychiatry*. 2020;11:74.

Dunk JH, Jones DS. Sounding the Alarm on Climate Change, 1989 and 2019. *New England Journal of Medicine*. 2020;382:205–07.

Dunk JH, Jones DS, Capon A, Anderson WH. Human Health on an Ailing Planet — Historical Perspectives on Our Future. *New England Journal of Medicine*. 2019;381:778–782.

Earls M. Despite Climate Change Health Threats, Few Medical Schools Teach It. *Scientific American*, 27 December 2019. Available at: https://www.scientificamerican.com/autho r/maya-earls/

Finkel ML. A Call for Action: Integrating Climate Change into the Medical School Curriculum. *Perspectives on Medical Education*. 2019;8:265–66.

Health Foundation. 2019. *Mortality and Life Expectancy Rates in the UK*. Available at: https://www.health.org.uk/publications/reports/mortality-and-life-expectancy-trends-i n-the-uk?gclid=Cj0KCQiA1-3yBRCmARIsAN7B4H39ArKPPF_ojBqLaDzllkN-75 bMyKPhlrHK1M3w4Tp0GU_PTBPGzgUaAmRqEALw:wcB

Howard B. Climate Change in the Curriculum. *AAMC News*, 10 October 2019. Available at: https://www.aamc.org/news-insights/climate-change-curriculum

Kahn R. 2010. *Critical Pedagogy, Ecoliteracy, Planetary Crisis: The Ecopedagogy Movement*. New York: Peter Lang.

Kirschgaessner S, Holden E. Naomi Seibt: "Anti-Greta" Activist Called White Nationalist an Inspiration. *The Guardian*, 28 February 2020. Available at: https://www.theguard

ian.com/environment/2020/feb/28/naomi-seibt-anti-greta-activist-white-nationalis
t-inspiration

Leaf A. New Perspectives on the Medical Consequences of Nuclear War. *New England Journal of Medicine.* 1986;315:905–12.

Leaf A. Potential Health Effects of Global Climatic and Environmental Changes. *New England Journal of Medicine.* 1989a;321:1577–83.

Leaf A. Health in the Greenhouse. *Lancet.* 1989b;1:819–20.

Leaf A. 1996. *Autobiographical Memoir and Oral History: Interview with Arnold S. Relman.* Boston, MA: Harvard Medical School.

Marzouk S, Choi H. 2019. What Does the Next 25 Years Hold for Global Health? *Med Box.* Available at: https://medbox.org/document/what-does-the-next-25-years-hold -for-global-health#GO

Maxwell J, Blashki G. Teaching About Climate Change in Medical Education: An Opportunity. *Journal of Public Health Research.* 2016;5:673.

Mercer C. Medical Students Call for More Education on Climate Change. *C.M.A.J: Canadian Medical Association Journal.* 2019;191:E291–92.

Offill J. 2020. *Weather.* London: Granta.

Orr DW. 1992. *Ecological Literacy: Education and the Transition to a Postmodern World.* New York: State University of New York Press.

Piazza T. 2009. *City of Refuge.* New York: Harper Perennial.

Picketty T. 2014. *Capital in the Twenty-First Century.* Cambridge, MA: Harvard University Press.

Pinar WF. 2006. *The Synoptic Text Today and Other Essays: Curriculum Development after the Reconceptualization.* New York: Peter Lang.

Pinar WF. 2011. *The Character of Curriculum Studies: Bildung, Currere, and the Recurring Question of the Subject.* New York: Palgrave Macmillan.

Pinar WF. 2012 2nd ed. *What is Curriculum Theory?* London: Routledge.

Rappleye E. US Healthcare Is World's 7th Largest Producer of CO_2. *Becker's Hospital Review,* 20 April 2018. Available at: https://www.beckershospitalreview.com/populat ion-health/us-healthcare-is-world-s-7th-largest-producer-of-co2.html

Salas RN, Malina D, Solomon CG. Prioritizing Health in a Changing Climate. *New England Journal of Medicine.* 2019;381:773–74.

Schieber A. 2019. *Climate Change Curriculum in Med School is a Waste of Time of Money.* Heartland Institute. Available at: https://www.heartland.org/news-opinion/news/c limate-change-curriculum-in-med-school-is-a-waste-of-time-and-money

Solomon CG, LaRocque RC. Climate Change – A Health Emergency. *New England Journal of Medicine.* 2019;380:209–11.

Van der Niet AG, Bleakley A. Where Medical Education Meets Artificial Intelligence: "Does Technology Care?" *Medical Education,* 20 February 2020. Available at: https://on linelibrary.wiley.com/doi/abs/10.1111/medu.14131

Vollmann WT. 2018. *Carbon Ideologies Vols. I and II.* New York: Penguin Random House.

Wallace-Wells D. 2019. *The Uninhabitable Earth: A Story of the Future.* London: Allen Lane.

Wellbery C, Sheffield P, Timmireddy K, et al. It's Time for Medical Schools to Introduce Climate Change Into Their Curricula. *Academic Medicine.* 2018;93:1774–77.

World Health Organization (WHO). 1998. Climate Change and Human Health – Risks and Responses. *Summary.* Available at: https://www.who.int/globalchange/summary/ en/index2.html

5 Political emergency

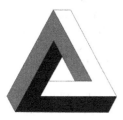

Conservative backlash to identity politics or "political correctness"

Under National Socialism in Nazi Germany, Hitler inaugurated what Paul Rabinow and Nikolas Rose (2016: 304) called "a complex mix of the politics of life and the politics of death", where:

> Nazi doctors and health activists waged war on tobacco, sought to curb exposure to asbestos, worried about the overuse of medication and X-rays, stressed the importance of a diet free from petrochemical dyes and preservatives, campaigned for whole grain bread and foods high in vitamins and fiber, and practiced vegetarianism.

Yet, the same philosophy of active health free from contamination saw Jews, Gypsies and black people as contaminants paving the way for "the paths to the death camps". The same authors (ibid.: 323) see in contemporary global democracies "a new political economy of vitality", where "cystic fibrosis groups cut across national and class barriers as do their caregivers; models of patient activism spread and are taken up and reinterpreted from Bangladesh to Toronto", while depressed people form a "global category" in a "new biopolitics of mental health" advertising grassroots support structures that transcend race, ethnicity, class, gender and age classifications. Such "expert patient" and "lay self-help" networked cultures advertise to some extent the demise of medical paternalism.

Many doctors too are not just anti-paternalistic, but are also social activists. Charles van der Host (2014: 1958) notes that "in April 2013, North Carolina health care professionals began joining diverse other activists in 'Moral Monday' protests aiming to change the minds of the governor and state legislators about expanding Medicaid under the Affordable Care Act", an act of "civil disobedience". Merlin Chowkwanyun and Benjamin Howell (2019: 1870) describe a "revival of activism among U.S. medical students" as part of a "dissenting tradition in medical training". But in the same period that this "revival of activism" is occurring, there is a not unexpected counter-resistance from conservatives.

After the horrors of the Nazi Holocaust, a group of social scientists (Else Frenkel-Brunswik, Daniel Levinson, and Nevitt Sanford) under the leadership of Theodor Adorno (Adorno et al. 1950), a Jew who had fled Germany to live in America, wrote a book to gather thoughts about what makes an authoritarian psychological type. They formulated a cluster of traits: conventionalism, anti-intellectualism, superstition and occultism, power and toughness, destructiveness and cynicism, tendency to project one's faults onto others, scapegoating and exaggerated concerns over sex. To this we can add the most obvious traits: nationalism, separatism and racism. This profile is readily seen today in white, gun-toting, right wing populist militia groups worldwide.

But left wing totalitarian regimes too display authoritarian style. For example, while Cuba is lauded for educating an extraordinary number of doctors per head of population, and many of them will practice globally in challenging contexts, the medical education system is hierarchical and infused with militaristic rhetoric. Cuban medical texts are overtly political, showing how socialist medicine must be practised and then ideologically interpellating doctors into society. Such structures emphasize militaristic hierarchies, subordination to overt power and self-discipline. The Cuban "revolutionary doctor" is described as a "health militant" (Rigol et al. 1994: 28). Indeed, Cuban medical school curricula typically include mandatory military training and identity construction as an insurgent fighting imperialism and injustice.

In support of the system, however, we should note that the state demands that doctors be authentic – simple and honest – in their dealings with others, at the other end of the scale from the authoritarian diktat. In a later chapter, I have a concluding section on Cuban doctors, noting too that they do notably good work internationally (de Albornoz 2006). Medical workers are said to be Cuba's main export, with over 20,000 working out of the country at any one time, mostly in needy and deprived locations.

A cousin to the authoritarian personality is the narcissistic personality, oblivious to the concerns of others resulting in objectification, self-aggrandizing and never admitting to fault or error. Psychoanalysts typically see this presentation, once the distinguishing mark of surgical culture, as a pathologized product of lack of extensive and intensive play as children, where the person was never able to practice a range of social interactions that challenged self-centredness. Productive play sets the stage for learning democratic habits. As adults, narcissistic types always have second chances at learning how to socialize adequately through "adult play" (or better – "work" as aesthetically fulfilling) as the humanities and arts, where fantasy is not just allowed but encouraged, and where objectification is discouraged (Nussbaum 2010). This, again, is a primary role for the medical humanities in medical education.

In an opinion piece in the *Wall Street Journal*, Stanley Goldfarb (2019: unpaginated), a physician and retired associate dean of curriculum at the University of Pennsylvania's Perelman School of Medicine, complains about "woke" medical schools where "curricula are increasingly focused on social justice rather than treating illness". "Woke" is invoked here in a disparaging way. It is an African American term referring to vigilance (staying awake, or "woke") to acts of discrimination. We should expect that progress in mixing medicine and politics would attract snide remarks from naysayers.

Goldfarb's nostalgia for a golden age of medical education lost to so-called woke interests is badly misguided as the state of American medicine shows. There is a serious fault-line running through American medical education that has a knock-on effect for the health system. As William Hsiao (2020: 96, 97), a Harvard economist, notes: "There are many statistics that illustrate the flaws of the U.S. health-care system", where "The United States is the only advanced economy that does not offer universal health care coverage". This in itself should be enough to provoke widespread protest amongst medical educators. Where Americans spend nearly twice as much per capita on healthcare than other advanced post-industrial economies, in comparison with European, Japanese, Australian and Canadian societies, Americans have "lower life expectancy, higher infant mortality rates, and a higher prevalence of heart disease, lung disease, and sexually transmitted diseases", where income inequality feeds health disparities.

Hsiao notes also that around 30% of the capital spent on healthcare per annum in America is wasted – just as vast amounts of food and energy are wasted. This amounts to $1 trillion a year bleeding out from the healthcare budget. Fraud and abuse in insurance claims, high administrative expenses and duplication of services all add to this waste, yet, again, many Americans do not have any or adequate health insurance. Affordable and effective universal healthcare in what is the world's most advanced economy is a puzzle to those of us who look on from a free at the point of service nationalized healthcare system (paid by taxation, but the system – apart from 25% that is privatized – runs as not-for-profit). In contrast, Hsiao (ibid.: 99) notes that in America, "health care still remains primarily a private-sector activity driven by the profit motive".

Daniel E. Dawes (2020) meticulously tracks the development of President Barack Obama's "comprehensive health care reform" initiated in March 2009 as a model for "the political determinants of health". The late Senator Edward Kennedy took on the task of promoting such reform as a personal mission, as he himself was dying from a brain tumour. By July 2009, under pressure from opponents of reform, the president referred to "health care reform", dropping the descriptor "comprehensive", and by August 2009, this had mutated to "health insurance reform". This became popularized as "ObamaCare". Dawes shows how political machinations practically wrecked the plan for healthcare for all, and how, since Donald Trump's election as president in 2016, strenuous efforts have been made to sabotage and dismantle the proposal. But Dawes does not get at the root reason why universal healthcare is so disliked in America – where it is perceived as government meddling in an individual's business. This is part of a hysterical element in the American psyche that so treasures individualism that it equates such liberty with the right to citizens carrying guns, despite the consequences for high levels of gun crimes. The right to bear arms – the 2nd Amendment – was ratified in 1791 and in that context can be understood. But in the current era, following the 2nd Amendment, constitutes one of America's major health hazards, where

> more than 30 years of public health research supports thinking of guns as sta-tistically more of a personal hazard than a benefit. Case-control studies have repeatedly found that gun ownership is associated with an increased risk of gun-related homicide or suicide occurring in the home … For homicides, the association is largely driven by gun-related violence committed by family members and other acquaintances, not strangers.
>
> (Pierre 2019)

We saw in the previous chapter that the American Medical Association (AMA) is now a strong supporter of introducing the climate emergency into the under-graduate curriculum. But the AMA was not always so liberal. In the late 1940s, President Harry Truman tried to introduce a universal healthcare insurance, but this was blocked by the AMA, who stirred up a bitter campaign to disparage Truman's plan as "socialized medicine", even calling it "un-American" and sup-porting "the Moscow party line" (Hsaio 2020). In the mid- to late-1940s, UK doctors responded initially in the same way to early proposals for the National Health Service (NHS), fearing they would lose private work.

Stanley Goldfarb (2019) chastises the American College of Physicians for supporting stricter gun controls, where medicine has "stepped out of its lane". Let's again address this prejudice with facts. Particularly in emergency medicine, American doctors are called upon to treat injuries from firearms costing an esti-mated $230 billion annually, while there are 40,000 deaths annually from gun use, just behind deaths caused by opioid and other drug uses (rising from nearly 40,000 in 2011 to nearly 70,000 in 2019). Guns are the leading cause of death among children and adolescents and African American youth, and are impli-cated in 70% of over 8,000 suicides per annum in the elderly population.

It was the powerful National Rifle Association (NRA) and the pro-gun lobby who recently advised doctors to "stay in their lane" when issuing state-ments on gun control and safety, but Rebecca Cunningham and colleagues (Cunningham, Zimmerman and Carter 2019) report the "beginning of the end of the medical community's silence on the issue of firearm research and safety". (There are many advocacy groups for gun control: http://library.ship.edu/c. php?g=21651&p=126895). In the USA, Physician Political Action Committees (PACs) are common. There is however a "disconnect" between PACs' member-ship positions and gun control action (Schuur, Decker and Baker 2019). Doctors too are reluctant to upset the NRA and wider gun lobby. This echoes an earlier era where doctors were not outspoken enough about tobacco use as they remained in some cases financially supported by the tobacco industry.

Goldfarb also notes disapprovingly: "During my term as associate dean of curriculum at the University of Pennsylvania's medical school, I was chastised by a faculty member for not including a program on climate change in the course of study", where "such programs are spreading across medical schools nationwide" as if this were an unwelcome infection. Skeptics such as Goldfarb, meanwhile, might take heed of analyses such as that of Alice Hill and Leonardo Martinez-Diaz (2020: 107) who suggest that "lost productivity due to climate-related illness are projected to consume an estimated $500 billion per year by the time a child born today has settled into retirement".

Medical schools are chastised for "inculcating social policy" when they should be teaching students to "cure patients". Goldfarb blames "A new wave of educational specialists" who are "increasingly influencing medical education" and who emphasize "social justice" topics "at the expense of rigorous training in medical science". This in turn, claims Goldfarb, comes of a mindset that "abhors hierarchy of any kind and the social elitism associated with the medical profession in particular". Further, "The prospect of this 'new,' politicized medical education should worry all Americans" claims Goldfarb, who then lays the blame on social learning theorists, again infecting medical education: "Theories of learning with virtually no experimental basis for their impact on society and professions now prevail. Students are taught in the tradition of educational theorist Étienne Wenger, who emphasized 'communal learning' rather than individual mastery of crucial information".

This actually runs counter to the evidence base for the effectiveness of teams. For example, changes in operating theatre practices that embrace the mandatory global Surgical Safety Checklist must include collaborative briefing and debriefing of lists, found to improve surgical outcomes (Gawande 2009; NHS England 2019). As noted several times in this book, evidence shows that more democratic team structures in healthcare have better patient outcomes, also improving patient safety and worker satisfaction (Borrill et al. 2000).

Of course it is easy to spot the source of Goldfarb's prejudice, and this links back to the politicization of healthcare in America. The emphasis upon the heroic individual, the heart of Protestant-Capitalist ideology (as argued by Max Weber), leads to a prejudice against nationalized and centralized healthcare, or collaborative rather than individualistic practices of learning. Democracy is translated back to the freedom of the individual (and the right to bear arms) rather than progressed forward to collective responsibility (and peaceful negotiation towards compromise, however tough). Thus, as Hsiao (2020) points out, Medicare for All proposals are rejected as policy interference in the right to choose how one's healthcare will be managed. But of course those who need the care the most are the ones who are not in a position to choose.

Goldfarb's doomsday polemic properly attracted a largely hostile online response. More than 150 alumni of the Pennsylvania's School of Medicine bothered to strongly refute his claims. On Medscape (2019), Penn Med graduate doctors said: "We are compassionate, socially responsible, and grounded in the deep-rooted belief that doctors are vehicles for social justice. … we believe that social justice should not only have a place, but a central place, in the medical school curriculum".

While scientific medical practices can rise above party politics, medical provision is necessarily the subject of ideology. But this is not a one-way process, with active politics shaping a passive medicine, as medicine too can speak back to political systems with its own ideological agendas. For example, as noted here, in 1948, UK senior doctors actively resisted the formation of the National Health Service (NHS), realized as a Labour Party (socialist) vision. A resolution had been passed at the 1934 Labour Party Conference by Dr Somerville Hastings, then president of the Socialist Medical Association, to set up a state health service. Consultants further threatened withdrawal of labour over the suggestion that they should relinquish their private (and financially lucrative) work. But should we be concerned about doctors' party politics? In the UK certainly, one's political affiliations are generally thought of as a private affair. But doctors' voting habits should be of interest, even concern, to patients and colleagues.

The voting habits of doctors

While doctors are not traditionally supposed to allow their political beliefs to influence their medicine, this is evidently not the case. I am sure that Stanley Goldfarb provides excellent personal care for his patients, but his value system clearly affects his views on medical pedagogy, and this has a knock-on effect on how he might help shape the character of his students. We have scant evidence concerning links between doctors' political affiliations and their work, but what we have is telling.

In an age of patient-centred medicine and inter-professional teamwork with "flattened hierarchies", we might expect that democratic habits are taught at medical school and linger into later practice. The knock-on effect of this is that you might expect doctors to lean towards a socialist or left wing politics that promotes equality and equity or a social justice agenda. As Yannis Gourtsoyannis (2019), a doctor working in the UK, says: "As an NHS doctor, it's my public duty to vote Labour" (socialist or left wing). But doctors do not necessarily support a socialist or collaborative agenda. After all, many are in profit seeking businesses, embedded in neo-liberal capitalist economies. Pharmaceutical and medical equipment companies are vying for sales, while hospitals are no longer places of "hospitality" but "managed" independent companies desperately cutting corners to save costs.

In an article entitled "Your Surgeon Is Probably a Republican, Your Psychiatrist Probably a Democrat", Margot Sanger-Katz (2016: unpaginated) notes voting patterns in the USA by medical specialty, where "In surgery, anesthesiology and urology, for example, around two-thirds of doctors who have registered a political affiliation are Republicans. In infectious disease medicine, psychiatry and pediatrics, more than two-thirds are Democrats". Researchers know this from combining a listing of every doctor in the USA with party registrations of every voter across 29 states. This yields a dataset of 34,532 physicians. The data reveal that more than half of doctors who vote do so as Democrats, but a significant minority identify as Republicans. True to a stereotypical expectation, Republicans feature more heavily in surgery, while Democrats are the large majority in psychiatry.

Sanger-Katz reports that political leanings are probably already established as medical students and then reinforced on work-based rotations in the later undergraduate years. For example, a placement on infectious diseases may bring a medical student into contact with members of communities from under-privileged backgrounds that may become addicts with hepatitis C. Students veering towards family and community medicine are likely to be pre-disposed towards medicine as a social intervention to redress issues arising from inequality and under-privilege.

In North America, higher earning doctors such as surgeons are more likely to align with Republican than Democrat values, resisting practices of redistribution of wealth through taxation. Gender also matters; again in the USA, women doctors are more likely to align with Democrats than Republicans, and women now outnumber men in both recruitment to medical schools and medical practice worldwide, where "as women enter fields like pediatrics, obstetrics/gynecology and psychiatry, they may be making those fields more liberal" (ibid.). The political landscape amongst younger doctors has shifted to the left, partly, or mainly, because of the influx of women into medicine over just one generation. In general, "the partisanship of doctors looks very different from a generation ago, when most physicians identified as Republicans. The influx of women may help explain that change" (ibid.). In North America, doctors (the majority of whom were male) once ran their own businesses and took on the pro-business position of moderate right wing politics. Now, most doctors' work has been subsumed in large corporations and hospitals, and this has resulted in a shift to democratic values in challenging the large profit margins of corporations at the expense of employers (the doctors themselves) and consumers (patients).

Hippocrates meets the voting booth

So much for the distribution of affiliations, but does this mean anything for practice – does a doctor's ideological leaning affect his or her treatment recommendations? Ideology can indeed influence the treatment of patients in the face of doctors' commitments to treat all patients equally (ibid.). Eitan Hersh and Matthew Goldenberg (2016) looked at the relationship between doctors' political affiliations and choices of treatments culled from hypothetical cases. Doctors were asked to consider groups of hypothetical patients with a range of presenting symptoms. For most symptoms, all doctors would respond in pretty much the same way, but for three symptoms, responses from the doctors differed markedly. One hypothetical patient presented with a history of abortions and was seeking advice about another abortion. Where Democrat-leaning doctors asked: "what does the patient want?" and would give medical advice accordingly facilitating the patient's wishes, Republican-leaning doctors were more prescriptive. These doctors would wish to recommend counselling and warned of the dangers of mental health issues in the wake of an abortion.

A second patient who talked in a consultation about owning guns and presented with mental health problems would be advised by Democrat-leaning doctors about not keeping guns at all at home, where Republican-leaning doctors would recommend safe storage of guns. A third hypothetical case was a patient who was a habitual marijuana user. Democrat-leaning doctors would not judge the marijuana use per se, but tended to look at this in the overall context of the patient's mental health, where Republican-leaning doctors would actively counsel against marijuana use, stressing legal and health implications. Of course doctors across the board will differ, sometimes radically, in their treatment recommendations for reasons other than ideological bias, but this study is suggestive and invites further explorations. Where it would be very unusual for a patient to inquire about a doctor's political leanings prior to a consultation, if the patient is presenting with issues concerned with, say, reproductive health or drug use, the political leanings of the doctor may matter. Politics and ethics of treatment are then linked.

Politics in the medicine curriculum – still a novelty

The house journal of the American Medical Association (JAMA) advertises what appears to be a comprehensive list of topics covered by the journal. Authors are encouraged to "Customize your JAMA Network experience by selecting one or more topics from the list below". These are listed as Table 5.1 below. It is sobering to think of the breadth of this list and how slender it may have looked a century ago when Abraham Flexner (1910) published his landmark Carnegie Foundation Report on the state of medical education in North America and Canada.

Although "humanities" is listed, what is notable by its absence from this fulsome JAMA list is the topic of "politics". Topics that are taboo, or culturally repressed, still "hang around" in language but are kept *sous rature* (under erasure) (Heidegger 1962; Derrida 1967). Again, medicine has historically shown an outward face of keeping politics "under erasure": as politics. What is under erasure may be a trace or a deposit from a historically important period or idea, or it may be a "live" issue that is repressed or kept at arm's length. Politics in medicine has had this quality of "stink" about it. Politicians, meanwhile, have the stink on them, having no problem in explicitly shaping the face of medicine. Actually, medicine has always been political while seemingly in denial of this fact, as repeated throughout this book. More, medical *education* has deliberately avoided the political. It is time to examine the motives for this and the benefits for medical education of cultivating a more explicit but refined and thoughtful, relationship with the political.

Table 5.1 Journal of the American Medical Association (JAMA) topics

Acid Base, Electrolytes, Fluids
Allergy
Allergy and Clinical Immunology
Anesthesiology
Anticoagulation
Art of the JAMA Network
Bleeding and Transfusion
Cardiology
Caring for the Critically Ill Patient
Challenges in Clinical Electrocardiography
Clinical Challenge
Clinical Decision Support
Clinical Implications of Basic Neuroscience
Clinical Pharmacy and Pharmacology
Complementary and Alternative Medicine
Consensus Statements
Critical Care Medicine
Dental Medicine
Dermatology
Diabetes and Endocrinology
Drug Development
Electronic Health Records
Emergency Medicine
End of Life
Environmental Health
Ethics
Facial Plastic Surgery
Foodborne Illness
Gastroenterology and Hepatology
Genetics and Genomics
Genomics and Precision Health
Geriatrics
Global Health
Guide to Statistics and Medicine
Guidelines
Hair Disorders
Health Care Delivery Models
Health Care Economics, Insurance, Payment
Health Care Policy
Health Care Quality
Health Care Reform
Health Care Safety
Health Care Workforce
Health Disparities
Health Informatics
Health Policy
Hematology
History of Medicine
Humanities
Hypertension

(Continued)

Table 5.1 (Continued)

Images in Neurology
Imaging
Immunology
Implementation Science
Infectious Diseases
Innovations in Health Care Delivery
JAMA Infographic
Law and Medicine
Leading Change
Less is More
Lifestyle Behaviors
Medical Coding
Medical Devices and Equipment
Medical Education
Medical Education and Training
Medical Journals and Publishing
Melanoma
Mobile Health and Telemedicine
Narrative Medicine
Nephrology
Neurology
Neuroscience and Psychiatry
Notable Notes
Nursing
Nutrition
Nutrition, Obesity, Exercise
Obesity
Obstetrics and Gynecology
Occupational Health
Oncology
Ophthalmic Images
Ophthalmology
Orthopedics
Otolaryngology
Pain Medicine
Pathology and Laboratory Medicine
Patient Care
Patient Information
Pediatrics
Performance Improvement
Performance Measures
Perioperative Care and Consultation
Pharmacoeconomics
Pharmacoepidemiology
Pharmacogenetics
Pharmacy and Clinical Pharmacology
Physical Medicine and Rehabilitation
Physical Therapy
Physician Leadership
Poetry
Population Health

(Continued)

Table 5.1 (*Continued*)

Professional Well-being
Professionalism
Psychiatry
Public Health
Pulmonary Medicine
Radiology
Regulatory Agencies
Research, Methods, Statistics
Resuscitation
Rheumatology
Scientific Discovery and the Future of Medicine
Shared Decision Making and Communication
Sleep Medicine
Sports Medicine
Statistics and Research Methods
Stem Cell Transplantation
Substance Use and Addiction
Surgery
Surgical Innovation
Surgical Pearls
Teachable Moment
Technology and Finance
The Rational Clinical Examination
Tobacco and e-Cigarettes
Toxicology
Trauma and Injury
Treatment Adherence
United States Preventive Services Task Force
Urology
Users' Guide to the Medical Literature
Vaccination
Venous Thromboembolism
Veterans' Health
Violence
Women's Health
Workflow and Process
Wound Care, Infection, Healing

Bibliography

Adorno TW, Frenkel-Brunswik E, Levinson DJ, Sanford RN. 1950. *The Authoritarian Personality*. New York: Harper & Row.

Borrill C, West MA, Shapiro D, Rees A. Team Working and Effectiveness in Health Care. *British Journal of Health Care Management*. 2000;6:364–71.

Chowkwanyun M, Howell B. Health, Social Reform, and Medical Schools – The Training of American Physicians and the Dissenting Tradition. *New England Journal of Medicine*. 2019;381:1870–75.

Cunningham RM, Zimmerman MA, Carter PM. Money, Politics, and Firearm Safety: Physician Political Action Committees in the Era of "This is Our Lane". *JAMA Netw Open*. 2019;2: e187823.

Dawes DE. 2020. *The Political Determinants of Health*. Baltimore, MD: Johns Hopkins University Press.

De Albornoz SC. On a Mission: How Cuba Uses Its Doctors Abroad. *British Medical Journal*. 2006;333:464.

Derrida J. 1967. *Of Grammatology*. Baltimore, MD: Johns Hopkins University Press.

Flexner A. 1910. *Medical Education in the United States and Canada: A Report to the Carnegie Foundation for the Advancement of Teaching*. New York: Carnegie Foundation.

Gawande A. 2009. *The Checklist Manifesto: How To Get Things Right*. London: Profile.

Goldfarb S. 2019. Take Two Aspirin and Call Me by My Pronouns. *The Wall Street Journal*, 12 September 2019. Available at: https://www.wsj.com/articles/take-two-aspirin-and-call-me-by-my-pronouns-11568325291

Gourtsoyannis Y. 2019. As an NHS Doctor, It's My Public Duty to Vote Labour. *The Guardian*, 27 April 2017. Available at: https://amp.theguardian.com/commentisfre e/2017/apr/27/doctor-nhs-vote-labour-austerity-conservatives?CMP=share_btn_ tw&__twitter_impression=true&fbclid=IwAR1UMsnKZ0jP-lNA6yXhPRnxEN -Mkp0w9MbG3waJKAa_-fANUNrgujO9KXQ

Heidegger M. 1962. *Being and Time*. New York: Harper & Row.

Hersh ED, Goldenberg MN. Democratic and Republican Physicians Provide Different Care on Politicized Health Issues. *Proceedings of the National Academy of Sciences of the United States of America*. 2016;113:11811–16.

Hill A, Martinez-Diaz L. Adapt or Perish: Preparing for the Inescapable Effects of Climate Change. *Foreign Affairs*, Jan/Feb 2020, 107.

Hsiao WC. How to Fix American Health Care: What Other Countries Can – and Can't – Teach the United States. *Foreign Affairs*, Jan/ Feb 2020. Available at: https://www.for eignaffairs.com/articles/united-states/2019-12-10/how-fix-american-health-care

Medscape. 2019. *An Open Letter to Our Former Dean, Dr Stanley Goldfarb, From 150+ Alumni of the University of Pennsylvania School of Medicine*. Medscape. 20 September. Available at: https://www.medscape.com/viewarticle/918782

NHS England. Decade of Improved Outcomes for Patients Thanks to Surgical Safety. *Check List*, 21 January 2019. Available at: https://www.england.nhs.uk/2019/01/surgi cal-safety-checklist/

Nussbaum MC. 2010. *Not for Profit: Why Democracy Needs the Humanities*. Princeton, NJ: Princeton University Press.

Pierre JM. The Psychology of Guns: Risk, Fear, and Motivated Reasoning. *Palgrave Communications*. 2019;5:159.

Rabinow P, Rose N. 2016. Biopower Today. In: VW Cisney, N Morar (eds.) *Biopower: Foucault and Beyond*. Chicago, IL: University of Chicago Press, 297–326.

Rigol OR, Perez FC, Perea JS, et al. 1994. *Medicina General Integral – Tomo Uno*. La Habana: Editorial Pueblo y Educación.

Sanger-Katz M. Your Surgeon Is Probably a Republican, Your Psychiatrist Probably a Democrat. *New York Times*, 6 October 2016. Available at: https://www.nytimes.com/2 016/10/07/upshot/your-surgeon-is-probably-a-republican-your-psychiatrist-probabl y-a-democrat.html

Schuur JD, Decker H, Baker O. Association of Physician Organization–Affiliated Political Action Committee Contributions With US House of Representatives and Senate Candidates' Stances on Firearm Regulation. *JAMA Network Open*. 2019;2:e187831.

Van der Horst C. Civil Disobedience and Physicians – Protesting the Blockade of Medicaid. *New England Journal of Medicine*. 2014;371:1958–60.

6   An uncomfortable intimacy

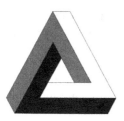

Medicine can both assimilate society and accommodate to it

The interplay of politics and medicine can be read as two sides of a coin: on one side the assimilation of society into medicine, or the "medicalization" of society to form a politically charged "pharmacracy" (Szasz 2003, 2007; Conrad 2007), and on the other, the accommodation to society by medicine through community-collaborative public health. Both are political projects but with differing goals. The medicalization of society represents a totalizing process of assimilation of a wide range of cultural activities and values into a medical model.

Here, medicine operates as a dominant discourse or is hegemonic so that a wide range of behaviours and experiences previously unlabelled become marked as symptoms – medical or health issues. For example, everyday angst becomes treatable "anxiety". Social behaviours are read as symptomatic ills of a social body that can be treated largely by pharmaceuticals. "Big Pharma" (Law 2006) colludes with, or even shapes, the medicalization project with a promise of profit. Szasz (2003) suggests that this leads to a "pharmacracy", a culture dependent upon prescribed drugs, where Big Pharma, embracing the most profitable and largest of global companies (Ledley et al. 2020), exerts undue power. Medicine and politics are inextricably mixed, as pharmaceutical companies also become major lobbyists, particularly in American politics.

In contrast to the assimilation model, the medical accommodates other discourses such as the psychological, sociological and anthropological, as one amongst a number of explanatory approaches. Here, the political and the medical have a benign relationship in which the medical is the listener and the political the speaker, often of the voice of the oppressed. Medicine offers its expertise in a collaborative gesture in support of common wealth and furthers its democratization.

Pharmacracy: Medicine assimilates society

Ivan Illich's (1974: 1) celebrated *Medical Nemesis: The Expropriation of Health* opens with a startling claim: "The medical establishment has become a major threat to health. The disabling impact of professional control over medicine has reached the proportions of an epidemic. Iatrogenesis, the name for this new epidemic, comes from *iatros*, the Greek word for physician, and genesis, meaning origin". Numerous commentaries have appeared on this work, most recently Seamus O'Mahony's (2020) review of how Illich's work looks 40 years on.

In an earlier review, Raymond Killeen (1976: 69) defended medicine against Illich's argument that it stripped laypersons first of the capability to tolerate illness and pain, and second of the capability to treat themselves where possible. Killeen warns that a polemic such as Illich's "is the kind of stuff that social planners and politicians will leap upon because it means inaction and a step backwards". In other words, politics is, unfairly, set square against medicine and is full of empty promises.

Jack Geiger (1976: 1), in a review in the *New York Times*, notes that Illich claims: "Modern medicine has made us sicker. Worse, it has created in us a worldwide addiction, as passive medical consumers, to 'therapeutic' relationships with monopolizing professionals and arrogant medical bureaucracies and institutions". While Geiger agrees with Illich that personal responsibility for healthcare must not be substituted with reliance upon professionals, he also reminds us that those professionals provide care as well as aiming for a cure. He sees Illich as promoting a "sterile individualism", a form of self-help, so easily exploited by small-scale entrepreneurs ready to peddle their snake oil in the "alternative medicine" market.

In the wake of Illich, perhaps the most acute observer of the medicalization of society, where medicine assimilates society, is probably the radical psychiatrist and psychoanalyst Thomas Szasz (2003, 2007), although he writes from the perspective of a radical libertarian who is highly critical of centralized government intervention and control, and, further, he argues largely about the medical shaping of mental health rather than somatic conditions. Such libertarianism in contemporary America proves to be a precarious position – while Szasz is not right wing, the territory he occupies is one shared by right-wing groups and "antivaxxers" (Shwetz 2020) and fuelled by conspiracy theories. For example, nearly a third of Americans believe that COVID-19 was produced in a Chinese laboratory (Noor 2020).

Szasz's "medicalization thesis" follows from earlier work in which he debunks modern psychiatry partly as a discipline that invents the conditions it treats. Thus, what were once personal or social issues are re-badged as medical conditions requiring therapeutic intervention. This may be one of personal choice but also of coercion. Szasz (2007) suggests that this is a double-edged sword:

"Medicalization is not medicine or science; it is a semantic social-strategy that benefits some persons and harms others". I will have more to say about the relationship between semantics and medical education later in this book, but here we can turn Szasz's critique on its head.

Szasz clearly means that merely by "labelling" an activity an illness, it takes on a different colouration. For example, what was once lauded as mild melancholia – the disposition of thinkers – now becomes treatable "depression", given a sharp profile as it is situated in an age of mania, inflation, psychological buoyancy through therapy and excessive consumption. But Szasz's argument too relies on semantics: for example, "pharmacracy" is a swollen neologism that smacks of control. Chronic pain sufferers, for example, bless the pharmacracy for the balm it can administer. Ivan Illich, in challenging medical dominance, does so from an extreme position of exhorting the qualities of suffering.

The sociologist Peter Conrad's (2007) *The Medicalization of Society* reinforces Szasz's view. Conrad has debunked the notion of "hyperactivity" (for example in Attention Deficit Hyperactivity Disorder or ADHD) that has led to a rash of diagnoses in children, even as young as seven, and an inflation of the stimulants-based pharmaceutical regimes that "treat" ADHD such as Ritalin and Focalin (Bleakley 2015, 2016) and the "geneticization" of conditions better seen as psychological or cultural. Conditions that are genetic – such as male pattern baldness – are not medical issues (illnesses) yet lead to stigma and searches for treatments or cures.

Conrad does not blame medicalization purely on medicine in league with Big Pharma, but sees some patient advocacy groups – otherwise normally lauded for their work – affirming and intensifying questionable diagnoses, often reinforced by media interests. He does not suggest that society as a whole is subject to medicalization as a totalizing assimilative strategy, but rather that medicalization happens in, rather than to, society. He notes, however, that the US pharmaceutical market constitutes 40% of the world market. Thus, rather than discussing the validity or invalidity of medical diagnoses, Conrad prefers to describe the "viability" of a dominant medical overview – for example in asking "could the issue (such as 'erectile dysfunction') be seen as a behavioural or even a moral one rather than a medical condition demanding a medical intervention?" Some conditions, such as Chronic Fatigue Syndrome (CFS) or myalgic encephalomyelitis (ME), sit in an uncomfortable position between biomedical legitimacy (an immune disorder) and psychological expression ("tiredness"). The illness then is "viable" but not necessarily valid. Patient advocacy groups fight for recognition of the illness as somatic, where the descriptor "myalgic encephalomyelitis" affords legitimacy, while psychotherapists advertise that they can "work with" those suffering from CFS, largely by-passing the somatic.

Szasz notoriously challenged medicine's totalizing of human behaviour that Foucault, as we have seen and will discuss further in Chapter 7, referred to as biopower exercised as a governmentality or surveillance – the absolute control of human habits through the organization of capillary power. Foucault described how the medical clinic comes to manage bodies and minds as a form of sovereign power expressing a power differential between doctors and patients based on both knowledge and privilege. At the same time, people become medicalized as they operate within fields of biopower such as health awareness, hygiene regimes, self-help and self-development, support groups and so forth. These organizations of capillary power can work with a dominant discourse (hygiene regimes) or against such discourse as forms of resistance (for example self-harming as an artistic performance strategy). Szasz sees medicalization as politicizing bodily and mental states: as both a top-down (medical experts categorizing previously non-medical conditions as medical) and bottom-up (biopower as self-policing) process.

As a psychiatrist, Szasz, following Michel Foucault's *Madness and Civilization* (republished in 2006 as *History of Madness*), is largely concerned with the medicalization of behaviour and mind. Foucault sees the rise in the classification of so-called mental illnesses as part of a widespread move to order in society through naming as a basis for the exclusion of the unwanted. For Szasz, the rise of psychiatry mirrored a shift in moralizing behaviour to pathologizing it, and this, in turn, again provided a basis to a profit-seeking pharmaceutical industry promising treatment of the very conditions they invent, hand-in-glove with capitalist medicine. In a medicalized society, where behaviour was previously judged for its ethical impact – virtuous or immoral – now it is judged as healthy or unhealthy, and often reduced to speculation about underlying neurological causes.

Where behaviour is symptomized, so cures or treatments are not far behind. Where a neural mechanism or a biochemical imbalance is invoked as a cause (even where the evidence for such a mechanism may be lacking or fuzzy), so a pharmaceutical may be developed or adapted from its original target to treat the condition. Rather than the condition and symptom preceding the treatment, the treatment may precede and create the condition – a world that Lewis Carroll's perverse Queen of Hearts knows well.

An example of this is the history of Ritalin, mentioned above, a super-amphetamine now commonly used to treat attention deficit hyperactivity disorder (ADHD). In the grandiose naming of the "disorder" we already see medicalization and medical inflation at work as political interests: ordering the flow of biopower and creating a form of governmentality sanctioned, as Szasz himself says, by mainstream psychiatry. Ritalin (the trade name) is methylphenidate, first synthesized in 1944 but not identified as a stimulant until 1954. First used to compensate for low blood pressure, Ritalin was named by the chemist Leandro Panizzon, who first synthesized it, after his wife whose nickname was Rita. It was not until the 1960s that the drug was used to treat so-called maladjusted children, as it was first used as a super-stimulant to redress the effects of narcolepsy and barbiturate-induced coma. The drug was also used to treat memory loss in the elderly. An extended-release version of the drug – trade name Concerta – was released in 2000.

The target for the drug then changes through trial and error, and the development of the application is hit and miss. At this point, a bifurcation appears – the drug may be medicalized and legitimated, or it may be criminalized and delegitimated. But the drug remains the same chemically. For example, the Swiss chemist Albert Hofmann first synthesized lysergic acid diethylamide (LSD) in late 1938 at the Sandoz (Novartis) laboratories in Basel, Switzerland, as an analeptic (a respiratory and circulatory stimulant). But it was not until 1943, when Hofmann accidentally absorbed traces of the drug through his fingertips, that he discovered its hallucinatory effects. For two decades, the drug followed the medicalization route as a legitimate pharmaceutical and was used in experiments by psychiatrists interested in treating psychosis. By the mid-1960s, due to widespread recreational use of the drug, it was criminalized and politicized (for "lefties" and "liberals").

Returning to the example of Ritalin, within the medicalization model, the condition that the drug treats gradually comes to be formed by those with commercial interests, against the grain of a host of side effects (anxiety, loss of appetite, weight loss, poor sleeping patterns and, more seriously, heart issues and psychosis). It is thought that Ritalin works by inhibiting dopamine and norepinephrine uptake at neuro-receptor sites, but this is not confirmed. Recreational and casual use of the drug is widespread, particularly among students, and ironically including medical students, as an aid to studying (Bleakley 2016). It is seen as performance enhancing rather than recreational. But we can clearly see the Queen of Hearts effect here in terms of power plays and the politics of medicalization. A hit-and-miss research process is aligned with what is effectively a false target: "hyper-activity" in children is turned from a managed behavioural condition to a psychiatric symptom with a suspected neurological cause.

As this biopower is organized and channelled, it comes to micro-manage increasing numbers of children's and teenagers' lives within a pharmacracy, where prescription drugs are normalized (Bleakley 2015). Meanwhile, as a form of resistance, an outlaw band is formed with those who use the drug for cognitive enhancement. This group ironically involves doctors and, as noted, medical students (Beyer, Staunton and Moodley 2014) – some studying well into the night to answer examination questions (maybe even in their psychiatry tests on the uses of amphetamines in treating ADHD!). The politics of medicine can be like an ouroboric serpent eating its own tail.

In the pharmacracy, behaviours previously seen as virtuous or wicked, wise or unwise are now dealt with as healthy or sick – to be controlled as if they were health issues. This is not to say that children do not suffer from "attention deficit" or "hyperactivity". Rather it is their totalizing as medical conditions that has changed historically, where such behaviours before may have had a much higher threshold of tolerance and be seen as merely confusing or troublesome. Once, "depression" was "melancholia", a condition of deep introversion often admired. Now it is stigmatized and widely treated. Again this is not to say that depression cannot be debilitating, but reactive depressions such as mourning should not be subject to medicalization but allowed to run their course. As mentioned earlier, even death is now a medical condition, as Illich was at pains to point out.

More, politicians are now handed power as the architects and dispensers of healthcare, where, claims Szasz, "politicians define disease". This cuts two ways – it gives politicians power, but, as Szasz points out, it also provides people with a convenient scapegoat, suspending personal responsibility. A knock-on effect too is that it is easier for people to reach for a pill than, say, engage in a change in lifestyle. This benefits the pharmaceutical companies and offers them a means of governmentality feeding profits.

Morality is muddied and muddled by pharmacracy. For example, we criminalize mind- or mood-altering drugs, creating a black market, as these form a resistance to a pharmacracy's power flow, beyond the control of the pharmaceutical companies. Criminal organizations fill the gap vacated by Big Pharma. In turn, we medicalize mood (depression, anxiety, hyper-elation) and provide mood-altering drugs as "cures" or at least as relief, where Big Pharma has vested interests. As Szasz (2001: unpaginated) argues, we are "preoccupied by diseases, literal and metaphorical" as

> we extend the idiom, imagery and technology of medicine to every aspect of life. Virtually every human problem thus appears to be a disease and every remedy for it is viewed as a treatment. The result is that democracy, limited government, and the rule of law are replaced by "pharmacracy," unlimited government, and the rule of medical discretion.

Szasz's argument is powerful but has a serious flaw – as noted earlier, and like Illich's sentiment, it is based itself on a political idea, that of self-help and individualism ("individual liberty and personal responsibility" in Szasz's [ibid.] own words), and the rejection of centralized government interference in personal liberty, that permeates American life. This is the Protestant-Capitalist mentality described by Max Weber as the marriage of the Protestant work ethic and the Capitalist spirit, shaping "personal responsibility" (and rejecting collectivism). Thus, Szasz (ibid.) concludes:

> An old American proverb warns: "Protect me from my friends, I will take care of my enemies". A foe that threatens to harm you is easy to resist. A friend eager to help you – even though you could, if you tried hard enough, help yourself – poses a more subtle danger. Therein lies pharmacracy's threat to individual liberty and personal responsibility.

Szasz's view offers a powerful rejoinder to those who say that medicine is under the thumb of politicians. For Szasz, medicine is not politicized; rather, politics are medicalized.

Rudolf Virchow: Medicine accommodates to society

A more positive view of the relationship between medicine, society and power to that of the recent critics of medicalization is found in the work and legacy of the 19th-century German doctor and polymath Rudolf Virchow (1821–1902), who said, "Medicine is a social science, and politics is nothing more than medicine on a grand scale" (Meili and Hewitt 2016). For Virchow, there is clinical medicine within its own cultural confines. But then there is (capital M) Medicine as a metaphor – a way of seeing and diagnosing – that can be applied to society in a way that does not totalize but is responsive. Medicine here draws on its method to accommodate to various social issues and provide help and insight where needed. This sensitive approach, advertised by Virchow's own work, is the legacy of public health as a democratic social intervention, a responsive politics.

It is in this accommodating sensitivity and responsiveness that medicine in the public sphere can be seen as an effect of the humanities and arts as much as of science and technology. Friedrich Nietzsche (and later Gilles Deleuze) famously viewed artists as "diagnosticians of culture". Drawing on a medical analogy, artists see symptoms in culture and suggest artistic interventions that are often radical. Szasz's notion of pharmacracy can be read as an articulation of the assimilating effects of capitalist biopower, particularly as a psychiatric trope, but ignores the qualities and intensities of forms of productive resistance inherent to medicine, detailed in Chapters 7–9. Virchow's model of public health, as we shall see, articulates an aesthetic and ethical resistance to a totalizing medicine in democratizing health interventions. Virchow's "moral medicine" suggests that political systems have ethical obligations to challenge social inequalities and inequities and to provide platforms for patient advocacy. More, such interventions must not be blunt but elegant, sensitive and sensible.

As commentators such as Ryan Meili and Nigel Hewitt (2016) point out, as much as 75% of medical issues globally are public health concerns or socially determined – such as tainted water, lack of food and shelter, displacement, outcomes of environmental disasters and so forth. Yet, as noted, medical students spend very little time studying public health and policy issues. As Meili and Hewitt say, medics treat the child who has been fished out of the river downstream but fail to engage with the reasons why the child fell into the river upstream in the first place. The authors make a plea for a more intensive and extensive development of upstream medicine.

In the UK, a project called "Well North", piloted by Public Health England, links upstream thinking with volunteer and community services to target vulnerable people. Known and trusted figures such as the local postmen and women are briefed to assess and report back on vulnerable persons in the community. Acting in the role of carers, such community members, as "caristas" (from "baristas"), offer warm care by networking with a variety of social care, medical and community services, to best fit the vulnerable person into a network of care and concern. This is what communities used to do well, but the specialization of services has destroyed the fabric of many communities by de-powering citizens and setting up boundaries between care specialties. The most vulnerable often fail to check in to see their general practitioners on a regular basis because they are cowed by the power differential. One of the effects of the Well North scheme is to restore confidence to patients to do simple things like asking more questions of their doctors and gaining clarification where necessary.

"Upstreamism" works too in a model proposed by a medical doctor in California, Rishi Manchanda (2020). He has proposed a new category of doctors and healthcare professionals called "upstreamists" who are nakedly political in the sense that they are committed to equity, equality and advocacy through activism as policy stimulus. They go upstream to where symptoms are rooted by putting together wider social pictures from patients, visiting them in their homes, work and leisure locations; making medical interventions outside of formal clinics and hospitals, where this can nip a problem in the bud; forming trust with communities; and networking with politicians and legislators in affecting policy. Manchanda, co-founder Laura Gottlieb and colleagues at HealthBegins forecast recruitment of 25,000 upstreamists by 2020.

Upstreamists can also work out of a clinic. Recognizing that income is a key determinant of health, the Centre for Effective Practice in Canada developed a "Clinical Tool for Poverty" (https://acfp.ca/cfpc-launches-a-clinical-tool-for -primary-care-providers/). This helps doctors screen for poverty, better diagnose risk and intervene by helping patients to maximize access to benefits. A database is built up that allows simultaneous consideration of a patient's medical conditions and social needs.

The sausages duel

Rudolf Virchow was an ardent democrat and pacifist. He co-founded a liberal socialist party in direct opposition to Germany's "Iron Fist" conservative chancellor Otto von Bismarck, arguing that Bismarck had inflated the military budget, diverting funds that could be used for the public good. The chancellor took it as a personal insult: Virchow's insistent challenge angered Bismarck so much that Bismarck challenged Virchow to a duel. As the challenged, Virchow would get to choose the duelling weapon. An apocryphal story has Virchow cleverly embarrassing Bismarck by accepting the challenge but substituting something quite different from the sword or pistol that Bismarck imagined. The "duel" would involve two pork sausages. One was normal while the other was stuffed with *Trichnella* (a parasitic roundworm) larvae. The challenge was to eat one sausage each. One of the men would thus be infected. A bemused – and presumably suitably disgusted – Bismarck declined the challenge.

I recount the story partly to remind us of Virchow's genius for "thinking otherwise" as innovation and improvisation. Whether or not the "sausages duel" is an apocryphal story, there is a lesson here for medical education. Where Bismarck represents a conservative will-to-stability characterized by lack of ambiguity and imagination, Virchow demands "thinking outside the box", or pursuing an innovative "line of flight". Despite his bravado, Bismarck cannot entertain the risk that Virchow literally brings to the table, where Virchow introduces into the argument what Helga Nowotny (2015) calls "the cunning of uncertainty" – tolerance of risk and ambiguity is inherent to expanding our horizons, as discussed in Chapter 10. Uncertainty, as it were, cunningly plans on our behalf a breaking of boundaries, and discovery follows. But discoveries in medicine must be, says Virchow, for the common good. Medicine must be democratic.

Virchow saw that democratic social and political reform was essential to the health of a population, where symptoms are grounded in both inequities and inequalities. Medicine cannot escape ideological shaping and should serve democratic ends. Science without social application is hollow: "If medicine is to fulfill her great task, then she must enter the political and social life. … The physicians are the natural lawyers of the poor, and the social problems should largely be solved by them" (in Buchman et al. 2016). Ensuring public health required radical action through "full and unlimited democracy" and "education, freedom and prosperity". More, Virchow brought both a vivid imagination and enthusiasm to the political encounter, as he intertwined the political with the aesthetic (form, elegance) and the ethical (values).

A group of upstreamists practising in Canada – Sandy Buchman, Robert Woollard, Ryan Meili and Ritika Goel – describe social accountability in action as a legacy of Virchow:

> Screening for poverty. Providing health care to uninsured migrants. Advocating for a national pharmacare program. These are but 3 examples of how family physicians are currently actualizing social accountability in Canada at the individual (micro), community (meso), and system (macro) levels.
>
> (Buchman et al. 2016: 15).

Both obligation to treat and accountability as both professional and citizen formulate a contract with patients and their communities, the underlying principle of which is social justice. Importantly, medical education is at the heart of this, where "The history of medicine in the 20th century could be described as an uncritical and unrequited love affair with specialization and technology. This has led to the unfortunate separation of personal and population health, and of health professional schools and schools of public health", so that now "our educational and health systems must produce the optimal number of physicians and other health care providers, as well as achieve the appropriate ratio of family physician generalists to other specialists".

As we consider in these early chapters *why* medical education should embrace politics, and the necessity for a shift from downstream hospitalism to upstream community care and activism, we need to consider what primary historical forces are blocking such a transition. Drawing on Yrjö Engeström's work, I frame this as an "anchor effect" in which medical education is pulled back into a conservative "will-to-stability" rather than pulling up the anchor and sailing forth into the territory of "possibility knowledge" or innovative pedagogies. Here, new seed concepts may be formed and expanded, as "spearheads" for a new medical education shaped by global issues such as the climate emergency and lessons drawn from the novel coronavirus pandemic. Further, in medical education there is a stubborn anchoring to traditions of individual learning, knowing and activity rather than social or collaborative learning, knowing and activity. Having plotted out the *why*, later chapters show how medical education can embrace both politics and aesthetics simultaneously through curriculum reconceptualization, with the medical humanities as a medium for change, offering mediating sets of artefacts acting as the second stimulus in double stimulation learning, an example of which is sketched below, with a social justice prompt to counter structural racism in traditions of dissection (Bleakley 2020b) and accompanying anatomy texts.

FIRST STIMULUS
LEARN ANATOMY (FUNCTIONAL) ---------- REPRODUCE FOR ASSESSMENT
                                        APPLY KNOWLEDGE IN CLINICAL SETTING

SECOND STIMULUS
MEDICAL HUMANITIES --------- RE-THINK ANATOMY CRITICALLY, AND "DEEPLY"
                              APPRECIATIVELY: FROM AESTHETIC, ETHICAL,
                              HISTORICAL, ETC. PERSPECTIVES (E.G. WHOSE
                              BODIES HAVE BEEN USED FOR DISSECTION
                              HISTORICALLY? WHY DO DERMATOLOGY TEXTS NOT
                              SHOW BLACK OR BROWN SKINS?)
Double stimulation in an anatomy lesson: Countering structural racism

Self-help

Traditions of self-help permeate mainstream medical education, the centre of gravity of which for over a century has been North America. This has led to a bias of individualism over collectivism. The Scottish doctor, author and reformer Samuel Smiles, who trained in medicine at Edinburgh, published *Self-Help* in 1859. Smiles was critical of materialism, but he also thought that poverty was a product of irresponsibility and was avoidable. Ironically, Smiles, one of 11 children, was supported through medical school by finances provided by his mother after his father had died from cholera. In the 1840s, Smiles engaged deeply with political reform, arguing for democratic principles including the rights of women. But by the 1850s, he had stopped campaigning for general political reform as he vigorously promoted the idea of self-sufficiency. *Self-Help* sold 20,000 copies in the first year of publication, and by the time of Smiles' death in 1904, the book had sold over 250,000 copies.

Orison Swett Marden (1848–1924), an American physician and polymath, had degrees in law, science and arts as well as medicine. Orphaned at the age of seven, as a teenager Marden fortuitously came across a copy of *Self-Help* and was smitten with Smiles' ideas. Marden wrote his own self-help book – *Pushing to the Front*. Published in 1894, it was the first and most influential popular psychology self-help book in America. By 1925, it had run to 250 editions and became a global bestseller. Spurred on by the initial success of his book, Marden founded a magazine called *Success* in 1897, with a circulation of 500,000. It was indeed a runaway success as the first motivational self-help journal.

By then, Marden had left medicine and hospitals to enter the hospitality industry, running several hotels and a holiday resort, and eventually employed over 200 people to run his periodical. In 1916, he became the first president of

"The League for the Larger Life" in New York, an organization whose mission statement was "to spread a knowledge of the fundamental principles that underlie healthy and harmonious living" and "to assist the individual in the solution of personal problems". The "pop" psychology, personal development culture was established, grounded in the wider values of the American "frontiersman" mentality of heroic-individualism, strong work ethic (Protestantism's main secular value) and opportunistic capitalism.

The UK's *Observer* newspaper recently reported a boom in sales of self-help books, particularly pertaining to mindfulness, with sales of 3 million in 2019 (Walker 2019). In France, nearly 15 million self-help – or health and wellbeing improvement – books were sold in 2018, compared with 10 million cookery books and nearly 3 million books on gardening, animals and nature (https://www.statist a.com/statistics/734218/self-help-books-sales-volume-by-category-france/). The self-help or personal growth market in the USA is now turning to "life coaching" and is worth $10 billion, predicted to rise to $12 billion by 2022 (https://blog.m arketresearch.com/the-10-billion-self-improvement-market-adjusts-to-new-gen eration). While more women than men read self-help books, more men than women write them (https://qz.com/1106341/most-women-reading-self-help-bo oks-are-getting-advice-from-men/).

Stressing the "frontiersman" virtues of resilience and persistence (core to "self-help") and the Protestant work ethic, Orison Marden recounted how his first manuscript copy of *Pushing to the Front* had been destroyed in a fire when one of his hotels burned down. He immediately wrote three new versions and sent them simultaneously to three different publishers – each wanted to publish the book. Again, Marden, inspired by Samuel Smiles, had created the self-realization movement that today we know by descriptors such as "personal growth", and that has exploded through YouTube and social media, and may just be medicine's greatest ally as a public health intervention.

Marden was almost certainly influenced by a 19th-century American movement called "New Thought", formed initially by the ideas of Phineas Quimby. Drawing on ideas from a number of religious denominations, the New Thought movement's doctrine was that health is a product of "right thinking", and conversely, sickness a product or "wrong thinking". In short, the individual is in charge of his or her fate and responsible for his or her actions and bodily states. Biopower was reduced to the nakedly personal and brazenly commodified.

The Scottish-American industrialist and philanthropist Andrew Carnegie (1835–1919) made a fortune from producing steel. He was a staunch believer in independence, the Protestant work ethic and self-help, and admired Marden's work in particular. Carnegie set up a charitable Foundation to re-distribute around 90% of his considerable fortune (around $65–70 billion in today's money). There was, however, a dark side to Carnegies beliefs that also characterized Samuel Smiles' philosophy – those who could not help themselves were seen as either weak or lazy and should be allowed to perish. This twisted version of Darwinian "survival of the fittest" offered a cruel injunction to the physically or mentally challenged or impaired, or to those stuck in a poverty trap or cycle.

Marden's and Carnegie's shared value system would come to describe a cultural style and trait among North Americans that would shape educational systems and pedagogical practices, focused on the self and self-improvement. Its main proponent would be John Dewey, born in the year that Samuel Smiles' *Self-Help* was first published (1859) and a contemporary of both Marden and Carnegie. Dewey was a firm believer in democracy, but more in autonomy: self-determination and self-realization – a pedagogy of the individual spirit. Democracy started with the rights of individuals and freedom of expression. Dewey believed that autonomous or self-determining persons would naturally subscribe to the common ideal of democracy, as participative engagement for the common good. This, in the context of North American competitive capitalism, has proved to be illusory. "Self-help" readily becomes "every man for himself".

The darker competitive side of Samuel Smiles' legacy has dominated North American pedagogy, and this has bled into medical education, including Western European versions. The individual – and the cult of individualism expressed competitively – has been the primary driver for medical pedagogies. There is a complex of factors at work that characterize this style of learning and being, resulting in an identity: a worldview characterizing success as a result of self-help, extreme individualism, the cult of strong leadership and the heroic and conquering frontiersman (gendered male). More, the obverse of the coin is the main motivator: as success is self-reliance, so failure is described as reliance on others. Recall Stanley Goldfarb's invective recounted in the previous chapter and published in the *Wall Street Journal*, where, in medical education: "Theories of learning with virtually no experimental basis for their impact on society and professions now prevail. Students are taught … 'communal learning' rather than individual mastery of crucial information". Goldfarb frames such collectivism as moral slippage and failure.

The self-help philosophy of Marden, the pedagogy of Dewey and the philanthropy of Carnegie converge in the work of Abraham Flexner, a Classics graduate who was an ambitious educationalist and who originally ran his own school. For the origins of modern medical pedagogy, we must go back over a century to the politics of Flexner and his hugely influential reports on medical education in North America and Canada (Flexner 1910), and later, in Europe (Flexner 1912).

Flexner's political worldview

The shape of modern medical education can be ascribed to the work of this one man, a Classics scholar turned educationalist: Abraham Flexner (1866–1959). Flexner was a contemporary of Orison Marden, his educational inspiration was John Dewey, and the funding that allowed his vision of medical education to be realized was gained originally from the legacy of Andrew Carnegie in the form of the Carnegie Foundation for the Advancement of Teaching.

Modern medical education has its origins in a text published in 1910 that is usually treated for its historical interest but is in fact a text of political and ethical interest: Flexner's *Medical Education in the United States and Canada: A Report to*

the Carnegie Foundation for the Advancement of Teaching. Flexner was not a doctor but, as noted, had studied Classics and was an educationalist. The Carnegie
Foundation, however, did not want a doctor to carry out the on-the-ground
research and subsequent writing of the report, but somebody who would be dis-
passionate. Many considered Flexner to be the most important educationalist of
his era, even more so than his contemporary John Dewey (1859–1952), whose
educational methods Flexner greatly admired. On his death, the *New York Times*
front-page obituary said of Flexner: "No other American of his time contributed
more to the welfare of his country and of humanity in general". Not everybody
agreed. An American doctor, Lester King (1984) called Flexner's report "probably
the most grossly overrated document in American medical history", pointing out
that recent medical historical scholarship has placed Flexner among a network of
many equally important factors influencing medical education of his time.

Flexner was the sixth of nine children born to German Jewish immigrant parents in Louisville, Kentucky. His father Moritz was a hat seller and his mother
Esther a seamstress. His eldest brother Jacob supported Flexner through his first
degree at Johns Hopkins University in Baltimore. Jacob, a pharmacist, later
trained as a doctor, while Flexner's older brother Simon became a renowned
pathologist and bacteriologist. Flexner taught Greek and Latin at High School,
and – on the back of private education tuition from wealthy donors – set up his
own experimental school in which lessons were not compulsory and students
did not enter for exams. Yet many went on to attend prestigious universities and
colleges, and the school gained a reputation for educational innovation. Flexner
married one of his former students, Anne Crawford, who had become a teacher
and playwright. She had a Broadway success, and the profits financed Flexner
to close his school and study full time for a Master's degree in Psychology from
Harvard, and then to spend a year-long sabbatical in Germany at Berlin and
Heidelberg Universities, where he decided that the German educational system
was the finest in the world.

The wealthy Carnegie Foundation asked Flexner in 1908 to conduct the
planned survey of the quality of medical education in North America and
Canada. The president, Henry S. Pritchett, had read Flexner's recently published
(1908) critique of higher education, *The American College: A Criticism*, in which
Flexner attacked in particular large lecture teaching as a "cheap" and "wholesale"
way of turning education into cruder management of learning. Flexner was taken
by surprise at the invitation, as he knew nothing about medical education and
had never set foot inside a medical school. When he did, what he saw shocked
him. From January 1909 to April 1910, Flexner visited all 155 medical schools
in North America and Canada, some only briefly and some of them twice, clock-
ing up 175 visits. Most visits – the results were published in 1910 – revealed the
medical education of the time to be largely a totally unacceptable way to prepare
doctors for practice.

Admissions policies were poor, haphazard or non-existent. Curricula had no
formal shape. Pedagogies went unexamined. Resources were lacking – 140 of the
155 schools had no library; schools were poorly equipped and had no link with

nearby hospitals. Yet the certificates received upon completion of studies licensed graduates to practice medicine. Most importantly, there was an over-production of doctors (Flexner claimed four to five times as many doctors were being trained in North America as in Germany per head of population). Only one school – Johns Hopkins in Baltimore – required entrants to possess a prior degree. Flexner took this institution as his standard for future development of medical schools.

As fee-paying private institutions, medical schools were more interested in profits than standards, often recruiting their students from industrial occupations. Flexner had apparently uncovered a scandal. Fifteen thousand copies of his report were printed and distributed free of charge, causing widespread alarm. By 1922, of the 155 schools, only 81 remained. Flexner himself had called for a maximum of 31. He initiated four major changes: medical schools would be university based; faculty would be involved in research, both scientific and educational; students would be recruited only after obtaining a first undergraduate degree in sciences; and they would learn through a standardized curriculum of two years of anatomy and bench science, followed by two years of clinical study through the university's attachment to hospital settings.

In a comprehensive history of North American medical education, Kenneth Ludmerer (1999) argues that Flexner did not suddenly initiate modern medical education and that his observations of medical schools often suffered from a lack of appreciation of how far many schools had come since inauguration – especially those that catered for women and minority groups. Appalled by the laxity of home-based medical education, some – more thoughtful, inquisitive and morally sensitive – American doctors had gained experience in Germany, where medical students underwent a rigorous education, first socialized as anatomists (through cadaver dissection) and then bench scientists before engaging in clinical medicine. Ludmerer (ibid: xxii) shows that the Flexnerian revolution had antecedents since the mid-19th century "when a revolution occurred regarding how medicine should be taught". The revolution was not confined to medicine, but was one of ideas and adventures in pedagogy based on a social contract. Capitalist society, driven by entrepreneurs, would provide the climate for generation and subsequent flourishing of schools and universities, including medical schools. In turn, doctors educated in these schools would engage in a social contract in which they committed not only to serving communities, but also to developing the highest possible standards of research and professionalism within their field. As Ludmerer says, this was a "financial, *political*, and moral" exchange (ibid., my emphasis).

Financial capital from private sources flowed in to medical school development, not in dribs and drabs but in huge quantities, reflecting Flexner's new influential role at the Carnegie Foundation and then the Rockefeller Foundation; as Ludmerer (ibid: xxiii) notes, in 1910, a leading medical school may have had a budget of around $100,000, but by 1940 that would have swelled tenfold, to $1 million.

More sinister is whether or not Flexner had consciously decided to come down heavily on those schools that catered for women and minorities. They were the most vulnerable, short of funding and then equipment and expertise. Nowadays, we would see this as a good reason to support them and invest in them to counter both inequity and inequality, but the climate in Flexner's time was different. It did not seem to matter to Flexner that women would be dispossessed of the opportunity to study medicine – a condition that persisted until relatively recently. However, there were certainly open motives for discouraging people of colour from studying medicine. Flexner suggested that black doctors should only work with black patients, using the spurious argument that such doctors might infect white patients with illnesses carried only by people of colour.

Flexner's view about race issues was complex. In a letter from 1930 concerning the recruitment of staff at Princeton University, Flexner's belief in offering opportunities to all individuals is clear: "It is fundamental in our purpose, and our express desire, that in the appointments to the staff and faculty as well as in the admission of workers and students, no account shall be taken, directly or indirectly, of race, religion, or sex". Further, while Flexner was Jewish, he never openly spoke out against anti-Semitism and was strangely quiet when Hitler came to power. In the 1930s, when high-profile Jewish intellectuals and scientists emigrated to America, Flexner was often involved in employing them through his role as founding director of the Institute for Advanced Study at Princeton, where his biggest "catch" was Albert Einstein.

As Michael Nevins (2010) argues, Flexner's achievements in pedagogy and medical education have been lauded, while his infamous character flaws of irascibility and narcissism have been noted, but his values and beliefs, despite his 1940 autobiography and an update in 1960, remain opaque – complex, contradictory and difficult to decipher. He must have been conflicted over his love for the German educational system, his Jewish ancestry and what he was seeing in Germany as Hitler came to power, but he never made this plain. Nevins asks why Flexner did not openly come out against the institutionalized anti-Semitism that was reflected in the popularity of the eugenics movement in America during the first half of the 20th century.

Medical schools as businesses

The German sociologist Max Weber (1864–1920) was a contemporary of Marden, Carnegie, Dewey and Flexner. First published in 1905, but not translated into English until 1930, and then probably unknown to the spearhead figures in American self-help and self-sufficiency thinking, Weber's *The Protestant Ethic and the Spirit of Capitalism* put forward a radical idea. Goethe's 1809 novel *Elective Affinities* took the idea – prevalent at the time – that certain chemicals were attracted to other chemicals and would react with these and not with others. Goethe took this as a metaphor for human passions and relationships. We still use the term "chemistry" to describe such affinities. Weber poached Goethe's idea to explore social and intellectual bonds. He was puzzled as to why market-driven capitalism was so successful in the Western world and suggested that this can be explained by capitalism's affinity with the central ethic of Protestant belief: "getting ahead" through self-help and independence or what we might now call a "work ethic".

A small group, the Protestant "Elect" (based in Calvinism) could gain entry to Heaven in the afterworld if they showed two traits in this world: first, the ability for commerce and subsequent profit; and second, the willpower to not spend profits on yourself, but to either save and re-invest, or engage in philanthropy. Weber argued that Protestant Calvinism, in particular, popular in Scotland, England, Germany and the Netherlands, mapped on to the rapid development of capitalist economies in these European countries when compared to Catholic-dominated countries such as Spain, France and Italy. Calvinism encouraged hard work in this life with reinvestment of profits (rather than what was seen as frivolous spending) to set up salvation in an afterlife. More, buying in to this predestination eased any conscience about social and economic inequality in this life; that could be put down to laziness or indulgence. Subsequent historians, notably Fernand Braudel, have challenged Weber's thesis, claiming that the roots of capitalism can indeed be found in pre-Reformation Catholic Church communities where both wealth and power were concentrated.

We have seen that Flexner's fieldwork inquiry and subsequent report uncovered a common model amongst North American and Canadian medical schools. Whatever their quality and standing, they were all profit-seeking private institutions or businesses. Paradoxically, drawing more on John Dewey's idea of independent learning than on democratic engagement as the primary pedagogy for medical education, Flexner's purging and reconceptualizing of medical education drove curricula deeper into capitalist ideology, where knowledge and skills were obtained through individual effort and retained as personal capital. With Flexner's initiative, the political body of North American (and then Western European) medical education is laid bare. In short, the dominant model of learning remained individualistic and not social, and competitive and not collaborative, certainly up to the dawn of the 21st century (Bleakley, Bligh and Browne 2011). Where did this situating of medical education leave socialist models?

Soviet learning theory

In the previous chapter, we saw Stanley Goldfarb, a conservative physician and medical educator, complaining that "the prospect of this 'new,' politicized medical education should worry all Americans", laying the blame at the feet of social learning theorists: "Students are taught in the tradition of educational theorist Étienne Wenger, who emphasized 'communal learning' rather than individual mastery of crucial information". Poor Étienne Wenger (now Wenger-Trayner), who came from a medical family but decided to study psychology, and never wrote about medical education until late in his career. Wenger's work, with his colleague the anthropologist Jean Lave, was focused on craft apprenticeships in areas such as butchery and non-medical community midwifery, and identity construction amongst "non-drinking alcoholics" in Alcoholics Anonymous (AA) groups.

Goldfarb should know better – all junior doctors learn in "communal" settings such as teams on ward rounds, crash teams in resuscitation scenarios or surgical teams in the operating theatre. While individualistic learning theories are poorly equipped to explore clinical team dynamics, Lave and Wenger's community of practice model also falls short. It describes how a learner engages with, and is socialized into, a community of practice as a passive recipient. The learner is then not an agent of change, and how communities of practice change, adapt, expand and innovate remains unclear. Lave and Wenger's model however does illustrate Marx's view of the difference between the use and exchange value of labour as a commodity. Where labour's output is valued as a means of entry into a community of practice, the apprentice experiences a subjectification or a making of identity. But where labour's output becomes a commodity simply for exchange value, then the apprentice experiences objectification and subsequent alienation.

Cultural-Historical Activity Theory (CHAT) and Actor-Network Theory (ANT) (Bleakley 2014) significantly extend the reach of communities of practice models in exploring processes of development and innovation beyond mere absorption into a community. Goldfarb, I guess, would not welcome medical students' and junior doctors' challenges, but would wish that they are absorbed neatly and quietly into tradition without promising revolution. We have to thank the psychologist Michael Cole (1989, 1997) for introducing collectivist Soviet Learning theory to North America, just as Yrjö Engeström (1987) played the same foundational and pioneering role in Europe (and then joined with Cole in America).

John Dewey's dilemma was how to fuse rabid autonomy and capitalism (the American way) with democracy, to give equal weight to "mind" and "culture". How should the individual mind and habits of the heart survive in commitment to collaborative, democratic progress? Dewey's answer was to integrate culture into the individual mind, as a commitment to collective endeavour without losing individual rights and freedoms. But this path morphed into what Kenneth Galbraith (1992) would later deride as a "culture of contentment". As individuals gained more money, power and prestige, they would abandon collectivism for self-interest, drifting away from the common good. The less successful would be cast adrift. The socialist way is to sacrifice individualism for what the collective can afford the individual. This is achieved through division of labour and parallel resistance to commodification of labour – but such a division must offer a level playing field so that all can contribute to realize the potential of their capabilities, while profit from labour is shared back equally amongst all who participate. This, for example, is a fundamental principle of problem-based learning.

Cole, a University of California San Diego communication and psychology professor, was drawn to the work of the pioneering Soviet psychologists Lev Vygotsky (see Fu 1997) and his student and collaborator A.R. Luria, who wrote: "the determining factor in the psychological development of the child and in the creation of the complex mechanism of the psyche is the social development of the child". In the early 1960s, Cole spent a year at Moscow University as an exchange student. He later became a translator and editor of Luria's writings and, for over three decades, was the editor of the journal *Soviet Psychology*. Cole's political interests came partly from the influence of his father, Lester Cole, a Hollywood film screenwriter who held left-wing views and was under surveillance during the height of the McCarthy era. He refused to answer questions when interviewed about his possible Communist affiliations, along with a group of Hollywood directors and writers who became known as the "Hollywood Ten".

Again, we see assimilation and accommodation at work; in the Protestant-Capitalist individualistic model, advertised as the "American Way", there is resistance to accommodating collaborative principles if the individual gains traction for personal good. In fact, the Protestant view is that such success will be rewarded in the afterlife. A puzzling fact of American life in a scientific era is that a majority of the population holds strong religious views. Life is then assimilated into this personalistic worldview (Bellah et al. 2008). In atheistic socialism, faith rests with the potential of collaborative humanity who accommodate to the wider good. Returning to our example of the doctor and medical educator Stanley Goldfarb, we can see how a conservative individualism would be blinkered to the value of collectivism and rail against new-fangled social learning theories in medical education. Following Luria's maxim that "the determining factor in the psychological development of the child … is the social development of the child", if Goldfarb had been born in Cuba, he would probably have followed a quite different set of values as a doctor.

Cuban doctors

Cuban medicine is essentially political, formed through a socialist interpellation and focused on global social justice agendas. Cuba has one of the highest levels of doctors per capita of any country – 6.7 per 1,000. This is a staggering figure, as globally there are only 1.13 doctors for every 1,000 people. The UK has 2.8 doctors per 1,000 people, the USA 2.6 and Canada 2.2. Cuba's Latin American School of Medicine is the largest medical university in the world. Importantly, Cuban citizens have an average higher life expectancy than those from the USA.

As a result of over-production of doctors, Cuba has established a global network of the provision of medical workers, particularly for emerging nations and for emergencies (De Albornoz 2006). In the press at the time of writing are accounts of Cuban doctors helping with the coronavirus pandemic worldwide. However, within Cuba, doctors are relatively poorly paid and medical facilities are often outdated, with the lack of access to key equipment and supply of essential drugs. The State is also authoritarian and freedom of expression is curtailed, where "public criticism of the government is a crime in Cuba" (Hirschfeld 2007). Indeed Katherine Hirschfeld's PhD thesis ethnography scoping the Cuban healthcare system recorded "serious complaints about the intrusion of politics into medical treatment and health care decision-making", where "there is no right to privacy in the physician–patient relationship … no patients' right of informed consent, no right to refuse treatment, and no right to protest or sue for malpractice". Medical care in Cuba, concludes Hirschfeld, can be dehumanizing.

Of course, from the Cuban point of view, they would want to know about Hirschfeld's politics and potential biases. For example, her criticism of the seeming lack of medical ethics in the Cuban system – "There is no right to privacy in the physician–patient relationship in Cuba, no patients' right of informed consent, no right to refuse treatment, and no right to protest or sue for malpractice. As a result, medical care in Cuba has the potential to be intensely dehumanizing" – is written from an individualistic perspective. As Hirschfeld goes on to say, "values such as privacy and individualism are rejected by the socialist regime as 'bourgeois values' contrary to the collective ethos of socialism".

Ideological interpellation can be damning, from both the right and left. Cuban doctors notoriously carry out uplifting medical work globally in underprivileged communities and in post-disaster and conflict zones. But at home, says Hirschfeld, typical totalitarian tactics are used to massage health data for the positive effect such as "deliberate manipulation of health statistics, aggressive political intrusion into health care decision-making, criminalizing dissent, and other forms of authoritarian policing". She also notes that a small number of earlier ethnographies of the Cuban healthcare system were poorly designed and executed and failed to scratch the surface to reveal ideological biases, or the extent of corruption such as a vigorous black market exchange for medications.

Politics in medicine and the medicalization of politics can, through chronic ideological interpellation, appear as propaganda and dissimulation. The challenge for contemporary medical education is to establish democratic habits in medical students. This, in turn, is grounded in resisting the commodification of medical student labour and the objectification of their persons. The mirror image to this is that medical students must learn to resist the historical habit of medical culture to both commodify and objectify patients within a neo-liberal capitalist frame. Such resistance to the dominant medico-political status quo is the mother of invention for progressive medical education. The following three chapters consider such forms of resistance to conventional medicine and medical education that are not externally generated, but embedded in clinical and medical-pedagogic cultures.

Bibliography

Bellah RN, Madsen R, Sullivan WM, et al. 2008. *Habits of the Heart: Individualism and Commitment in American Life*. Berkeley, CA: University of California Press.

Beyer C, Staunton C, Moodley K. The Implications of Methylphenidate Use by Healthy Medical Students and Doctors in South Africa. *BMC Medical Ethics*. 2014;15:20.

Bleakley A. 2014. *Patient-centred Medicine in Transition: The Heart of the Matter*. Dordrecht: Springer.

Bleakley A. 2015. *The Medical Humanities and Medical Education: How the Medical Humanities Can Shape Better Doctors*. Abingdon: Routledge.

Bleakley A. Bargaining with Hypnos: Sleep Deprivation in Junior Doctors as Durational Misperformance. *Performance Research*. 2016; 21: 49–52.

Bleakley A. 2020. *Educating Doctors' Senses Through the Medical Humanities: "How Do I Look?"* Abingdon: Routledge.

Bleakley A, Bligh J, Browne J. 2011. *Medical Education for the Future: Identity, Power and Location.* Dordrecht: Springer.

Buchman S, Woollard R, Meili R, Goel R. Practising Social Accountability: From Theory to Action. *Canadian Family Physician.* 2016; 62:15–18.

Cole M. Cultural Psychology: A Once and Future Discipline. *Nebraska Symposium on Motivation.* 1989;37:279–335.

Cole M, Engeström Y, Vasquez O. 1997. *Mind, Culture and Activity.* Cambridge: Cambridge University Press.

Conrad, P. 2007. *The Medicalization of Society: On the Transformation of Human Conditions into Treatable Disorders.* Baltimore, MD: Johns Hopkins University Press.

De Albornoz SC. On a Mission: How Cuba Uses Its Doctors Abroad. *British Medical Journal.* 2006;333:464.

Engeström Y. 1987. *Learning by Expanding: An Activity-theoretical Approach to Developmental Research.* Helsinki: Orienta-Konsultit Oy. Available at: http://lchc.ucsd.edu/mca/Paper /Engestrom/Learning-by-Expanding.pdf

Flexner A. 1910. *Medical Education in the United States and Canada: A Report to the Carnegie Foundation for the Advancement of Teaching.* New York: Carnegie Foundation.

Flexner A. 1912. *Medical Education in Europe: A Report to the Carnegie Foundation for the Advancement of Teaching.* New York: Carnegie Foundation.

Foucault M. 2006. *History of Madness.* Abingdon: Routledge.

Fu D. Vygotsky and Marxism. *Education and Culture.* 1997;XV:10–17.

Galbraith JK. 1992. *The Culture of Contentment.* London: Sinclair-Stevenson.

Geiger J. Medical Nemesis. *The New York Times,* 2 May 1976, Section BR, 1. Available at: https://www.nytimes.com/1976/05/02/archives/medical-nemesis-the-20thcenturys-lea ding-luddite-turns-to-medicine.html

Hirschfeld K. Re-examining the Cuban Health Care System: Towards a Qualitative Critique. *Cuban Affairs.* 2007;2(3). Available at: http://www.cubanaffairsjournal.org

Illich I. 1974. *Medical Nemesis: The Expropriation of Health.* London: Calder & Boyars.

Killeen RNF. A Review of Illich's Medical Nemesis. *Western Journal of Medicine.* 1976;125:67–69.

King L. XX-The Flexner Report of 1910. *Journal of the American Medical Association.* 1984;251:1079–1086.

Law J. 2006. *Big Pharma: How the World's Drug Companies Control Illness.* London: Constable.

Ledley FD, McCoy SS, Vaughan G, et al. Profitability of Large Pharmaceutical Companies Compared with Other Large Public Companies. *Journal of the American Medical Association.* 2020;323:834–43.

Ludmerer KM. 1999. *Time to Heal: American Medical Education from the Turn of the Century to the Era of Managed Care.* Oxford: Oxford University Press.

Manchanda R.2020. *What Is an "Upstreamist" in Health Care?* Institute for Healthcare Improvement Open School. Available at: http://www.ihi.org/education/IHIOpenScho ol/resources/Pages/AudioandVideo/Rishi-WhatIsAnUpstreamist.aspx

Meili R, Hewett N. Turning Virchow Upside Down: Medicine is Politics on a Smaller Scale. *Journal of the Royal Society of Medicine.* 2016;109:256–58.

Nevins M. 2010. *Abraham Flexner: A Flawed American Icon.* New York: iUniverse Inc.

Noor P. Coronavirus Conspiracy Theory Laboratory Report. *The Guardian,* 13 April 2020. Available at: https://www.theguardian.com/us-news/2020/apr/13/coronavirus-consp iracy-theory-laboratory-report

Nowotny H. 2015. *The Cunning of Uncertainty.* Cambridge: Polity Press.

O"Mahony S. 2020. Medical Nemesis 40 Years On: The Enduring Legacy of Ivan Illich. In: A Bleakley (ed.) *Routledge Handbook of Medical Humanities*. 114–22.

Shwetz K. 2020. The Chaotic Narratives of Anti-Vaccination. In: A Bleakley (ed). *Routledge Handbook of Medical Humanities*, 185–91.

Szasz T. Beware of Pharmacracy. *Independent Institute*, 21 August 2001. Available at: https ://www.independent.org/news/article.asp?id=276

Szasz T. 2003. *Pharmacracy: Medicine and Politics in America*. New York: Syracuse University Press.

Szasz T. 2007. *The Medicalization of Everyday Life. Selected Essays*. Syracuse, NY: Syracuse University Press.

Walker R. Stressed Brits Buy Record Number of Self-Help Books. *The Guardian*, 9 March 2019. Available at: https://www.theguardian.com/books/2019/mar/09/self-help-book s-sstressed-brits-buy-record-number

7 Resistance: Part I

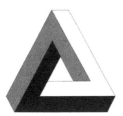

Grasping the nettle

Wherever power is exerted or manifests itself, forms of resistance – as a coun-ter-power – will spring up. Typically, resistance is exerted against injustice. Defined as "the refusal to accept or comply with something", resistance has its origin in the Latin *resistere*: "to make a stand". A stand can be active (strikes, street marches) or passive (such as refusing to move when provoked: "move on, there's nothing to see here!"). As in the physics definition, where resistance is the degree to which any substance prevents electricity from flowing through it, resistance can be a refusal to be persuaded or affected – shocked, mocked or victimized.

Mass resistance movements are typically "underground", associated with destabilizing tactics during the occupation by an invading force. I know of no better account of this than Peter Weiss's (2009: 9) novel *The Aesthetics of Resistance*, set in Germany just before World War II and in Spain during the Spanish Civil War (a trilogy, of which only the first two parts have been pub-lished in English, in 2009 and 2020). Weiss shows how resistance movements can draw inspiration for their political stances from aesthetics. The novel opens with a group of young men in Berlin in 1937 forming a communist resistance cell against the Nazis (later they also fight in the Spanish civil war against Fascism). They gain their political inspiration from studying ancient Greek sculptures in museums, for example depicting the struggle of the gods – led by Zeus – against the Titans, expressing "not the struggle of good against evil, but the struggle between the classes". What they quarry from the ancient Greek statues is not just the mythical gods and the allegories they promote, but the back-stories of the workmen – usually slaves working underground by lamplight – who quarried the marble, hewing out the stone and carrying it on their backs to the sculptors' workplaces, inhaling stone dust, their lives short and brutal, their labour dispensable to the aristocracy.

In this chapter, I extend the discussion of kinds of power set out in Chapter 1, but now with the focus on patterns of resistance to such power. As set out in Table 7.1, I will discuss how power can express itself as forms of resistance that are not only restricted to conflict but also include embrace, engagement, expansion, determination and so forth. Resistance is as much a flow to be negotiated as a power to be fought. One might see the arts in general as forms of resistance to conventions and not primarily as embellishment or decoration, while science provides a primary form of resistance to woolly thinking and assumption without evidence – the latter the badge of contemporary populist politics.

Table 7.1 Kinds of political resistance within medicine and medical education discussed in Chapters 7–9

Kinds of resistance	Example
1. Biopower	The power to seek another form of life as resistance against a dominant power (e.g. medicalization); to administer and produce life, e.g. gender re-assignment; using the body in radical performance art as biopolitical labour.
2. Truth telling (parrhesia) 2.1 Whistleblowing 2.2 Narratives of resistance	2.1 The Bristol paediatric heart surgery scandal. 2.2 Students reporting and reflecting on seniors' professionalism lapses.
3. Democracy and common wealth 3.1 Teamwork pursuing possibility knowledge – teeming, negotiated knotworking, work as a rhythm	Democratic structures of resistance such as a medical student parliament; and public, deliberative and hybrid forums with dialogic democracy (e.g. as a public engagement art event). 3.1 Teamwork as a complex, adaptive system
4. Advocacy	Actively identifying and helping patients and patient groups who cannot help themselves or find insuperable barriers to seeking care (e.g. patients with refugee status or temporary residence; treating the homeless; and translation services).
5. Dissensus	Thoughtful non-compliance. Pedagogies of dissent.
6. Activism 6.1 Direct action 6.2 Community action	6.1 UK junior doctors' strike (withdrawal of labour) 2015–16. 6.2 During the coronavirus pandemic, local community groups shared resources and collaborated to make personal protective equipment (PPE) for use by frontline healthcare workers.

Table 7.2 Kinds of political resistance within medicine and medical education not discussed in Chapters 7–9 but widely discussed in the sociological medical education literature

Kinds of resistance	Example
Anti-colonialism and anti-racism	Challenging structural and institutional racism in health inequities and inequalities
Anti-gender discrimination Feminisms Gender identity (LGBQT)	Countering casual sexism on medical students' work placements
Anti-stigma (e.g. disability, poverty)	Countering cumulative micro-aggressions aimed at disadvantaged patients or patient groups

Biopower

According to Michel Foucault (1976: 33), at the time of the French Revolution, politics and medicine were identical: "The first task of the doctor is therefore political: the struggle against disease must begin with a war against bad government". Bad governments provide no public healthcare and fail to address disparities that imperil the health of the poor and disadvantaged. The idealism of the Revolution was intertwined with the health of a nation. Freed from subjection to an aristocracy, democracy first promised universal health and lifestyle improvement, and the medical profession would oversee this. The "normal" and the "pathological" would be defined medically, and bodies and minds would be governed accordingly. For Foucault, "There is, therefore, a spontaneous and deeply rooted convergence between the requirements of political ideology and those of medical technology" (ibid.: 38).

This is biopower operating at the level of the population as forms of medicalization, that Foucault came to call "governmentality" – a totalizing outlook in which the state or public body takes responsibility for every citizen's private body. For Foucault, this state of affairs is not to be judged morally, but rather tracked historically to better understand the present and available options. In fact, for Foucault, the centralized provision of public health services is not an oppressive "medicalization" in Thomas Szasz's terms, as a deprivation of liberty and a frustration of self-help. Rather, it is largely progressive.

The coronavirus pandemic illustrates the good and the questionable about centralized public health governance. Mainly, governments came up with strategies and decisions, advised by scientists such as epidemiologists and public health experts, and the public followed the advice given where it was perceived as subscribing to safety. However, states of emergency were called, where governments could take decisions without recourse to debate and vote. For example, in the UK, despite a not-for-profit national health service, profit-seeking private sector companies were brought in to run activities such as testing, tracking and tracing without the normal procedures of tendering. The public's view of the pandemic was shaped in a characteristic way, through metaphors of war ("fighting the virus"), and security ("stay at home", "lockdown") – another face to governmentality, that of benign propaganda. If we are under siege, then a siege mentality operates where we pull together as if at war and seek shelter. Another set of metaphors for the pandemic would not necessarily have promoted a "Dunkirk spirit".

According to Foucault (1980: 144), biopower, or "biopolitics", is a technology of power related to health that "has to qualify, measure, appraise, and hierarchize". It is primarily recognized, as noted, in the face of modernity's development of governmentality, where government and public bodies come to increasingly enter into the lives of citizens to shape and control bodies and their health. Biopower operating through the individual body is never free from the collective body of politics. People may take responsibility for their being or not, but they are monitored, surveilled and advised by the government. At the level of the individual, as happened across the USA in particular during lockdown, some individuals would perceive that their liberties were being stripped by government edict, and demonstrations for individual liberties, against the central government and state government lockdown measures, occurred. State governmentality met self-help as individual resistance. And then the Black Lives Matter demonstrations, following the callous killing (indeed, a modern-day lynching) of George Floyd, brought into focus how the biopower that is the policing of citizens' bodies pushing to the limit the boundaries of the law can meet the biopower that is the public right to expression within the law. This set off waves of protest or resistance globally against perceived racial injustice. Biopower then pings around like billiard balls as states and individuals engage.

The biopower that Foucault described – as both bodily-based and population-based – has been extended to include biopowers of technologies such as surveillance and communication through social media. So George Floyd's death at the knee of a police officer is caught on a mobile phone camera by a bystander and goes viral. This seeds global mass shock and protest. Power extends from body to public body to the technological extensions of the body through popular communication technologies. Resistance rebounds to the site of the killing so that the officers involved are brought to justice, now eyed by the court of the global populus, especially black people suffering from longstanding structural inequities and inequalities.

In the wake of George Floyd's tragic death, in Bristol in the UK, a statue of Edward Colston, a 17th- to 18th-century merchant slave trader, is pulled off its plinth by protesters and dumped in Bristol Harbour. Despite the fact that Colston was a philanthropist and gave readily to develop the city of Bristol, his wealth was built on slavery. Biopower now extends to social activism as productive of political change, certainly in terms of waking up the general public to the issue of black lives mattering.

As a background to the global protests, statistics show that black, Asian and minority ethnic (BAME) groups are disproportionately represented in coronavirus deaths. This is not a genetic issue, but a direct consequence of structural racism. BAME groups are more likely to suffer from social deprivation (such as poor housing, poor diet, higher exposure to air pollution, lower educational attainment leading to insecurities in employment) that has a direct impact on health. The street artist Banksy, whose home is in Bristol, suggested on Instagram a compromise between protesters and those who saw toppling the statue as an act of vandalism: "We drag him out the water, put him back on the plinth, tie cable round his neck and commission some life size bronze statues of protesters in the act of pulling him down. Everyone happy. A famous day commemorated". This social media posting (Banksy has over a million and a half followers) too is an act of resistance and of biopower, for contemporary conceptions of biopower must include artefacts, such as public statues, through which each of us makes sense of our private embodiment, and which reflects tensions and contradictions in the public body.

Banksy's protest posting suggestion was not taken up by Bristol city council, where the statue of Colston was fished out of the harbour and will be displayed in a museum with a contextual narrative. The current mayor of Bristol, who is black, expressed mixed feelings about the statue, caught between civic duty to preserve the city's history and personal outrage at the affront that the statue celebrating a slave trader brings. Meanwhile, still in Bristol, a far-right nationalist poured bleach onto the bronze statue of the black poet, actor and playwright Alfred Fagon as a statement of white supremacy. If we take the body of the city, the polis, as open to symptomizing and treatment, then here we have a whole series of moves and counter-moves advertising biopower as forms of resistance couched in liberal reformist and arch conservative political guises. Every act of resistance becomes a way of either healing or deepening the infirmities of the public body.

Foucault's model of biopower, as a productive power (particularly through resistance, and particularly productive of identities contra the commodification of labour), was developed as a counter to the historical insistence upon the decisive, controlling power of authority, such as the church or the king, exercised as the sovereign power that could deal death over life, or excommunicate. Such sovereign power is one of total domination. Foucault (2008), however, points out that such machinations of power are not just national or state issues, but happen at the local or "capillary" level in differing contexts in differing ways: a landlord subjugates his tenants, a violent husband terrorizes his wife, an employer demeans and sexually harasses an employee, a member of a constituency sends an offensive and threatening email to the local member of parliament and so forth. But these are still examples of power as repressive. Again, for Foucault, most power exchanges and flows are productive, particularly of identities.

Power is not just a commodity that some have and can exercise, and others lack. Rather it is something that exists throughout life and is mobilized or rendered immobile in a variety of ways such that any one person may be dominant in one context but submissive in another. Power plays out at this level, particularly in intimacy and sex. At a bodily level, power is not just something pressing on something else, but something pressing back by the nature of its presence, such as voluntary bodily expressions, or an involuntary rush of adrenaline, a blush, the acceleration of heartbeat, a flexing of muscle, an in-breath and so forth. Biopower is then both impressive (offering biological feedback to the body and the embodied mind), and expressive – of desire, personality and invention. Biopower, at its most subtle, is a blush in embarrassment or recognition of desire. It is an erection of the clitoris or penis in anticipation of either intimacy or self-pleasure.

Biopower can operate as a symptom (a tic, sudden loss of inhibition as an early sign of dementia) or an internalized control (inhibiting a need to spit in public). In turn, such biopower can produce subjectivities as *subjection*, or the power to produce and administer life. Again, this is not necessarily oppressive but productive. Subjection to mass vaccination, drinking clean tap water, reporting symptoms of illness to a general practitioner, getting regular dental check-ups, maintaining bodily hygiene, controlling alcohol consumption, watching one's diet – all of these benefit not only individuals but society as a whole.

Citizenship offers a powerful identity. Biopower then embraces bodily habits of hygiene that have others in mind. This leads to the second type of biopower discussed above, one that governs at the level of the population, institutionalized in public health and one that also allows for aesthetic expression through *fashion* and trends such as hairstyle, piercing and tattooing. Biopower as governmentality at the public level is, say, a government edict for social distancing, and at the personal level is, say, washing our hands at regular intervals. The two levels are readily illustrated also as compliance expected at the public level of a doctor's pharmaceutical prescription as compliance, and at the personal level of use where non-compliance is a choice.

Production of subjectivities through the exercise of biopower can act as forms of resistance, as the power to seek another form of life away from perceived convention. This may be based on illogical conspiracy theory, as with the anti-vaxx movement (Shwetz 2020), or may be a genuine desire for "aesthetic self-forming" such as voluntary piercings and tattoos. Here, subjectivities are actively formed rather than accepted in docile states. Medicine and biopower are clearly closely linked, where medicine is a totalizing biopower in a pharmacracy. Here, we "think" the body medically and symptomatically rather than ontologically, in terms of existence. The body is first reduced to machine-like status for ease of disciplining. Second, the body becomes a canvas for a symptom rather than an expression of character, where we are all hypo-chondriacs (literally meaning "under the cartilage or breastbone"), worried about our heart rates or ease of breathing, or a host of aches and pains blown out of proportion by the excessive biopower coursing through the brain – mainly as "imagination" of symptom – with its obsessive self-concern.

A cynic might say that any political party will aim to harness biopower instrumentally, as a form of control disguised as efficiency. Again, biopower then regulates and disciplines. Governments globally were surprised at the degree of co-operation that the public showed with rules of lockdown during the first wave of the Covid-19 pandemic, where internalized norms – legitimated by science – largely displace external rules of law. This position is supported by datasets presented by politicians as "we're following the science", where such politicians are actually bending the science to their own ends, for example, by advertising that "targets" are being met in testing, without giving any detail about how many tests fail, are lost or give false results.

Foucault actually dropped the term "biopower" in his later writings for the term "governmentality" (Cisney and Morar 2016). He coined the generic descriptor "biopolitics" in recognition that public health matters subject to medicalization were eclipsed by politics at the level of policy and political interpretation, now subject to party-political, ideological interests. As an example, referred to above, during the early stages of the coronavirus outbreak in the UK, the right-wing, neo-liberal Tory government chose to outsource testing, at a cost to the taxpayer, to private companies with commercial interests (profit incentives), rather than to National Health Service (NHS)-run laboratories (such as pathology labs), where profit incentives are not considered. Had a Labour government been in power, the socialized NHS services would have been the first choice.

Foucault (2008) makes a distinction between three functions and levels of power: (i) security of a territory through sovereignty; (ii) maintaining an institutional hierarchy through discipline; and (iii) ensuring security through the management of risk and safety. Medical education has a concern with the politics of all three levels by introducing formal patterns of resistance. In (i), learning patient-centred practices questions the historical medicalization of society. In (ii), learning interprofessional team practices as fluid "knotworking" (Engeström 2008, 2018) – see Chapter 8 for an exposition of "knotworking" – questions the historical hierarchies established in healthcare; and (iii) while maintaining a patient safety climate, a culture of productive risk must be established for the medicine to develop; this demands education for the tolerance of ambiguity best offered by core, integrated medical humanities provision. These three forms of curricular resistance to normative medical socialization can produce subjectivities of a doctor as an agent of democracy.

Foucault's model of biopower, morphing into "governmentality", fails to make clear how conceiving of power as circulating across life helps us to distinguish between the use of power to bolster conventions and use of power as forms of resistance to conventions – such as challenge and outrage as political, moral and aesthetic stances. Further, there are no specifics in Foucault's model to help us to chart ways of resisting gender, race, ethnicity, poverty and disability or special needs inequities. This is puzzling, as Foucault's gay identity, which he chose never to discuss in public, must have shaped his theoretical dispositions.

While seeing the value of Foucault's turn away from repressive sovereign power to productive capillary power, Giorgio Agamben (1998) suggests that we must not ignore the continuing power and presence of divisive sovereign power strategies that create a "bare life" of mere existence in the case of poverty, the homeless, prisoners, prisoners of war, the dispossessed, the scapegoated, refugees, political exiles, victims of homophobia, trafficked women forced into prostitution, organ donors forced by poverty and so forth. Agamben asks: "have we not learned anything from the Holocaust?" – or from subsequent genocides.

For psychoanalytically oriented theorists such as Judith Butler (1997), Foucault's description of biopower is necessary but not sufficient, falling short where it fails to engage with psychoanalytic notions of rational conscience clouded by the irrational or unconscious. As the forces of governmentality shape identities, this is accompanied by emotional reactions such as shame and guilt, and these interact with, and re-stimulate, repressed childhood memories, some traumatic. These shape a moral conscience. For example, doctors' erotic or sexual feelings towards patients are tightly controlled by a professional and ethical expectation that such feelings should not be acted out, as the patient is considered to be vulnerable while in the care of the doctor. A significant period of time should elapse before any suggestion of acting upon deep feelings such as falling in love with a patient that is reciprocated, as the patient's response may be clouded by unacknowledged positive transference. However, the stimulation of erotic feelings in the present, as psychoanalytically oriented theorists such as Butler know, is entangled with repressed desires from the past that may or may not be re-constructed in the present as fantasies or memories. Personal parental psychodynamics are readily projected onto one's cultural "parent", such as the doctor. Further, the study of such psychodynamics is not a standard part of medical students'" education in the spheres of professionalism and clinical communication, a situation that I interrogate in Chapter 14.

As the flow of intimate feelings in both doctor and patient that may be exercised as forms of power and resistance, biopower is accompanied by the institutional-medical sovereign power ruling of ethics and professional behaviour. But psychoanalytic theorists such as Judith Butler remind us that the vicissitudes of biopower are not just to be tracked as surface phenomena understood through cultural history, as Foucault's model suggests. Rather, personal history creates another layer for concern. The psychic life of desire and control offers a deeper layer of conscience to the layer described by Foucault of the flows of capillary power. For example, unconscious or tacit impulse may drive a horse and cart through the forces of governmentality (ethics of medicine codified in professionalism), so that "desire" trumps governmentality as a form of power in its own right. Such libidinal power is irrational, where governmentality is a technical-rational process encompassing bureaucracy and its counter-resistances, such as non-compliance. A good example of this is Donald Trump's compulsive lying. His exercise of governmentality at a personal and collective level is trumped by the irrational life of the personal psyche and goes unchecked by his associates who become part of the symptom complex through collusion.

In such irrationality, "conscience" is occluded or over-powered. Biopower is then sandwiched between Agamben's reminder of the continuing power of the sovereign state, religious state or autocratic individual as a cruel oppressor, and the irrational, unconscious life of desire that runs beneath reflective bodily life. While, in turn, this sandwich of powers and resistances is further complicated by how our lives are enmeshed in globalized and instant technologies that extend our cognition. Since Foucault (1977) first warned of the creeping power of governmental surveillance in *Discipline and Punish: The Birth of the Prison*, we are now enmeshed by a biopower that collapses space (we are everywhere at once) and contracts time to instants of gratification.

Returning to conscious governmentality, this is often described by historians as a web of everyday discourse such as manners, forming glue for social cohesion and stratification. The idea that "manners maketh man" can be traced to the 14th century, but it is a very modern notion in the sense of Foucauldian models of power. Cultivating a civil self need not depend on external authority or sovereign power but rather on self-control and self-forming as one's own self-imposed discipline. The historical conditions of possibility for rules of "civility" to emerge have been tracked across cultures, such as 18th-century Britain (Barker-Benfield 1992), and early- to high-modern Japan (Ikegami 2005). In medical education, "civility" is now called "professionalism" – a code of conduct (Smith 2018) that is often re-iterated but rarely critically examined.

Power running through a system is also institutionalized, as noted above, as surveillance – the "soft" side of politics as extensive bureaucratic control. We are all stitched into a complex bureaucratic web in which our records, including medical records, are kept. These become commodities and capital. Medical records can be traded to offer ways in which, say, pharmaceutical companies can target for advertising purposes.

While politics (primarily policy) is commonly exempted from the medicine curriculum, and where medical students want "the cold dope" of functional medicine (diagnosis and treatment) with no frills, we find that actually medicine and politics at the level of biopower and governmentality are inseparable and equally distributed between conformity and intractable resistance. Life and death are medicalized, from birth certificates to death certificates signed by doctors, and even life after death is medicalized as autopsy reports, cadaveric dissection and famous "cases" recurring over generations of learners in medicine. Decisions are made by psychiatrists on whether or not a person should be "sectioned" (excluded from civic life on the basis of incapacity, and then reduced to "bare life"); by public health doctors on whether or not a person should be quarantined; by general practitioners on whether or not a person is fit for work or for travel; and by obstetricians on how and where births should be conducted. But these decisions must first be filtered through politics and law to become policy.

Truth telling (parrhesia) and whistleblowing

In 2007, the Indian government charged an Indian paediatrician and public health specialist, Binayak Sen, with sedition. He was called a Maoist. Paradoxically, "sedition" was a law created by the British colonial government to gain control over the local population. Sen was sentenced to life imprisonment. He had worked tirelessly to expose inequities in healthcare suffered by indigenous people in India, or *adivasis*, the most marginalized of groups who lived in dire poverty. Sen had worked to educate local people in community healthcare practices, as "barefoot" practitioners, where the Indian government had not provided reliable healthcare. After organized protests, in 2011 Sen was released from jail, after spending some time in solitary confinement, but no apology was forthcoming and his original appeal is still pending today. Meanwhile, Sen has been celebrated internationally for his work in human rights, civil liberties and peaceful protest in the tradition of Ghandi.

Once, in the 1930s and 1940s, smoking was "physician tested", approved by medicine. Tobacco was advertised in medical journals ("More doctors smoke Camels than any other cigarette".). While we have finally come to see the health dangers of tobacco smoking, there is a long history of the tobacco industry lobbying the medical community through political channels to suspend advertising the link between smoking, lung cancer and other illnesses. Finally, the US Surgeon General produced a report in 1964 linking smoking with lung cancer, laryngeal cancer and chronic bronchitis. Nevertheless, tobacco companies continued to lobby the political and medical communities up to the late 1990s, maintaining that links between smoking and ill health were "controversial". A UK doctor, Judith Mackay, had been calling out tobacco companies since the 1960s after studying links between smoking and illness in Hong Kong under British rule. But the government refused her evidence, and she received threats, also being called "psychotic human garbage", and a "power-lusting piece of meat" by tobacco company representatives.

Steve Biko, a black medical student in South Africa, began a social movement to fight apartheid in the 1970s. Apartheid meant that black doctors were not allowed to treat white patients or even examine their bodies at autopsy. Biko tried to expose systemic and systematic inequities but was surveilled by the government and banned from political activism. Ignoring the censure, Biko was detained by police in 1977 as a "terrorist" and beaten. He sustained a brain haemorrage and died alone in a jail cell. In 1985, Wendy Orr, a government doctor, blew the whistle on sustained and systematic torture of black prisoners by white police. She was threatened with losing her job but took Biko's and others' cases to the South African Supreme Court, where it was thrown out. Orr later became the commissioner for the Truth and Reconciliation Commission of South Africa, where multiple abuses were recounted in detail and considered as punishable injustices for the first time.

Appointed as a new consultant anaesthetist at the Bristol Royal Infirmary in 1989, Stephen Bolsin noted that a higher than the normal number of babies were dying from heart surgery than the national average, and he suspected that cardiac heart surgeons' practices were outdated and lax. An investigation subsequently revealed poor practices reinforced by inward-looking habits where the surgeons effectively formed an old boys' club. Mortality rates fell from 30% to less than 3% as a result of his whistleblowing intervention, which came to a head in 1995. In his wake, the *Kennedy Report* recommended sweeping changes in clinical governance in UK hospitals, challenging lack of transparency and surgical cabals. Bolsin himself was frozen out by his colleagues and emigrated to work in Australia, where he was a pioneer in the patient safety movement.

Sen, Biko and Bolsin are three amongst many stories of resistance as activism and whistleblowing. After direct activism, whistleblowing is the next most powerful form of resistance as speaking truth to power. This requires moral courage that the ancient Greeks called *parrhesia*, "truth telling" or "fearless speech", and existentialists call "authenticity" (Bleakley 2014). Such moral courage is a virtue. The blowback from whistleblowing can be serious, such as blacklisting and excommunication by colleagues (Marshall and Bleakley 2017). While the good work of medicine is often productively shaped and progressed by policy, it is also readily tainted by political interference. In totalitarian regimes, doctors mainly remain quiet in the face of political scandal for fear of retribution. Those who do speak out may be gagged or written from the record. The Chinese authorities arrested, interrogated and reprimanded Dr Li Wenliang, the Wuhan-based doctor who first spoke out about the possibility of a coronavirus epidemic, for "spreading rumours". He later died from catching the virus and was then exonerated. Dr Ai Fen, a woman doctor and head of emergency medicine in Wuhan Central hospital, also blew the whistle on state suppression of knowledge about the speed and potency of infection. At the time of writing, she is reported as "missing" (Reporters Without Borders 2020; Patel and Rao 2020).

But in democracies too we need whistleblowers; time and again during the coronavirus crisis, we saw healthcare staff speaking out about lack of personal protective equipment (PPE) and other resources, and in the next breath, hospital management issues a rebuttal or squeezes out an excuse, while the staff in question are rebuked and told not to talk to the press. And in democracies too we are not free from the excesses of capitalism, where medicine is for profit and becomes habitually over-productive and over-consumptive rather than lean: over-diagnosing, over-testing and over-treating (Welch, Schwartz and Wolosin 2011). Medicine, as commodity, is tainted by the zealotry of the free market, for-profit neo-liberal capitalism. It is abundantly clear that such an economic model does not provide the conditions for good universal healthcare, but rather has created gross health inequality. Ironically, supposed lifestyles of "choice" for many involve high carbohydrate, high cholesterol foods that are comforting, cheap and convenient, leading to an epidemic of obesity, heart problems and type 2 diabetes.

Each of the examples that open the section above advertises a form of resistance against an external authority or power. The resistance contradicts, subverts, inverts or deflects the power, opening up a new perspective on the issue. For example, the Bristol paediatric heart surgery scandal is fully investigated and a surgical cabal is broken, leading to improvements in the surgical provision, patient safety and public transparency. Such transformative effects of lines of resistance show how medicine and politics are intimately engaged. But more, they show that innovations or solutions can be elegant and fair. Politics in medicine also engage in aesthetics and ethics. For example, whistleblowers' narratives do not just show justice at work, as examples of principles-based ethics, but also virtues-based ethics and habits of the heart; also, such accounts are often interesting literary texts in their own right. In this context, the work of resistance is also necessarily rhetorical or persuasive (Bleakley 2006).

But resistance can also be subtle, and illustrates what the cultural and literary theorist Homi Bhabha (1985) calls "sly civility". In the context of British colonialism in India, Bhahba notes that subtle and everyday forms of resistance, as opposed to street-based political activism and civil disobedience, were embodied in gestures of tongue-in-cheek servility and civility – outwardly polite but with elements of sarcasm or parody, subservient gestures of mild irony, or "backstage" banter. Sly civility is a common politically subversive tactic in clinical settings subject to oppressive managerialism, such as the governmentality of state-set "targets" and outcomes for clinical work.

For example, the UK government issued guidelines for the maximum amount of time a patient should wait in a hospital emergency department before a doctor sees them, and this is echoed by similar guidelines globally. Hospital management enforces such conditions, where breeches of the maximum waiting time can lead to the hospital's emergency department being downgraded and losing funding. Such departments in the UK are severely underfunded and understaffed after years of government-imposed austerity, and departments are often overwhelmed at certain times of the year such as winter when influenza infections peak. Emergency departments have developed tactics to avoid breeching, such as putting patients on trolleys and taking them to corridors at the "breeching hour" and then returning them as fresh admissions (Allard and Bleakley 2016).

Students reporting professionalism lapses, micro-aggressions and other bad behaviour from seniors

What do students think of professionalism lapses, micro-aggressions and other bad behaviour that they see in senior doctors, acting as both teachers and role models, in work-based learning clinical settings? More, what can they do about this if they feel some moral outrage? Students interviewed in several medical schools across the world report lapses in professional behaviour by their senior doctor teachers, such as ritual humiliation of students and sexist comments by male tutors towards female students (Monrouxe et al. 2014; Monrouxe and Rees 2017; Shaw et al. 2018). Reports also describe the objectification of patients and displays of arrogance by doctors towards nursing staff. Such behaviour was common even 20 years ago, but students had expected that it had all but disappeared and were concerned by its continuing presence. While they were happy to anonymously report such professionalism lapses to researchers, they were mostly unable to confront the senior doctors engaging in this behaviour.

Drawing on data gathered from 808 UK and Australian medical students, using audio diaries, focus groups and interviews, Lynn Monrouxe, Charlotte Rees and colleagues (Monrouxe and Rees 2017) tease out the anatomy of resistance against perceived transgressions. Resistance is defined as "a reaction against confining social structures". This definition is rather woolly and all embracing, demanding clarification at every point: what kind of "reaction"? What is meant by "confining"? Where "social structure" is all embracing, what kinds of structure are we talking about – authoritarian regimes, tame hierarchies, mock "teams", etc.?

An argument is made that "medical students encounter traditional medical and interprofessional hierarchies as they learn to become doctors. These create a power disparity that may prevent their empowerment and ability to resist". An "interprofessional" hierarchy is a contradiction in terms. Inter-professionalism is achieved when hierarchies are flattened across previously multi-professional settings. The "power disparity" that medical students may feel in these settings would surely not "prevent" their "ability to resist" – in fact, resistance is only made possible by the existence of the power disparity.

Despite this shaky framework, the data gathered speak volumes about students' experienced uncertainties in clinical settings. Where they perceive "professionalism dilemmas" – or "situations that contradict their ethical, moral, and professional understandings of appropriate medical practice" – this can lead to "direct and indirect, verbal and bodily, instantaneous and delayed forms of resistance to counter the professionalism lapses of their seniors". Students show patterns of resistance to "hegemonic practices" including patient and student "abuse", lack of hygienic practice and slippage in obtaining patient consent. The authors claim:

> Through these various acts of resistance (and their narration), medical students may promote the subtle transformation of the dominant medical structure either consciously or unconsciously. They may do this through reflecting on acts of resistance to professionalism lapses, making sense of their moral position and the development of their professional identities, by encouraging others to also resist through sharing resistance narratives, and finally, by altering the professional conduct of their seniors.
>
> (Shaw et al. 2018: 45)

We might conclude from this that medical education, once an apprenticeship or socialization into a community of practice, can now be read as (potentially and radically) a politicized resistance. Such resistance is on behalf of patients and serves to construct an identity as a patient-centred trainee doctor. Simultaneously, the medical student resists potential commodification of his or her labour, leading to objectification. The resistance is then productive, as another step towards democratizing medicine. The following chapter picks up this thread.

Bibliography

Agamben G. 1998. *Homo Sacer: Sovereign Power and Bare Life*. Palo Alto, CA: Stanford University Press.

Allard J, Bleakley A. What Would You Ideally Do if There Were No Targets? An Ethnographic Study of the Unintended Consequences of Top-Down Governance in Two Clinical Settings. *Advances in Health Sciences Education*. 2016;21:803–17.

Barker-Benfield GJ. 1992. *The Culture of Sensibility: Sex and Society in Eighteenth-Century Britain*. Chicago, IL: University of Chicago Press.

Bhabha HK. Sly Civility. *October*. 1985;34:71–80.

Bleakley A. "You Are Who I Say You Are": The Rhetorical Construction of Identity in the Operating Theatre. *Journal of Workplace Learning*. 2006;18:414–25.

Bleakley A. 2014. *Patient-Centred Medicine in Transition: The Heart of the Matter*. Dordrecht: Springer.

Butler J. 1997. *The Psychic Life of Power: Theories in Subjection*. Palo Alto, CA: Stanford University Press.

Cisney VW, Morar N (eds.) 2016. *Biopower: Foucault and Beyond*. Chicago, Ill: University of Chicago Press.

Engeström Y. 2008. *From Teams to Knots: Activity-Theoretical Studies of Collaboration at Work*. Cambridge: Cambridge University Press.

Engeström Y. 2018. *Expertise in Transition: Expansive Learning in Medical Work*. Cambridge: Cambridge University Press.

Foucault M. 1976. *The Birth of the Clinic: An Archaeology of Medical Perception*. London: Routledge.

Foucault M. 1977. *Discipline and Punish: The Birth of the Prison*. New York: Random House.

Foucault M. 1980. *The History of Sexuality: Vol I. An Introduction*. New York: Vintage Books.

Foucault M. 2008. *The Birth of Biopolitics: Lectures at the Collège de France 1978–1979*. London: Palgrave Macmillan.

Ikegami E. 2005. *Bonds of Civility: Aesthetic Networks and the Origins of Japanese Culture*. Cambridge: Cambridge University Press.

Marshall R, Bleakley A. 2017. *Rejuvenating Medical Education: Seeking Help from Homer*. Newcastle: Cambridge Scholars Publishing.

Monrouxe L, Rees C, Dennis I, et al. Professionalism Dilemmas, Moral Distress and the Healthcare Student: Insights from Two Online UK-Wide Questionnaire Studies. *BMJ Open*. 2014;5(5). Available at: http://dx.doi.org/10.1136/bmjopen-2014-007518

Monrouxe LV, Rees CE. 2017. *Healthcare Professionalism: Improving Practice Through Reflections on Workplace Dilemmas*. Hoboken, NJ: Wiley Blackwell.

Patel NA, Rao A. Doctors Have Been Whistleblowers Throughout History. They've Also Been Silenced. *The Guardian*, 8 April 2020. Available at: https://www.theguardian.com/education/2020/apr/08/coronavirus-doctors-whistleblowers-history-silenced

Reporters Without Borders. 2020. *Whistleblowing Doctor Missing After Criticizing Beijing's Coronavirus Censorship*. 10 April, Updated on April 14. Available at: https://rsf.org/en/news/whistleblowing-doctor-missing-after-criticizing-beijings-coronavirus-censorship

Shaw MK, Rees CE, Andersen NB, et al. Professionalism Lapses and Hierarchies: A Qualitative Analysis of Medical Students' Narrated Acts of Resistance. *Social Science & Medicine*. 2018;219:45–53.

Shwetz K. 2020. The Chaotic Narratives of Anti-Vaccination. In: A Bleakley (ed). *Routledge Handbook of Medical Humanities*, 185–91.

Smith R. Medical Professionalism: A Key to a Better Health System and More Satisfied Doctors. *BMJ Opinion*, 6 December 2018. Available at: https://blogs.bmj.com/bmj/2018/12/06/medical-professionalism-a-key-to-a-better-health-system-and-more-satisfied-doctors/

Weiss P. 2009. *The Aesthetics of Resistance Vol I*. Durham, NC: Duke University Press.

Weiss P. 2020. *The Aesthetics of Resistance Vol II*. Durham, NC: Duke University Press.

Welch HG, Schwartz LM, Woloshin S. 2011. *Over-Diagnosed: Making People Sick in the Pursuit of Health*. Boston, MA: Beacon Press.

8 Resistance: Part II

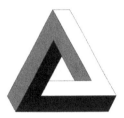

Democracy, "teams" and common wealth

The key act of resistance to normative healthcare provision worldwide is the same as the key act of resistance to political domination by minority authorities worldwide, as autocracies, "hard" or "soft". First, contemporary medicine may claim to be "authoritative" rather than authoritarian, and healthcare systems may claim to be multi-professional. But we should be aiming higher – for fully democratic structures, including authentic inter-professionalism. Second, hospitals – rather than communities – act like magnets for medical education, as we have seen, and they tend to work with hierarchical management and clinical structures.

The result is that students get drawn away from community-oriented medicine where they can learn about, and how to address, health inequities and inequalities through democratic habits. In Cuban medical education, for example, students spend most of their time in the community rather than hospitals, but this is set in a wider authoritarian structure, as we have seen. In the opening to this chapter, I take the issue of democratizing medicine as an example of resistance to lingering historically determined hierarchies while being careful to note that of course democratic structures cannot be imposed autocratically.

In Shakespeare's late play *The Tempest* (probably written in 1610–11), Prospero, the usurped Duke of Milan, causes a shipwreck that strands several of his enemies on the island that he himself was exiled to 12 years earlier with his daughter Miranda. Among those from the new shipwreck is an old and wise councillor, Gonzalo. As the villains Antonio (the brother of Prospero and usurper of his Dukedom) and Sebastian (Alonso and Prospero's second brother) try to get their bearings on the island along with Gonzalo, so Shakespeare uses the "island" as a blank slate on which to project political fantasies – those of the two brothers as Machiavellian, cynical, pessimistic and dystopian; and those of Gonzalo as idealistic, optimistic and utopian.

Where Gonzalo (Act 2 Scene I) sees fertile land, fit for a "plantation", the cynical brothers see only ground fit for weeds: "nettle-seed" and "docks, or mallows". Gonzalo sees the island as a template for the "commonwealth", a reference to the English colonizing of Jamestown in Virginia (1607), with a view to setting up a democratic utopian community. Antonio and Sebastian see infertility, where the ground is not worth breaking, while Gonzalo sees breaking new ground as a challenge worth embracing.

In this exchange, Shakespeare rehearses a tension between the psychological types (and their worldviews) that the psychologist William James (1907), 300 years later, would call "tough-minded" and "tender-minded". The tough-minded Antonio and Sebastian are cynics, sceptics and pessimists who feel no guilt in exploiting others for their own purposes. The tender-minded Gonzalo is a principled optimist and idealist. But more, Gonzalo's vision of the commonwealth is one of collaborative democratic participation, where Antonio and Sebastian are by contrast competitive and wilful individuals. To redraw Shakespeare's metaphor, such individualism aligns with a vision of an unfertile, weed-strewn earth, where Gonzalo's earth is productive. Gonzalo is a model for resistance to an established order – an authority or an autocratic condition – promising positive change, a revolution.

The earth we have chosen in the West is rampant, free market capitalism, which promised to benefit all as economies grow. Neo-liberal capitalism promised that, as the wealth of the top earners increased, so this would trickle down to benefit all. The reality, as Thomas Piketty (2014), amongst others, has argued, is that the thinnest top slice of the population, as the extremely wealthy, have floated away in terms of an income bubble of unimaginable size, while the least wealthy have sunk into a poverty trap. As the tide of economic growth has risen, it has failed to raise all the boats with it. Shadowing wealth distribution are health and life expectancy. The wealthy live longer and have better overall health than the poor, and the burden of a country's health service remains with caring for the poor and disadvantaged. Illness is linked to social inequity and inequality.

Through Shakespeare, Gonzalo's cameo appearance in *The Tempest* linking the fertility of the land, or natural resources, to politics (the power arrangements that extract and distribute those resources) is an important reminder that we have lagged in our appreciation and understanding of how politics, ecology and health can be joined up to realize the value of democratic engagement. As important is the vehicle for Shakespeare's message – art, theatre, dramatic realization or aesthetics. The realization of a joined-up message between politics, ecology and health is better as an aesthetic gesture than a functional and blunt one. In realizing the medicine curriculum as a political text, the senses and a sense of form and beauty should be deeply engaged, as medical practice is enacted dramaturgically, as theatre.

Medicine, embedded in wider healthcare, is necessarily collaborative work, whether it is just patient and doctor or patient and nurse in a primary care setting; an operating theatre or ward team; or several tighter and looser associations of health and social care professionals, aided by lay carers, working around a patient's needs. In seeking ever-greater efficiency, healthcare has sought help from organizational and industrial psychologists. They have focused, at the organizational level (such as hospitals), on developing more efficient management of human resources through programmes of "leadership" and "teamwork". These have become mantras for "progress". But they have often acted in divisive ways, reinforcing unproductive hierarchies and de-powering "shop floor" workers, even doctors at a high level of experience.

Ivan Illich (1973) warned half a century ago, in *Tools for Conviviality*, that as industrial and medical technologies developed, so a common wealth of power to construct dwellings, grow food and look after health would be stripped from the general populus and would rest not just in the hands of experts, but more in the hands of the managerial class who organized expertise. This went beyond a standard Marxist reading by noting that what is then stripped from the populus is a common wealth of solidarity – first, "convivial" living (friendliness); and second, the aesthetics and ethics or value system that form convivial living. Jacques Rancière (2013) too has devoted his life's work to articulating and archiving a working class aesthetics and arts culture, recovering or restoring historical examples. Conviviality, suggests Illich, is endangered as once shared knowledge and skills grounded in basics of living – again, providing shelter, growing food and generating community-based basic healthcare and illness prevention – are, as it were, not only "privatized" and professionalized, but then managerialized.

Central to the rise of the human resources technologies has been the theorizing and packaging as a commodity of the very idea of conviviality, or what Roland Barthes (2013) calls "how to live together", the glue for which is "generosity" (Basil 2019). The package is then marketed as "improving teamwork", including "leadership" and now "followership" skills or behaviours. This thinking has permeated medical education, where the curriculum becomes an economic text. But it has a political dimension too, embracing neo-liberal capitalism, turning "team training" packages into commodities – marketable items for profit. In the following section I map out some of the contradictions in this approach and how the approach in general can be positively resisted, partly by re-configuring what we mean by "teams" and by restoring conviviality to grassroots workers – although I resist using Illich's term "tools" for conviviality as I believe that instrumentalizing "teamwork" ("toolboxes"), or turning aesthetic possibilities into the functional, is the first step towards commercializing and commodifying teamwork training.

"Teams" as things and "teeming" as process

Acts of resistance need not be radical disjunctions such as sharp identity shifts we call "radicalization", or major political shifts such as coups, but rather gradual processes of change – morphing, and the subtle "achieving ensemble" (Bleakley,

Allard and Hobbs 2013). Such slow processes can, however, cumulatively constitute a paradigm shift. The unit of analysis for understanding such slow morphing of work structures is historical. Much contemporary research and conceptual approaches to work groupings, commonly called "teams" – although this may be a misnomer – relegate the temporal dimension to team structure in giving dominance to the spatial.

"Teams" are generally not historicized as "process", but rather reified as objects frozen in time. For example, one identifiable shift in medicine and healthcare, the move to democratize practices (commonly, but crudely, described as "flattening hierarchies"), remains to be tracked temporally, or historically. "Team" is often treated as a magic bullet and this is a global phenomenon in healthcare, where deification follows reification. For example, Amir Babiker and colleagues (Babiker et al. 2014: 9), in the context of paediatric care teams in the Sudan, suggest:

> Identifying best practices through rigorous research, which can provide data on optimal processes for team-based care, is subject to identification of the core elements of this system. Once the underlying principles and core values are agreed and shared, researchers will be able to more easily compare team-based care models and commissioners will be able to promote effective practices.

Indeed, the authors do identify the core principles for effective teamwork, as "Shared goals ... Clear roles ... Effective communication ... Measurable processes and outcomes ... (and) Leadership". This is a common enough mantra, of which we should be sceptical. Teams in this view are built of parts, instrumentally, like a machine, and can then be tested for efficiency. Their engine oil is logic and clarity, and there must be a driver, a leader, at the helm. Indeed, this smacks of imperialism – the global mass marketing of American-based business and management models of "efficiency" in the service of increased productivity. But healthcare work is far too messy and unpredictable to be encapsulated by such efficiency models.

In this section, I briefly compare and contrast three approaches to challenging and dismantling historically accumulated hierarchical structures of power across healthcare groups through a discussion of "team working": (i) Michael West and colleagues' approach adopted by parts of the National Health Service (NHS), UK; (ii) Yrjö Engeström and colleagues' approach in Helsinki, Finland, to Expansive Learning in healthcare; and (iii) the celebrated French thinker and cultural theorist Roland Barthes' semiotic approach to social existence, or "how to live together", treated here as "how to work together".

Teams reified

Michael West (West et al. 2014) is the leading figure in the UK in theory and practice of team behaviour, bringing an organizational psychology mindset to healthcare practice. Through his work with the King's Fund, a health charity and independent think tank that feeds into NHS England, West has influenced authors such as Beccy Baird and colleagues (Baird et al. 2020) on "How to build effective teams in general practice". This approach begins with reducing a "team" to a noun, a thing, thus again reifying "team". As team becomes object, so team members are in danger of being objectified, treated as parts of the machinery of the team (as mentioned above). In this model, a "team" is built of individuals and is judged by how well it manipulates or controls the environment through dictated practices. For example, there is great emphasis currently on building "resilience" into team members under unusual conditions of stress produced during the coronavirus crisis.

However, it is not what a team is that matters, but what it does. Yrjö Engeström (2008, 2018) sees "team" as process rather than thing, coining descriptors such as "teeming" and "knotworking", turning the noun into the verb and qualifying adverbs ("negotiated knotworking"), where "the notion of a knot refers to rapidly pulsating, distributed, and partially improvised orchestration of a collaborative performance among otherwise loosely connected actors and activity systems" (ibid.: 86).

Baird and colleagues (2020) also talk of "teamworking", but their emphasis is as much on the constituents of the team, the team members, as the team's activities, where in general practice and primary care networks, "new roles are being introduced, creating multidisciplinary and multi-agency teams". So, the roles create the teams rather than the activity of "teeming" creating the roles. For Engeström, teams are constituted on pre-existent human sociality and are shaped through artefacts, including language and symbols. For Roland Barthes, a coming-together of people is best understood as a semiotic embodiment – a fleshed-out symbol of the need for humans to congregate with purpose: "Black Lives Matter" – it's a collective, a plurality, a pre-existent sociality.

In West and colleagues' models, teams need clarity of purpose, as Baird et al. (2020) reiterate: "A small number of meaningful objectives" and "Clear roles and responsibilities among team members". Time out needs to be built into teams for reflection. This would suggest a will-to-stability, or continuity, rather than tolerance for risk or ambiguity. Here already is a glitch – as the authors say, primary care teams may embrace "occupational therapists, psychologists, mental health nurses, health coaches and dieticians", as well as "Managers, administrators, data analysts, care navigators, prescribing clerks and receptionists". Yet, "Working with the same care team every day also helps build trust between clinical staff". How can this scattering of the wider professional elements serving the patient be made to cohere? As Engeström (2018: 88) suggests: "stable teams do not seem to be a sufficient answer to the challenge of coordinating complex arrangements of multiple lines of substantially different services that do not rely on each other's assistance and advice on a daily basis".

So, a contradiction is inherent in this model – a wish for team stability, requiring a core "micro" team, in the face of a reality of a sprawling set of associations amongst a number of community and primary care health providers and their administrative teams, requiring some management and co-ordination. The hope to bring this sprawling mass to functional order and stability is surely a misguided aim. This is an open, dynamic, complex adaptive system and not a closed, linear system that can be tuned and re-tuned. Complex systems have multiple "attractors" that provide forms of stability and allow them to shift to new levels of organization, but they must be apprehended as fluid, liquid or in process, able to jump to new levels of complexity through re-organization without falling into chaos. Such open systems cannot be regulated instrumentally like a closed system (Bleakley 2010, 2014).

For proponents of stability, creating psychological safety through generative dialogue is essential to the functioning of teams, but still we have the "mind the gap" problem that separates sprawling, loosely associated health and administrative practitioners across several groups with their separate identities, called "cross-boundary teamworking" by West and colleagues (Wells 2015) and "boundary crossing" by Engeström and colleagues (Akkerman and Bakker 2011). The difference in approaches is that Wells uses instrumental semiotics, talking of providing a "toolkit" for team members, where a boundary is an obstacle to be overcome, or a problem to be solved. A boundary is then an inconvenience, rather than a convenient semiotic for flagging "specialty" within an emergent inter-professionalism and thus maintaining hard-won identity in an increasingly fluid world of work.

Within the paradigm that I am ascribing to Michael West's approach to teamworking, Beccy Baird and colleagues also construct the paradox of fleshly human agency seen through an instrumental lens, so that while "Teamworking models will be most effective if they are co-designed with patients and carers … There are lots of toolkits that can help with this work providing guidance on everything from how to recruit patients to emotionally mapping their experience". Just as team process can be measured, so patients' emotional experiences can be mapped. The semiotic (thinking that we have Roland Barthes looking over our shoulders in this section) of "toolkits" is surely revealing. Again, team process is in danger of being commodified, where market-led exchange value (team scoring high on functional scales) replaces intrinsic use value (team members are experts in negotiated knotworking and boundary crossings in uncertain and fluid contexts).

Akkerman and Bakker (2011) describe boundary crossing as creating an opportunity out of a contradiction by the "understanding of boundaries as dialogical phenomena". Boundaries here are not problems to be solved but opportunities to be exploited, such as four potential learning mechanisms that can take place at boundaries: identification, co-ordination, reflection and transformation. These mechanisms show various ways in which sociocultural differences and resulting discontinuities in action and interaction can come to function as resources for development of intersecting identities and practices.

The co-ordination, maturing to collaboration, of associations between largely dis-connected groups is called "teaming" or "teamwork on the fly" by Amy Edmondson at Harvard University, where teaming's temporary nature is inevitable. Edmonson (2013) suggests that most innovative work cultures are fast paced and flexible, where stable teams are not appropriate for context, yet in her 2013 article nevertheless describes the "three pillars" of a "teaming" culture (as "curious, passionate, and empathic"). Again, a contradiction – mobile, liquid, fast paced teams require firming up through "pillars". A will-to-stability holds firm: back to teams as things, and the need for toolkits to fix them, lest they collapse. Until relatively recently, clinical teams were referred to as "firms": a semiotics of embracing, business-like and cohesive.

Suddenly, West and colleagues' model of teamwork does not sound so radical and may not even constitute a democratizing move as it fixes the very notion of "team" itself in a will-to-stability rather than projecting to the realms of "possibility knowledge" (Engeström 2018). The team is not a product of ecological-perceptual affordance, grounded in, and subject to, context. Rather, the team is built from persons outwards, and it is the persons we must change in order to make the teams work or cohere. This ignores historical (temporal) and spatial factors. For example, anybody who has been on a teaching ward round in a hospital setting with a senior clinician leading a clinical team of other doctors and nurses, plus say three medical students in tow, knows that the space around the patient's bed, as the curtain is drawn for privacy, dictates how the team works.

If there is a will-to-stability, including a shared cognitive model, across teams, how do such teams cope with unexpected and unusual events? The coronavirus pandemic has thrown up a particular issue for healthcare. As healthcare organizations are placed under unusual pressures, habitual practices, structures and rhythms of work have been constantly disrupted through high levels of sickness and turnover. Here, you might expect that teamwork specialists would look to engagement with process models of flow, liquidity or fluidity that stress adaptation above cohesion. Scott Tannenbaum and Eduardo Salas are amongst the foremost team researchers in the USA. In "Managing Teamwork in the Face of Pandemic: Evidence-Based Tips", Tannenbaum and colleagues (2020) also show an instrumental bent in considering how teams might adapt to extraordinary challenges where the title advertises "tips" (rather than, say, strategies). Again, the semiotic frame is telling.

Chief among such "tips" from Tannenbaum and colleagues is for teams under unusual pressure and stress to maintain a "shared mental model", achieved through briefing, debriefing and periodic "huddles". The model of the team is again one of working out from the minds of the individual members to engage a common script. As noted, there is another view, characterizing Activity Theory, that the team is a product of ecological affordance. Here, the "mind" is not formed collectively by the team, or is "in" the team, but rather is afforded by the environment or context of the moment. The team's activities are shaped according to environmental contexts and cues. The "shared mental model" is the confluence of adaptations. This view stresses the importance of adaptability and flexibility: innovation and experimentation in the face of fast moving contexts.

West and colleagues' work is stained to some extent with the American curse of stubborn individualism – a running critical theme in this book – in the face of the power of collectives, where the stress is on the importance of "leadership". The outstanding individual becomes the leader. Recent work stresses that leadership can change according to task, and that leadership can be collective. In a publication for the King's Fund Centre for Creative Leadership, Michael West and colleagues (2014) set out a manifesto for teamwork in healthcare that promotes the idea of "collective leadership" as a basis to "caring cultures". This can include "patient leaders". But surely the patient is the object of the team's work as an activity system, and then by definition is permanent "leader" as the focus of ecological affordance.

"Collective leadership" retains the primacy of the individual role masked as a democratic gesture and now embodied in a meritocracy. Indeed, individuals who cannot be leaders can study "followership" ("merit" follows a conventional hierarchy). Leadership embraces morality through virtuous qualities, again at the level of the individual. Thus, authentic democratic structures are subtly compromised. Hierarchies are not flattened but sneak back in through the back door of liberal leadership styles and perceived merit, as noted. Compulsive leadership is a form of imperialism. Roland Barthes (2013) gives the example of Daniel Defoe's Robinson Crusoe, who first enslaves a cat as a pet, then a goat and parrot, and finally the black Man Friday becomes the white man Crusoe's servant, maintaining white supremacy. The semiotics of this arrangement bleed out spatially, so that a "servant's quarters" can be set up in Crusoe's makeshift home.

West claims that "high performing" teams are "clearly defined teams" – the more stable, the better the outcomes. Such teams have:

- clear goals
- high levels of participation
- an ability to resolve conflict readily
- an ability to be reflexive, or self-reckoning and self-regulating
- an ability to manage status and hierarchies without conflict
- clear leadership

But what if "goals" are displaced by improvisation, participation is loose as team membership is fluid, conflict is utilized as a resource rather than "managed", reflexivity is replaced by experimentation, status and hierarchies come "pre flattened" and leadership is replaced by context-specific capabilities? West further distinguishes between "real" or authentic teams and "pseudo" teams, where real teams have shared objectives, task inter-dependence and self-regulation. Again, a "real" team is ordered – composed, coherent and self-knowing. Yet teeming and knotworking, or being in the rhythm of the event, are unpredictable and can offer bumpy rides precisely because they are responsive to bumpy terrain, but more, carry the imprint of bumpy historicity – legacies of contradictions. "Teams", of course, like particles at the sub-atomic level, can occupy two spaces simultaneously: the real and the imagined, theorized or simulated. Sometimes the theorized or simulated is mistaken for the real.

Yrjö Engeström's knotworking

Michael West and colleagues' approach is radical in the context of current team practices in NHS England, but looks conservative in relation to Yrjö Engeström and colleagues' movement from object-"teams" to process-"knots" within expansive learning; and, as outlined later, Roland Barthes' insistence on social activity as rhythmic and shaped semiotically. Linguistically and semiotically, West's teams, aiming for stability, can be seen as metonymic chains. Just as one word leads to another in a chain of associations (patient ... waiting ... room ... service ... changing oil: a chain semiotically signalling and invoking functional medicine as fixing or repairing the body), so a team is a chain of embodied roles, anchored by a leader. Even if leadership can be "distributed", nevertheless, the stable team requires such anchoring. A team that drifts is anathema to a model grounded in principles of stability.

For Engeström, the semiotics of "teeming", "negotiated knotworking", "learning by expanding" and "boundary crossing" suggest that the anchor has been raised. Signs have given way to symbols and metaphors. Teamwork activities drift, but not aimlessly; they encounter underwater rocks as contradictions but use these as means for transformation and do not founder on them; open seas offer wild currents and wide horizons, but these are taken as opportunities and improvisation is accepted as par for the course. While the voyage may be to the land of patient care and safety, this is always a horizon territory, ever changing, different for each patient's needs. Here, the challenge is how to turn co-ordination of differing clinical players and artefacts into, first, co-operation, and then communication or authentic collaboration – a transition from multi-professionalism to inter-professionalism.

In West and colleagues' model, while patients may be consulted, they mainly appear to be accessories to the team's core functioning, even though the activity is patient centred in principle. For Engeström and colleagues, the patient, as the object of the activity, constructs the activities around herself as a magnet or queen bee, demanding swarming. This shifts patient-centredness to patient-directed activity.

Following the work of Engeström and colleagues, I have previously written about "stable" team models critically and sceptically (Bleakley 2013), having spent a good portion of my academic research career studying clinical teams on wards and particularly in operating theatres, and working psychotherapeutically with general practice groups. Again, a major revolution in such work has been to translate "team" from noun to verb, from object to process. I borrow from Zygmunt Bauman to talk about "liquid" teamworking (ibid.). These terms describe fast moving, or pulsating, clinical contexts in which uncertainty is high and adaptation and improvisation are called for.

Engeström and colleagues describe exchanges between practitioners under such circumstances as "negotiated knotworking", and between teams as "boundary crossings". This inventive vocabulary advertises the importance of artefact as mediating activity and promotes the importance of a semiotic view of activity. While the sign (e.g. "team") is arbitrary, where the signified (the activity of teeming or knotworking) is meaningful, nevertheless the sign carries cultural value, as Barthes suggests. Signs are capital. In healthcare, "team" is invested with quality and weight, even though it is an arbitrary signifier for a concrete social process. But "teeming" and "knotworking", both serving as puns as well as serious descriptors of activities, have creative weight. They are artful and graceful. They signify buzzing, swarming, work-related activity, including gestural means of contact (tying and untying knots as temporary means of relating).

Such activities – loose and temporary – also defy habitual will-to-stability where "stable" teams are invoked. There is nostalgia in some parts of healthcare (especially surgery), where "stable" teams are talked about as the ideal forms, but the reality is that teamwork across healthcare has for some time been following the airline industry model, where teams are fluid, formed from a pool of players each of whom can, theoretically, be trusted for their capability at their level of experience. Stable teams can get into ruts, pursue habitual practices without reflection and work within fixed perceptual frames. Again, there is a will-to-stability rather than a forward looking to possibility knowledge.

Patient safety is relatively poor in medical contexts, particularly in surgery, as a result of poor teamwork, and this has been tracked to two factors: first, stable teams acquire bad habits (this was evident in paediatric cardiac surgery teams mentioned in the last chapter at the Bristol hospital where the anaesthetist Stephen Bolsin blew the whistle on bad practices that had led to an excess of mortalities over the national average). Second, stable teams tend to work with traditional role hierarchies, with medicine dominating nursing, where nurses often feel unable to challenge poor or perceived unsafe practices of doctors and surgeons (Bleakley 2014). Such teams are multi-professional and not inter-professional, where professions work and learn with, from and about other professions. In surgery, for example, such hierarchical arrangements extend from the "top" surgical team to "lower" supply teams such as surgical instrument cleaning team and even handover teams such as patient recovery.

Roland Barthes' "Living Together"

Our third figure, Roland Barthes (2013), has no truck with clinical scenarios, but is perceptive about the fundamentals of humans coming together for whatever purpose. Barthes' *How to Live Together* can be readily translated into "how to work together", and plays with the contradiction of the choice of solitary monastic life in the face of knowledge of social life. This contrasts sharply with the accounts in earlier chapters of the political isolation of individuals who are cast out, excommunicated or driven out as political refugees, casualties of war or environmental disaster – the figure in Roman law called *homo sacer*, not a "sacred" person but a "separate" person. Such a stigmatized person carries the contradiction that any citizen might kill him or her without retribution, while he or she also remains untouchable.

Where West and colleagues' work is grounded in organizational theory that foregrounds method in work studies, Barthes says that living together is "an attentiveness to forces" (ibid.: 4), or knowledge of power. It became all the more obvious during the coronavirus pandemic that living together is a health act governed by politics. For the first time for many people, the Western tradition of the will-to-act was suspended in "lockdown", as human contact was limited, so that people acted in the Taoist tradition of Wu-Wei – "non-doing" or purposeful inaction. There is, suggests Barthes, a desire to be social – phalanstery. A phalanstère was a type of building designed for a self-contained utopian community, ideally consisting of 500–2,000 people working together for mutual benefit, and developed in the early 19th century by Charles Fourier.

The desire to be social, says Barthes, is not a formation of a body, a gluing together of common types. Rather, it is finding a common *rhythm*. Social processes of democracy are not about identifying with those who are similar, but potentially dissimilar people finding a common rhythm. "Team" is not "in" the people who compose it, but "in" the rhythm to which they finally subscribe. Barthes himself finds such rhythm in literary accounts of "how to live together" as "novelistic simulations" of "everyday spaces". This is also a pun as "novelistic" means both illustrated in a novel, and "new". The bottom line is that the arts – literature – provide our best examples of how to do "teams" or work together.

The arts in performing ensembles can help us here. A string quartet or a jazz group finds its life in a common pulse. In idio-rhythmic life, one follows one's own way as in a monastic existence. Poly-rhythmic clusters occur where common tasks and modes of identification occur – such as local teams – where "swarming" is common, collective behaviour around a common task as individuals identify with the task rather than necessarily with each other in personality fixations.

In adapting Barthes' views on "living together" to the arena of patient care, we are reminded that "hospital" and "hospitality" have the same linguistic root. Under the roof of the caring community, can the patient expect what the ancient Greeks called *xenia*, or "guest friendship"? Healthcare is again an embodied semiotic exercise where a set of signs and symbols provide the media through which "care" is shaped and understood. How will a semiotics and linguistics be built that bridges patient and healthcare activities? This is a question that I address in Chapter 13, where I look at how medical language and symbols and lay language and symbols can meet.

While metaphors are usually located in linguistics rather than semiotics, they are cousins to signs and symbols. We undercut or devalue the experience of patients where we have already historically accumulated toxic medical metaphors undermining *xenia*, such as "illness as war" (particularly, martial metaphors in cancer care and treatment) that place the patient as both victim and fighter, when maybe they have no energy to fight (Bleakley 2017). Coronavirus patients have also been told that they are fighting an "unknown enemy". "Double blind" takes on a new meaning – first, you're in a war for which you did not sign up; and second, the enemy is invisible.

Healthcare practitioners "working together" and healthcare practitioners and patients "living together" present the challenge to medical care of finding the same rhythm as patients' presenting symptoms and lives. This is to be in tune with patients – empathic, sensitive and caring; having a sensibility for close noticing that follows patients' embodied symptoms, their words or descriptions and their wider life-forms – familial, social and cultural settings. Beyond necessary empathy and compassion, Anu Atluru (2016) draws on improvisational theatre and performance to suggest that "Thinking quickly and occasionally abandoning the medical-school script are critical for quality patient care". Atluru, a doctor and writer but also somebody who has taken the trouble to gain experience in improvisational theatre, says that how medical students are taught "communication skills" in simulated settings can be stifling, where live clinical contexts require "reacting" spontaneously and with intuition, rather than "acting" through a pre-defined script ("breaking bad news", for example).

Engestrom's (2018: 82) view of the work activities of teeming and negotiated knotworking coincide with Barthes' view of collaborative human activity seen as aligning rhythms, not roles: "In musical terminology, with expanding objects, time needs to be both composed and improvised ... Although improvisation is quick, it is above all rhythmically focused ... it is important to distinguish between rhythmically focused speed and mechanically forced haste". It is a common complaint of junior doctors, working flat out, that they do not have enough time. Perhaps they have not found both rhythm and reaction.

In West and colleagues' model, collectivity is "earned" as individuals move out from self to other. In rhythmic teeming, pulsing and knotworking, collectivity is assumed like a jazz group that can both play from scores and improvise with ease. The former teams are subject to schema to which the individuals adapt, where activity-oriented collectivism follows *rhuthmos*, a pattern or a fluid element ("liquid" teeming), modelled on the "rhythms of the waves", suggests Barthes. In such teeming, power is a productively channelled communal biopower, rather than exercised through authoritative hierarchies or forms of leadership.

Teams that do not work well may be a-rhythmic, or fail to find a rhythm in work. Barthes (2013: 9) gives an example of looking out of his window at a mother pushing a pram and walking with a young child. The mother walks at a certain pace and has her attention drawn to the pram, such that the young child cannot keep up. There is disjunction between the child's and the mother's rhythms. The child keeps stumbling and the mother gets frustrated. Barthes says the mother exerts "autarky", which is the characteristic of self-sufficiency. The term usually applies to political states, societies or their economic systems. Autarky exists whenever an entity or a state survives or continues its activities without external assistance or international trade. The mother becomes an island to the child even though she is holding her hand because they are out of step

– failing to establish, or start from, a position of collectivity. Sometimes a "team" can be a loose collection of monological types, failing to begin from the perspective of dialogue as assumed collectivism.

Coda

Yrjö Engeström (2018: 27) notes: "as one of the oldest, most prestigious, and most carefully protected professions, medicine carries within its very identity a tremendous historical ballast of individualism, compartmentalization, and hierarchical authority". We have seen how such factors impede adoption of processes of teeming and negotiated knotworking as the team is "achieved" as an instrumental entity within the linear mechanics of a closed system – seeking stability – rather than an open, adaptive, complex system often working at maximum complexity at the edge of chaos, especially in multiple healthcare provision contexts around a patient. Engeström (2018: 88) suggests that "stable teams do not seem to be a sufficient answer to the challenge of coordinating complex arrangements of multiple lines of substantially different services that do not rely on each other's assistance and advice on a daily basis".

One of the main flaws of standard approaches to team activity is that the focus on stable teams becomes the object of the activity rather than the patient the team serves. Further, members of the team have differing conceptions of patient care and safety that are not necessarily reconciled or seen as potentially productive contradictions. For example, historically, nurses view patients as subjects of care, whereas surgeons view them as objects of cure. Indeed, Engeström (2018) points out that doctors hold differing objects for patients, for example as disease, as consumer or unit (economic), as psychosomatic whole, as community member and as collaborator. AnneMaire Mol (2002), from an Actor Network perspective, takes this further where parts of the patient's body can be the "circulating" object of inquiry for differing medical specialties – such as a vascular surgeon operating on a blood vessel, a lab technician looking at a blood sample, a pathologist looking at a biopsy, a radiologist looking at a scan, a GP looking at the patient's notes and so forth. Thus, the "patient" is conceived differently across specialty medical inputs – the object (patient) is not coherent or presents as differing faces, a contradiction.

For proponents of stable teams, it is convenient to massage this contradiction by simply describing "the patient" as if the object of the activity were a coherent entity whose ontological nature was assumed, shared and understood by all practitioners. For Engeström (2018: 16), however, as noted many times, "Contradictions are the prime source of change and development in activity systems. Contradictions are not the same as problems or conflicts. Contradictions are historically accumulating structural tensions within and between activity systems". Indeed, such contradictions are inevitable, where practitioners "must learn new forms of activity that are not yet there. They are literally learned as they are being created" (ibid.: 17). The "literally" is telling – activities are concrete events that unfold, often in unexpected ways. Sometimes the "concrete" falls around

Table 8.1 Three approaches to collectivism and achieving ensemble

Michael West and colleagues	Yrjö Engeström and colleagues	Roland Barthes
Stable teams	Teeming	Living and working together
	Negotiated knotworking	Swarming
	Boundary crossing Expansive learning	
Forms of leadership and followership	Partially improvised, multi-level expansive exchanges	Hospitality
		Rhythm
	Timing	Leaderless
	Leadership as an emergent property of the system	Communal tasks
Patient-centred	Patient-directed	Common wealth, multitude and assembly
Schemata (form)	*Rhuthmos* (rhythm)	Novelistic
		Rhythm of the waves
Metonymic	Metaphoric	Semiotic (signs and symbols)

you, or worse, on your head. The whole prefabricated house of "teams" may turn out to be a house of cards, about to collapse (Table 8.1).

Bibliography

Akkerman SF, Bakker A. Boundary Crossing and Boundary Objects. *Review of Educational Research.* 2011; 81: 132–69.

Atluru A. What Improv Can Teach Tomorrow's Doctors: Thinking Quickly and Occasionally Abandoning the Medical-School Script are Critical for Quality Patient Care. *The Atlantic,* 24 August 2016. Available at: https://www.theatlantic.com/educati on/archive/2016/08/what-improv-can-teach-tomorrows-doctors/497177/

Babiker A, El Husseini M, Al Nemri A, et al. Health Care Professional Development: Working as a Team to Improve Patient Care. *Sudan Journal of Paediatrics.* 2014;14:9–16.

Baird B, Boyle T, Chauhan K, et al. 2020. *How to Build Effective Teams in General Practice.* London: King's Fund. Available at: https://www.kingsfund.org.uk/publications/effectiv e-teams-general-practice

Barthes R. 2013. *How to Live Together: Novelistic Simulations of Some Everyday Spaces.* New York: Columbia University Press.

Basil P. 2019. *Be My Guest: Reflections on Food, Community and the Meaning of Generosity.* Edinburgh: Canongate.

Bleakley A. Blunting Occam's Razor: Aligning Medical Education with Studies of Complexity. *Journal of Evaluation in Clinical Practice.* 2010;16:849–55.

Bleakley A. Working in "Teams" in an Era of "Liquid" Healthcare: What Is the Use of Theory? *Journal of Interprofessional Care.* 2013;27:18–26.

Bleakley A. 2014. *Patient-Centred Medicine in Transition: The Heart of the Matter.* Dordrecht: Springer.

Bleakley A. 2017. *Thinking With Metaphors in Medicine: The State of the Art.* Abingdon: Routledge.

Bleakley A, Allard J, Hobbs A. "Achieving of Ensemble": Communication in Orthopaedic Surgical Teams and the Development of Situational Awareness – An Observational Study Using Live Videotaped Examples. *Advances in Health Sciences Education.* 2013;18:33–56.

Edmonson AC. The Three Pillars of a Teaming Culture. *Harvard Business Review,* 17 December 2013. Available at: https://hbr.org/2013/12/the-three-pillars-of-a-tea ming-culture

Engeström Y. 2008. *From Teams to Knots: Activity-Theoretical Studies of Collaboration at Work.* Cambridge: Cambridge University Press.

Engeström Y. 2018. *Expertise in Transition: Expansive Learning in Medical Work.* Cambridge: Cambridge University Press.

Illich I. 1973. *Tools for Conviviality.* New York: Harper & Row.

James W. 1950(1907). *Principles of Psychology.* New York: Dover Publications.

Mol A-M. 2002. *The Body Multiple: Ontology in Medical Practice.* Durham, NC: Duke University Press.

Piketty T. 2014. *Capital in the Twenty-First Century.* Cambridge, MA: Harvard University Press.

Rancière J. 2013. *Aisthesis: Scenes from the Aesthetic Regime of Art.* London: Verso.

Tannenbaum S, Traylor AM, Thomas EJ, Salas E. Managing Teamwork in the Face of Pandemic: Evidence-Based Tips. *BMJ Quality & Safety.* 2020;1–5. Available at: https ://qualitysafety.bmj.com/content/early/2020/05/28/bmjqs-2020-011447

Wells G. *Crossing Professional Boundaries – A King's Fund Toolkit for Collaborative Teamwork.* 2015. The King's Fund. Available at: https://www.futurefocusedfinance.nh s.uk/blog/crossing-professional-boundaries-kings-fund-toolkit-collaborative-teamwork

West M, Eckert R, Steward K, Pasmore B. 2014. *Developing Collective Leadership for Healthcare.* The King's Fund. Available at: https://www.kingsfund.org.uk/sites/default/ files/field/field_publication_file/developing-collective-leadership-kingsfund-may14.pdf

9 Resistance: Part III

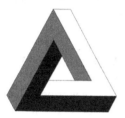

Patient advocacy

Patient advocacy is grounded in the assumption that some people will need others to speak up for them or to act on their behalf, either socially or legally. This may be because the patient is a child, or severely disabled, or elderly and suffering from memory loss or confusion, or suffering from mental health issues such as delusions, is homeless, or does not have healthcare insurance and so forth. In North America and Australia in particular, advocacy through laypersons is taken seriously as a career role and a lucrative business while maintaining a sense of dignity and commitment to social justice (Torrey 2015). But patient advocacy is a key role for healthcare workers too, and education in advocacy as a form of resistance to cultural and social inequities and inequalities is often missing or poorly represented in medical education.

As noted, Global Health Europe (2009) defines inequity and inequality thus: "inequity refers to unfair, avoidable differences arising from poor governance, corruption or cultural exclusion while inequality simply refers to the uneven distribution of health or health resources as a result of genetic or other factors or the lack of resources". From the point of view of equity, gross inequalities in standards of living between the very rich and the very poor are secondary to how we raise the standard of living of the very poor to a decent level, ensuring housing, food, healthcare and a living wage.

Medicine's social justice agenda is an expression of resistance against injustices arising from exercises of sovereign power or unethical flows of capillary power (such as using patients' medical data as a form of surveillance). Patient advocacy and social justice issues have been brought together under the umbrella term "political correctness" (PC), defined as: "The avoidance of forms of expression or action that are perceived to exclude, marginalize, or insult groups of people who are socially disadvantaged or discriminated against". You would think that this would be core to any decent health service and to all doctors. Advocates of course understand the positive and affirming nature of this definition within a democracy. However, it is a view that has come to be mocked by those with conservative political views.

Patient advocacy is assumed, and subsumed, in the broader reaches of this book. Hence, I devote a relatively small section to advocacy. For the most stimulating recent work on patient and community advocacy moving beyond critical thinking to engage ethics, activism and aesthetics in critical pedagogy, see the work in particular of Arno Kumagai (Kumagai and Lypson 2009; Kumagai and Naidu 2020a, 2020b), a diabetologist now based in Toronto who is a passionate advocate for health humanities and social justice.

A key aspect, maybe *the* key aspect, of democracy is provision of means for inclusion of those who find it difficult or impossible to speak for themselves. We immediately think of persons rendered powerless through physical or mental disabilities or other challenges. Jefferson Wong (2020), at the time of writing a final year medical student at Exeter University medical school in the UK, reminds us however of the way that all hospitalized patients can be potentially rendered powerless through a series of personally degrading rituals such as preparing for physical examinations. The patient is already made to feel vulnerable as they don an ill-fitting and flimsy hospital robe that does not tie properly. In the worse circumstances, a brusque and tired nurse briefly interviews and weighs the patient, who is then left sitting for a long period before a doctor arrives who does not introduce him- or herself and does not address the patient by name, mechanically running through the procedure the patient is about to endure. Wong (ibid.: 125) says:

> Beginning with the very first interactions with patients, patients are asked to remove their clothes and to re-dress in hospital gowns. This very act resembles the removal of civility for a "bare life" (Agamben 1995). People are told to remove their clothes and to wear a sheer cloth, which exposes the private areas of the patient. In public, people are very concerned with their appearance and would never tolerate such requests. But they are giving up this aspect of being civilised to be able to receive treatment. Furthermore, by removing their clothes, they are stripped of their individuality and culture. The clothes they are asked to wear have no flair or personality. The hospital gowns are void of any reference to who the patient is and where they come from.

Therefore, while my list opening this chapter referred to persons who are unable to speak for themselves and need an advocate, ironically, healthcare's potentially dehumanizing and objectifying routines, which Wong encapsulates so well, potentially place all patients in need of advocates. Medicine is of course not consciously bent on reducing the patient to "bare life" through objectification.

Nurses in particular often act as advocates for patients, rectifying an intrinsic power imbalance and not capitalizing on the patient's forced vulnerability. Alene Nitzky (2018), an oncology nurse, suggests six ways in which this can happen:

Advocating for patients

1. **Ensure Safety.** This applies during hospitalization, before and after treatment; but also when the patient is discharged – for example communicating with social workers about post-discharge assistance.
2. **Give Patients a Voice.** Literally, through providing a medical translator where the patient does not speak the host language; put medical terms into lay terms.
3. **Educate.** Help patients manage acute and chronic illness for example through advice on medications and self-care.
4. **Protect Patients' Rights.** Broker between family members where there is a disagreement about a treatment regime.
5. **Double Check for Potential Errors.** Checking handovers, documentation and prescriptions.
6. **Connect Patients to Resources.** Making links between the hospital and support in the community.

Advocacy is not speaking *for* the patient, but *on behalf of* the patient, empowering, supporting their rights, providing information and building capacity. The best advocacy brings patients, their families and community members into active participation in healthcare decisions and medical research, and activism and political lobbying where healthcare has failed. Distinctions are sometimes drawn between single-patient advocates and community advocates.

The patient advocacy movement has its origins in a contradiction in cancer care in the 1950s. In the USA, the National Institutes of Health (NIH) were concerned that patients should not be manipulated or ill-treated in any way by cancer research or by pharmaceutical companies associated with research, and so ethico-legal frameworks were set up to protect patients, or advocate for them. Stanley Farber, a Harvard-based oncologist and researcher, was particularly interested in childhood leukaemia, and coined the term "Total Care" to refer to treatment of the family of the child patient as a unit. However, while the NIH and Farber were extending this notion of empowerment beyond patients to families supporting cancer patients, there was also a counter-movement.

Anselm Strauss was working at the medical school at the University of California, San Francisco, in the early 1960s. He set up some fieldwork research looking at care of the dying in differing hospital specialties, and hired another sociologist, Barney Glaser, from Columbia University, New York, to help with the fieldwork. Both researchers had recently lost parents, and so the fieldwork touched a nerve.

What Strauss and Glaser (Glaser and Strauss 1967) found were differing expectations of death from relatives and healthcare staff. For example, on a premature infant ward where mortality rates were high, parents were often not aware of the impending death of their child. In an oncology setting, death was often over an extended period of time and staff had opportunities to keep family members in the loop about impending deaths. However, the communication between healthcare staff, patients and family members differed widely, embracing the following:

1. "Open awareness" (everybody is clear about the status of the patient).
2. "Closed awareness" (everybody is clear about the status of the patient, but patients and/or family members do not talk about death).
3. "Suspicion" (the doctors and medical staff are aware about the status of the patient, but although the patient and/or family members know that death is close, this information is not conveyed clearly to them).
4. "Mutual deception" (the doctors and healthcare staff tell the family that the patient should not be told about impending death). Such tactics had an important effect on the quality of care – where patients were kept in the dark about impending death, nursing would be limited to the bare minimum.

Nathaniel and Andrews (2010) describe such "mutual deception" and tactics of "closed awareness" as an "atmosphere of organized secrecy", where "family members purposely maintain the fiction that the dying patient might recover". Sadly, "This context does not allow patients to close their lives with proper rituals. Because of the organized deception, relatives' grief cannot be expressed openly". In short, this particular posture of medical culture showed an extraordinary level of inflation or hubris – where doctors extended their legitimate specialist technical roles into questionable forms of imperialism and authoritarianism as they adopt particular communication strategies, in turn manipulating family members' actions in diverting their natural concern and grief.

In other words, the capital of emotional response and grief held within the family comes to be owned and distributed by the medical profession according to its whims, rather than an open and transparent ethical framework. Medicine colonizes the voices of patient and family. This was in the mid- to late-1960s, and times have changed. It is now standard practice for those dying from cancer to be given their diagnosis and prognosis. However, while the specific culture that Glaser and Strauss explored may be seen as an historical anomaly, medicine's inflations persist in some quarters, particularly in surgical culture.

My father died from pancreatic cancer in 1970 – he was just 54 and I was 21, raw and confused. When the cancer found purchase – it started in the pancreas and rapidly spread – he plummeted from feeling out of sorts to a heart-rending fragility. After a short period in hospital he was transferred home – thin, bed bound, often in extreme pain, and eventually drifting in and out of long periods of deep, opiate-induced sleep. From diagnosis to death was less than six months. When he was diagnosed with terminal cancer, neither his family doctor nor the consultant oncologist revealed the diagnosis to him. They took my mother, my brother and myself aside, told us the diagnosis and prognosis, and asked us to not divulge anything to him. They told my father that he had complications from an operation on his gall bladder (that is how the cancer was first discovered) that would clear up in time (Bleakley 2020c).

I remember recoiling at the moral dilemma the doctors had set us – to not share the fatal diagnosis with my father but to spin a web of disguise through white lies – yet I joined the charade until the end. My dad, of course, knew that he was seriously ill, but the word "cancer" was never brought to the table. I was at the bedside when he drew his last breath. Laura Marks (2014) says: "Associated with the soul, animating the lungs, breath is that invisible and usually intangible entity that makes its passage known sonically": the hollow gurgling of the death rattle, then the sigh of resignation, and finally the wholesale withdrawal of noise – the void filled by the family's collective sobs. My father, in essence, had his last rounds of breathing controlled by medical culture and his close family, who colluded with that culture despite the awareness of the moral dilemma. His breathing was "occupied", to draw from Franz Fanon, who was an Algerian psychiatrist and resistance activist during the French colonial occupation of Algeria leading to the conflict and subsequent independence. Fanon (1970) described the occupied Algerian's breathing as "an observed, an occupied breathing. It is a combat breathing". A "combat breathing" because, as Fanon says: "You can observe my breathing, but you cannot occupy my breath" – the breath is the final barrier of occupation, the last gasp, but also the strongest part of resistance.

Three things in particular struck me about my father's medicalized death: first, the obscene pact of secrecy that we set up with the doctors based around subscription to the stigma that cancer carried; second, the irrational tenacity that we, as a family, showed in sticking religiously to that pact; and third, the oncologist's disturbing language register, describing the "invasion" of the cancer and how my dad had already "lost the war". I found the use of war metaphors particularly confusing because my father had no desire – or energy – to "fight" his illness. He was a combat veteran, serving in Egypt during the whole of World War II; he'd had his fill of war.

There are many advocacy institutions and groups (for example, the American Academy of Family Physicians [AAFP] has an advocacy section online: https://www.aafp.org/advocacy.html) and I will not extend the discussion to consider their merits, but it is worth mentioning their reach, especially as this bears on identity politics. For example, Blue Veins (http://blueveins.org/home/about) is a movement based in Pakistan with global reach. It was founded in 1999 and works on behalf and women and transgender persons to address health inequalities and social justice issues. With the motto "Awareness, Action & Advocacy", Blue Veins helps women, girls and the transgender community to realize capabilities through seeking support and intervention where injustice is evident.

Patient advocacy has been professionalized and turned into a market product, in the USA as "patient opinion leaders", sometimes as ex-patients, who may also have alliances with pharmaceutical companies. Advocates may also help with health insurance and medico-legal issues. Advocacy is important globally for the elderly in care homes to protect against potential abuses where there are no family members to take on this role. Both patient advocacy and health policy advocacy have become institutionalized educationally through award-bearing courses. This may sound all to the good, as surely patients or clients will ultimately benefit where the system is driven by justice. But there is a fly in the ointment.

As patient advocacy develops and is institutionalized, so there is a danger that medical education will see advocacy as something done by professional advocates or advocacy organizations and not by doctors and other healthcare staff. Medical students will miss out on building the foundation for an important future role. Delese Wear and colleagues (Wear et al. 2017) remind us of the importance of introducing advocacy to medical students, asking "whether medical education adequately prepares physicians to care for persons particularly affected by societal inequities and injustice who present to clinics, hospitals, and emergency rooms". They suggest: "medical school curricula should address such concerns through an explicit pedagogical orientation".

Anti-racist pedagogy and structural competency should be offered to address issues of "patients who are victimized by extremely challenging social and economic disadvantages and who present with health concerns that arise from these disadvantages". They note that medical and healthcare institutions can be complicit in ramping up social injustices rather than addressing them. More than a decade ago, Arno Kumagai and Monica Lypson (2009) had noted the need for medical education to include issues of social justice as core and compulsory provision. But, they note, this goes beyond "cultural competence" to "structural" issues that outstrip instrumental competence learning; and beyond "critical thinking" to engage with a Freirian critical consciousness. Medical students do not need to simply *know* about structural issues leading to health inequities and inequalities; they also need to know how to intervene and help.

This, says Kumagai and Lypson, is a question of "commitment" and must be learned in the field and not the laboratory or the lecture theatre. Centrally, they must learn how to engage in dialogue – genuine interchange. The medical/health humanities can offer a vehicle for such learning, for an education "of physicians equally skilled in the biomedical aspects of medicine and in the role medicine plays in ensuring social justice and meeting human needs".

Dissensus and critical inquiry

Dissensus (Rancière 2010), dissension or disagreement is the essence of resistance, but this is not just cussedness, perverse resistance or uninformed prejudice. Rather, dissensus arises from critical thinking – from deep reflection leading to disagreement. A constellation of terms hovers around the act of dissent: *thoughtful non-compliance*, *critical reflexivity* and *critical consciousness*. Indeed, whole systems of learning – pedagogies of dissent – are based upon the values that inform fairness and decency in human activity. It is imperative that medical students are taught how to think critically, and inevitably this will, and should, lead to positions of dissent that can be discussed within the formal curriculum.

Critical inquiry is the formal democratic mode of collective questioning of values, assumptions and evidence. This is grounded in the dual and contradictory Western tradition that simultaneously honours intuition (the Platonic model of insight into an illusory world of presence that hides a reality of archetypal forms that shape such presences), and rational argument (the Socratic method of formal questioning and testing through reason and logic). The tension between these two ways of knowing was formally resolved by Immanuel Kant's 1784 essay "Answering the Question: What is Enlightenment?" which ushered in Western Modernism. Kant argued for individuals to think for themselves, or "critically", and not have the Church or other authorities (the State) think for them through an irrational intuition based on faith. His resolution of the paradoxical relation between Platonic revelation and Aristotelian reasoning lay in the fact that for Kant, individuals' inability to think for themselves was not an intellectual issue, but an ethical one – that of summoning up moral courage to speak the truth. As noted earlier, in the ancient Greek tradition this was called *parrhesia* (truth-telling) and was directly opposed to rhetoric or persuasion. Its modern equivalent is existential authenticity.

Kant suggested that what stopped people thinking for themselves was political – the power of the Church's and the State's combined authority as a form of paternalism. Thinking for oneself, or thinking through with a critical mindset, was then a democratic gesture. Two emerging languages of the time raised important questions for Kant with regard to how an individual's critical consciousness (or "voice") could be raised. Just as Kant resolved the original tension between Platonic revelation and Aristotelian logical reasoning through syllogisms, so he raised another tension for modern times. As the word of the State in the service of the Church or the Church in the service of the State was challenged for independent thinking, Kant raised questions about how art and science would raise new modes of inquiry that could be debated by the now intellectually liberated citizen.

As art liberated itself from being in the service of the church, and as the new discipline of science questioned blind faith in formulating its ways of reasoning through evidence gained from controlled experimentation, so life itself became a series of acts of resistance or questioning. A new dialectic emerges: is art a revelation of truth that is different from science's reasoned facts? So the Modernist tension between fact and value (or quality) emerged.

The association of the leading British scientist of his time, Humphry Davy (1778–1829), with the poet Samuel Taylor Coleridge models how art and science were once considered inseparable. Davy taught Coleridge and Wordsworth how to set up a chemistry laboratory, while Coleridge gave Davy tuition in writing poetry. Early science dripped with aesthetics ("value") but this drained away to reside in the arts and humanities while science became instrumental and functional ("fact"). Where modern medicine identified as a science, so it embraced fact over value, and the art of medicine, as well as the arts in medicine, were sidelined. Where politics identified more with value than fact, so national and party politics too were sidelined, repressed and subjugated in medical education.

But such intentional purblindness has invited a reaction in the shape of various forms of resistance. Where politics has crept back into medicine, reinforced in particular by the coronavirus pandemic, so we see many outbreaks of activism such as protests against non-availability of personal protective equipment (PPE) (such as masks). Into this situation creeps farce. As noted earlier, PPE plastic facemasks tended to be modelled on male heads and so were too large for most women and found to be loose fitting. Women constitute the vast majority of the nursing and the auxiliary cleaning staff of hospitals. Structural gender bias – sexism – puts lives at risk.

Activism

Direct action

One of the oldest jokes about stereotyping of specialties in medicine is the impulsive surgeon mocking the stance of the reflective hospital or primary care physician: "Don't just do something, stand there!"

"Don't just stand there, do something!": direct action is the most powerful form of resistance, but one that doctors have resisted where it may lead to direct conflict with management and put one's job at risk. In this case, where there is a perceived injustice, the next level of political resistance is whistleblowing. For the citizenry in general, peaceful protest against perceived injustices, such as civil rights activism, follows Henry David Thoreau's 1849 essay "Civil Disobedience", in which Thoreau advised citizens to act with their conscience if a law or activity was perceived as corrupt, unjust or discriminatory.

Contemporaries of Thoreau, such as the Quaker activist Susan B. Anthony, supported social equality, standing up against slavery and the subjugation of women. In the wake of the Flexner Report of 1910, North American medical education would soon follow a different path. After closing (instead of helping to resource) the few medical schools catering for Black and women students, medical education followed a politically conservative and paternalistic path that discriminated against women and black and ethnic minority groups. As noted earlier, Flexner, a liberal in other respects and an innovative educator, also supported apartheid in medicine, suggesting a separation of treatment, where white patients would be treated by white doctors, and black patients by the few qualified black doctors.

Fitzhugh Mullan, who died in 2019, was a paediatrician and professor of health policy and management at George Washington University, Washington DC. He worked in the 1960s as a medical civil rights worker and was one of the first political activists in American medical education during the 1960s when he studied medicine in Chicago. Sixty years later, Mullan was still arguing for the incorporation of "social mission" in medical school curricula, beyond surface information about public health (Mullan 2019). To his credit, Dr David Sklar, the editor of the leading medical education journal *Academic Medicine*, decided to publish posthumously a commencement address that Mullan gave in 2018 at Yale University Medical School.

Mullan claimed that medical education must move beyond Abraham Flexner's vision, already over a century old, in which initial medical education closets itself in the dissection and biological sciences laboratories. Medical education must embrace the realities of the social world seen in clinical work as the effects of social inequities and inequalities on health. "Social mission" must not be relegated to an elective studied only by the more compassionate medical students, but must be core and compulsory provision. This begins with processes of selection to medical school.

Mullan notes that when he committed himself as a "civil rights" doctor in the 1960s, his class of 72 students had only one person of colour in it, and he was from Nigeria. Medical school, he says, was preparing him not for the future but for the past. In 1967, Mullan and several other students marched with Dr Martin Luther King at a civil rights rally in Chicago. Mullan's legacy can be seen in the few cases where doctors have been so outraged by their treatment by policy makers, politicians and management that they have decided to withdraw their labour – a rare and telling moment.

The UK junior doctors' strike

Doctors rarely withdraw labour as political activism. They recognize that patients must not be put at risk by an absence of workforce members. However, doctors are sometimes pushed to political activism where they perceive injustices that put patients at danger such as being asked to work unreasonable lengths of shifts leading to exhaustion and potential burnout. Junior doctors in England were put in this position in 2015–2016. In the NHS, "junior" doctor refers to the majority of the workforce, including all positions below consultant level. The withdrawal of labour was ostensibly about pay and conditions, but this hid deeper political concerns – a broad disagreement with the influence of the right wing Tory government that had accelerated privatization of up to a quarter of NHS provision (a publicly owned service), and had introduced austerity measures severely constraining healthcare provision.

Junior doctors in England earn relatively poor wages and are still paying off large debts incurred from borrowing for fees for their undergraduate medical degree studies. It is not until they gain seniority, ten or more years after starting medical school - specializing in a particular branch of medicine or surgery, or working as general practitioners - that income increases considerably. For English junior doctors, vocation and job satisfaction come before earnings. One way of boosting earnings in the early years is to work overtime, or extra shifts, but this can lead to exhaustion and poor performance, and may not be possible for doctors requiring childcare. A European Working Time Directive also limits the length of time professionals such as doctors can spend in any one shift.

A new contract for junior doctors had been subject to negotiations between the British Medical Association (BMA) and the National Health Service (NHS) since 2012. In 2015, the Tory government offered a deal in which basic rates of pay would be increased, but overtime pay between 7am and 10pm on every day except Sunday would be scrapped. The BMA calculated that junior doctors, relying on overtime rates to boost their salaries, would lose out on this deal. But there was a subtext to this pay negotiation. The Tory government of the day had introduced national austerity measures to save costs across public spending, and the NHS had been subject to crippling cuts to its income. Doctors were being asked to work long hours in an over-stretched system that badly needed an overhaul.

To place the strike in context, UK doctors are over-stretched. The UK NHS is low down in the league table for numbers of doctors per head of population, with 2.8 doctors per 1,000. Of the 33 countries in the Organization for Economic Co-operation and Development (OECD), the UK ranks 22nd in terms of doctors per head of population, where only Poland and Slovenia rank below the UK. The average across 33 countries is 3 doctors for every 1,000 persons. Austria has 5.1 doctors for every 1,000; and Switzerland, Germany, Norway, Italy and Lithuania have more than 4 doctors for every 1,000 (Moberly 2017).

On 12 January 2016, England's junior doctors came out on strike, with overwhelming public support, the first act of civil disobedience in the medical profession in 40 years. Emergency care was not withdrawn. A second withdrawal of labour took place on 10 February 2016, when 3,000 elective operations were cancelled. A third strike occurred on 26 April 2016, when both routine work and emergency cover were affected. Nearly 300,000 outpatient appointments were cancelled in hospitals, but the number of recorded deaths did not increase over normal levels. In the spirit of British compromise, an agreement on pay and conditions of work was finally reached in 2017. Neither side was happy. But the face of resistance in the UK National Health Service was changed forever, and medicine was now overtly politicized. The public remained largely sympathetic to the doctors' cause.

A coronavirus common wealth

Resistance in health arenas can come directly from the public body. A half century ago, in *Medical Nemesis*, Ivan Illich (1974) had already argued that globally the professionalizing of medicine and healthcare had come to de-empower the lay public of their ability to deal with a range of healthcare issues using resources within the community. He offered an anecdotal example of the stripping of power: rather than running out into the street to help somebody who has had an accident, the inhabitants of the houses peek through their curtains and wait for specialist paramedical services to turn up. While Illich's example is rhetorical – he wants to make a point but stretches credibility – he makes us think about the relative influences that medicine exerts as either an encompassing assimilative power or a sensitive accommodating partner.

In times of emergency or lockdown, the ability of the general public to inform and mobilize themselves without the help of experts and professionals is enhanced. This shows a positive side to resistance (to the numbing effects of expertise that Illich describes). Most obviously, the public can inform itself in a way that has never been possible before through social media and the Internet. This has led to a strengthening of expert patient and informed patient groups as well as support groups, particularly in mental health. There is of course an "invisible" group of carers, usually family members, who offer emotional support in the main, but also manage drug regimes and primary care and hospital visits (Allard, Wilson and Bleakley 2020). From the standpoint of assimilative medicine or medicalization, this can be perceived as a straightforward act of resistance to professional and expert power, or taken on only in the capacity of adjunct to medicine. But where medicine is accommodative, such lay expertise and community support is welcomed as equal partner.

The coronavirus epidemic brought out expertise in areas such as making medical Personal Protective Equipment (PPE) where there was an acute shortage. The *New York Times* (Jacobs and Abrams 2020) reports on lay "science geeks" making a basic ventilator from automobile parts, blood pressure cuffs and other readily available parts, which could be used in an emergency. 3-D printers have allowed artists and designers to make safety masks and plastic valves that allow two patients to use one ventilator simultaneously. This is being called "village medicine" based on a "national hive mind" constituted through open source Facebook groups. Sewing circles made surgical masks, while "One woman has come up with a respirator mask that uses a bra, coffee filters and citric acid". This mobilization of the masses to save the few was a great example of positive resistance to a political majority that was simply not mobilizing quickly enough in the USA in the face of exponential growth of infections.

Globally, what might have been called "cottage industries" sprung up as resistance markers to various governments' fumbling of the coronavirus crisis – reacting too late with poorly developed strategies such as failing to carry out widespread testing and tracing. George Monbiot (2020) saw the Covid-19 pandemic as a sign that global neo-liberal capitalism, based on a free market economy and limitless economic growth, may be faltering. Filling a gap for goods and services, cottage industries sprung up all over the world at a time when most people's work was temporarily suspended as the population went into isolation or exercised social distancing.

For example, groups of young people in India organized themselves to identify food supplies and get them to the most needy – those who have lost their jobs and are not being furloughed or compensated financially. Volunteer drivers in Wuhan, China, organized transport fleets to ferry equipment and supplies between hospitals. Communities in Johannesburg organized survival packs of sanitizer, water, food and toilet paper for isolated groups. Mutual aid groups the world over provided grassroots community-generated services for the elderly, needy and isolated. In Bristol, UK, a group called the "drug runners" ferried urgent pharmaceuticals to households where individuals could not get to the pharmacy or have them delivered.

David Bollier and Silke Helfrich (Free, Fair and Alive) (2019) called this collective global response to a health crisis the "commons". It reveals the multitude's common wealth, a grassroots resistance to governmental decision-making in a state of emergency, especially when the government was perceived to be inefficient or incapable, as "a social form that enable people to enjoy freedom without repressing others, enact fairness without bureaucratic control ... and assert sovereignty without nationalism". Monbiot called this "an insurgency of social power", in other words a loose-knit resistance or a form of "negotiated knotworking" (Engeström, Engeström and Kerosuo 2003) and networking that is temporary in focus, but lasting in terms of ideological impact. It was politics in the absence of State with a focus on emotional and social profit rather than material gain. It was a de-territorialized effort of care with no colonizing impulse or desire.

Endnote: Psychoanalytic resistance

These three chapters on resistance have to be limited in terms of available space. There is nothing here for example on feminisms as forms of resistance, and little on structural race inequities. These topics have large literatures. The reader will also note a bias towards positive readings of resistance, and of course resistance is an aporia, a contradiction, where it means both a positive pushing back in disagreement and a negative refusal. Sigmund Freud famously saw resistance as negative refusal, as an unconscious defence mechanism of the ego, as he saw patients refusing to accept and confront damaging implicit patterns of behaviour.

On the bigger scale, medical education still resists the compelling and recurring research evidence that by later years, medical students typically fall into patterns of objectification of patients and loss of empathy (cynicism). Doctors too are notoriously resistant to seeking help for their own symptoms, ailments and debilitating conditions, especially with mental health issues. As a result – and compounded by poor provision of psychological support, therapy and psychologically-oriented mentoring and supervision – there is a relatively high rate of anxiety, depression, burnout and suicide ideation amongst doctors (Peterkin and Bleakley 2017). In Chapter 14, I suggest a way that initial (undergraduate) medical education can address this, through the introduction of co-counselling and structured peer support groups to medical students, and, where possible, to multiprofessional student clusters. And finally, of course, resistance in the form of denial of the climate crisis is our biggest public emergency besides global poverty.

Bibliography

Agamben G. 1998. *Homo Sacer: Sovereign Power and Bare Life*. Palo Alto, CA: Stanford University Press.

Allard J, Wilson M, Bleakley A. 2020. Doctors need safe confessional and cathartic spaces: what we learned from the research project 'People Talking: Digital Dialogues for Mutual Recovery'. In: A Bleakley (ed.) *Routledge Handbook of the Medical Humanities*, 410–18.

Bleakley A. 2020c. Don't Breathe a Word: A Psychoanalysis of Medicine's Inflations. In: A Bleakley (ed.) *Routledge Handbook of the Medical Humanities*. Abingdon: Routledge, 129–35.

Bollier D, Helfrich S. 2019. *Free, Fair and Alive: The Insurgent Power of the Commons.* Gabriola Island, BC: New Society Publishers.

Engeström Y, Engeström R, Kerosuo H. The Discursive Construction of Collaborative Care. *Applied Linguistics.* 2003;2:286–315.

Fanon F. 1970. *A Dying Colonialism.* Ringwood: Pelican.

Glaser B, Strauss A. 1967. *Awareness of Dying.* New York: Aldine Publishing Co.

Global Health Europe. 2009. *Inequity and Inequality.* Available at: http://www.globalhea ltheurope.org/index.php/resources/glossary/values/17

Illich I. 1974. *Medical Nemesis: The Expropriation of Health.* London: Calder & Boyars.

Jacobs A, Abrams R. A Deluge of Suggestions to Fill Critical Needs. *The New York Times,* 2 April 2 2020, 8.

Kumagai AK, Lypson M. Beyond Cultural Competence: Critical Consciousness, Social Justice, and Multicultural Education. *Academic Medicine.* 2009;84:782–87.

Kumagai AK, Naidu T. 2020a. The Cutting Edge: Health Humanities for Equity and Social Justice. In: A Bleakley (ed.) *Routledge Handbook of Medical Humanities.* Abingdon: Routledge, 83–96.

Kumagai AK, Naidu T. On Time and Tea Bags: Chronos, Kairos, and Teaching for Humanistic Practice. *Academic Medicine.* 2020b; 95:512–17.

Marks LU. 2014. *Book Cover Commentary for D. Quinlivan. The Place of Breath in Cinema.* Edinburgh: Edinburgh University Press.

Moberly T. UK Has Fewer Doctors Per Person Than Most Other OECD Countries. *British Medical Journal.* 2017;357:j2940.

Monbiot G. Covid-19 Has Turned Millions of Us into Good Neighbours. *The Guardian,* 1 April 2020, 1. Available at: https://www.theguardian.com/commentisfree/2020/mar /31/virus-neighbours-covid-19

Mullan F. The Civil Rights Doctor, Revisited. *Academic Medicine,* 17 December 2019. Published ahead of print. Available at: https://journals.lww.com/academicmedicine/ Abstract/publishahead/The_Civil_Rights_Doctor,_Revisited.97350.aspx

Nathaniel AK, Andrews T. The Modifiability of Grounded Theory. *Grounded Theory Review.* 2010;9:65–75.

Nitzky A. 2018. Six Ways Nurses Can Advocate for Patients. *Nursing News,* 30 August 2018. Available at: https://www.oncnursingnews.com/contributor/alene-nitzky/2018 /08/six-ways-nurses-can-advocate-for-patients

Peterkin A, Bleakley A. 2017. *Staying Human During the Foundation Programme and Beyond: How to Thrive After Medical School.* Baton Rouge, FL: CRC Press.

Rancière J. 2010. *Dissensus: On Politics and Aesthetics.* London: Continuum.

Torrey T. 2015. *So You Want to Be a Patient Advocate?: Choosing a Career in Health or Patient Advocacy: Volume 1 (Health Advocacy Career Series).* USA: DiagKNOWsis Media.

Wear D, Zarconi J, Aultman JM, et al. Remembering Freddie Gray: Medical Education for Social Justice. *Academic Medicine.* 2017;92:312–17.

Wong J. 2020. Hospitaland. In: A Bleakley (ed.) *Routledge Handbook of the Medical Humanities.* Abingdon: Routledge, 123–26.

Part II
The contradiction cure

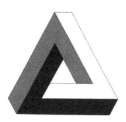

10 Contradictions cure

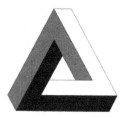

Men who give birth

Men who give birth may seem contradictory. But this is an exploratory contradiction – one that examines new territory, or living life with a twist, away from the norm and as an innovative leap and commitment such as a radical shift in identity. A powerful advert for such identity politics is the 2019 film *Seahorse*, telling the story of a transgender man who retained his womb and ovaries and put off corrective genital surgery, and, like a number of transgender men worldwide, was artificially inseminated and able to carry a child (Hattenstone 2019). To the conservative mind, such contradictions may feel uncomfortable. However, it is a basic premise of contemporary learning theories that contradictions are potentially generative in expanding capabilities.

Contradiction is not a symptom of something going wrong or being out of kilter, making us retreat to safety, but rather a cure for an excess of safety-as-conservatism, the curse of many medical education programmes. Contradictions, says Yrjö Engeström (2018: 16), are the engines for change in an activity system, showing "themselves in disturbances, often taking the shape of discursive manifestations such as dilemmas, conflicts, and double binds"; and should be distinguished from "problems or conflicts" that are not a product of "historically accumulating structural tensions within and between activity systems".

Medicine, outwardly confident, historically arrogant and brash, is also mostly compassionate. It is disconcerting then to find one of its most compassionate practitioners and educators, Tom Inui (2003), suggesting that: "(medical) students learn that medicine is a profession in which you say one thing and do another, *a profession of cynics*". Further, a lauded (now retired) British neurosurgeon, Henry Marsh (in Adams 2017), who has written two best-selling memoirs, says: "as soon as we have any interaction with patients, we start lying. We have to. There is nothing more frightening for a patient than an anxious or doubtful doctor". And to cap these conundrums, the late American writer Denis Johnson (1992), amongst the most perceptive of his generation, says through one of his characters: "It's always been my tendency to lie to doctors, as if good health consisted only of the ability to fool them".

What is the meaning of such deceptions? What might a medicine curriculum look like based on these principles of inauthenticity? Should we just throw in the towel and prepare medical students for a life of growing cynicism? Of course not! A principle of this book is that good medicine is grounded in existential authenticity (Steiner and Reisinger 2006). The Danish philosopher Søren Kierkegaard (1813–1855) first described "authenticity" as congruence between what one believes and how one acts. He believed that many people lead inauthentic existences, failing to "become what one is" (Kierkegaard 1989), and this was not a personal choice, but a product of what Louis Allthusser (2008) later called "political interpellation", where we are slotted into a social role that provides little meaning or satisfaction, producing feelings of both alienation and anomie, while Michel Foucault (1977) has detailed how we are "pinned" through techniques of mass surveillance as a form of discipline. Such "massification", to draw on Kierkegaard's term, leads to conditions of "despair", to draw on his most famous term. We saw this in an earlier chapter discussing "deaths of despair" (Case and Deaton 2020) in white, working class Americans becoming addicted to opioids. For Kierkegaard, the key symptoms of despair are a feeling of objectification (rather than formulating a strong identity or subjectivity), or becoming an "item" to others; and one of "spiritlessness". Meaning could be found in identifying with something lasting, outside oneself, as a spiritual condition.

Martin Heidegger (1889–1976) followed Kierkegaard's model of grounding existence in values that authentically inform activity and sense of self, but substituted "nature" for Kierkegaard's Christian Godhead. Heidegger (1962) suggested that authenticity is a felt experience of "indwelling" place, or a sense of identity with the natural world in which there is also congruence between values, thought and action. Ironically – and another lesson in contradictions – Heidegger was infamously a Nazi sympathizer. Authenticity has a major flaw – in aligning values, thought and action, what if the values base itself is corrupt and anti-democratic?

Medical humanities and double stimulation

Another contradiction, or a fault-line, is illustrated in the reception of the work of the groundbreaking Russian psychologist and educationalist Lev Vygotsky (1896–1934). While Vygotsky himself saw his work as grounded in Marxist orthodoxy, he was for years demonized by the ruling Communist Party as a developmental psychologist who would not wholly embrace collectivism, but lionized the individual (Fu 1997). Meanwhile, in direct contrast, his work has been resisted in North American circles in particular, where it has been viewed as a collectivist and not an individualistic psychology.

At the Institute of Psychology in Moscow in the 1920s, Vygotsky and a graduate student, Leonid Sakharov, carried out observational work on children's cognitive development. If children were given contradictory problems to address (first stimulus) that were beyond their current cognitive capacity, but were provided with sets of materials (second stimulus) to expand their thinking, they were able to use the second stimulus to creatively work to a new conceptual level of understanding. This was not a controlled experiment. Rather, while the activity was expanded, the outcomes of interactions with the second stimulus were unpredictable.

This principle, introduced in earlier chapters, was called "double stimulation": how do you use aids at hand to address issues or problems that are beyond your current comprehension (Sannino and Laitinen 2015)? Indeed – and irritating for those bound to instrumentalism advertised for example in inflexible learning "outcomes" – the second stimulus may be available to you in the environment and appear serendipitously. Instead of sticking with what you know, how could possibilities be opened up for knowing? This conceptual leap advertised the value of mediating artefacts and found objects, while learning is also enhanced through collaboration. Collaboration not only helps to iron out potentially sterile paths for learning, but also generates potentially fruitful lines of uncertainty, or what Deleuze and Guattari (2013) refer to as "lines of flight".

Learners work with a zone of proximal development (ZPD), an expanding zone of possibility: with one foot in what you already know and can do, and another stepping out into the unknown, with help from capable others. What is out of reach today becomes attainable alone tomorrow, as new challenging collaborative activities occur. Vygotsky's colleague, the psychologist Alexei Leont'ev, said that such "scaffolded" activity serves to: "realise a person's actual life in the objective world by which he is surrounded, his social being in all the richness and variety of its forms" (Leont'ev 1977). This serves as a good definition of expanding learning by doing. Of course, the ZPD may be mishandled, providing learners with a step too far through poor facilitation, as explored more in Chapter 14.

The arts characteristically act in the role of second stimulus in double stimulation. A good example is found in the work of Marcel Duchamp and his infamous "readymades", such as his notorious porcelain urinal. Duchamp entered the piece in a show in New York in 1917, signing it "R. Mutt" – it was not shown, formally not rejected but placed on one side by the curatorial team who were anxious about its public reception and perplexed about its status as "art". Placing a readymade in the space of an art gallery as an object for aesthetic contemplation charges the object as second stimulus to make us think about what an object of "art" might be. Duchamp said that the art is not representative of something, but is literally re-presented by placing it in a gallery setting (with the aura of expectation that comes with the "white cube" space), signing it, giving it a title, tilting it or modifying it in some small way. Such re-presented objects included a bicycle wheel, a bottle rack, a snow shovel and a coat-rack. The object may indeed be beautiful in its own right, or remind us of the power of industrial craft and the artisan, but its primary power now rests in its conceptual or semiotic presence as a symbol.

Double stimulation helps you break out of "meaningless situations", suggested Vygotsky (1987), or transform them. We now refer to this as "transformative agency", as a mode of reconfiguration of elements of learning within an activity, where agency is distributed across the medium of stimulation (or the context for change) and the individual as learner. By "meaningless", Vygotsky meant conflictual or contradictory, where paradoxically "meaningless" masks the "meaningful". The major contradiction of double stimulation itself is that it looks like an "out of the frying pan into the fire" situation – where the contradiction that is the first stimulus is not necessarily resolved by the second stimulus, but rather is used as a springboard to expand tolerance of that contradiction in a new level of learning that itself comes to pose challenges. This looks like wilful game-playing to a hard-boiled rationalist, but it is "readymade" Hegelian dialectic, an ever-moving evolutionary process that Marx turned on its head as a philosophical ideal to describe a concrete historical-material process of successive waves of innovation.

Addressing – as it does – contradictions, and generating further contradictions, this dialectical process is not wholly "wilful" – where Sannino and Laitinen (2015) describe double stimulation as "human beings' ability to wilfully transform conflictual circumstances with the help of auxiliary means", but again has potentially random or chance features such as serendipity. Central to double stimulation is the raising to awareness of conflict between motives and values that is impossible to "solve" rationally, mainly because it is situational rather than universal.

The power of double stimulation as a means of expanding activity is again advertised by Duchamp's readymades or "found objects", as the precursor of two new waves of art – Minimalism and Pop Art – that have dominated gallery art since the mid-20th century, culminating in Jeff Koons' sale of *Rabbit* – made in 1986 and inspired by a child's inflatable toy – at auction for $91.1 million in 2019. This is the highest price ever paid for a piece of art at auction.

Minimalism as a mindset is an important second stimulus for medicine, shaping the culture without explicit reference to the art world. The stripped-back, white walled, antiseptic clinic is the "white cube" of the gallery (O'Doherty 1986); the artwork on show is a continuous performance piece, tightly scripted. Doctors too use stripped-back technical language to present "cases" and record patients' progress or regress in shorthand, minimal notes; are coached by their seniors to be tightly focused in presenting cases; and where the audience is largely confined to beds, patients are reduced to spectators of scripted medical performance, and also stripped of complexity as a form of both objectification and surveillance ("observation").

My interest here in double stimulation is to progress the argument made in Chapter 2 that the medical humanities' main collective role – as artefactual mediator in the activity of medical education – is to act in various ways as a second stimulus in double stimulation. The above paragraph offers an illustrative example of illuminating medicine through the arts. But I will further illustrate this fruitful connection through a short discussion about learning anatomy – historically, perhaps the key curriculum component of early years medical education prior to later years' immersion in work-based clinical learning. The medical humanities act to address a fundamental contradiction in medical education, just as they serve to raise another set of contradictions. However, what they do provide is a way of "thinking otherwise" about medical practice and medical culture, offering an education into tolerance of ambiguity – essential for good practice. In this sense, the medical humanities (and arts) act as a "super" second stimulus, at once both raising contradictions for expansion of learning and providing the means through which such contradictions, as ambiguities, can be tolerated and progressed or expanded.

Learning anatomy with the medical humanities as second stimulus

Where extensive anatomy learning was once a central aspect of the first two years of any medical student's experience, the past 30 years have seen a hot debate about how much anatomy medical students need to learn, and how it should be taught. In a previous book on educating the senses in medicine (Bleakley 2020), I looked at the issue of learning anatomy through cadaver dissection, a powerful tradition in medical education. Indeed, Michel Foucault (1976) argued that the history of the development of modern medicine and medical education is intimately connected with the ordinarily taboo process of "opening up a few corpses" for pedagogical purposes.

That anatomy can be learned at an adequate level and for the purposes of most medicine other than surgery, without cadaver dissection – particularly if students are given opportunities to attend autopsies – leads medical educators to see the traditional way of learning anatomy as primarily a rite of passage rather than an educational necessity. Foucault argued that the medical "gaze" – the particular ways that doctors "look" upon their patients in diagnostic and treatment modes – was a direct result of literally gazing into the opened corpse in dissection, now transferred metaphorically to the ways that doctors gaze at living patients. The gaze acts as if penetrating their bodies to see the effects of diseases, as lesions, in order to gauge causes, as diagnoses. However, a collaborative gaze informed and shaped by patient-centred and inter-professional values and practices has now eclipsed such an individualistic, paternalistic and masterful gaze (Bleakley and Bligh 2009).

Learning anatomy through cadaver dissection has also been eclipsed in many medical schools globally (North American and African medical schools still subscribe to both educational and initiatory values of dissection), in some cases replaced by more limited prosection, and in some cases because of the difficulty in obtaining cadavers as the numbers of donations drop off. But a counter-view has emerged that is pedagogical. A new wave of learning a more functional "surface and living" anatomy – while learning depth anatomy through clinical imaging, virtual reality and plastinated models – has been established as a more engaging medical education. This can still engage tactile learning where palpation and percussion are used in surface and living anatomy teaching.

More, the body is appreciated as a living and expressive form. Pedagogically, "embodiment" replaces "body", so that students learning through surface and living anatomy come to appreciate the body before explaining it, and then resist an inexorable drift to objectification that has haunted traditional medicine and medical education. Such objectification, grounded in the cadaver dissection experience and potentially later ramped up through an organ-based or systems-based rather than holistic curriculum (Dubin 2016; Mannino and Pregler 2018), affords a primary ground for existential inauthenticity, as indicated at the opening of this chapter.

One of the main criticisms of learning anatomy through dissection is the "precession of the simulacrum" argument put forward by Jean Baudrillard (1983) to describe how phenomena in everyday life are misperceived where perception is "prepared" by a simulation. An example is dummy surveillance cameras. We behave as if they were real and watching us. Medical students may "see" in their dissections what they are prepared to see from studying the anatomy atlas rather than what is there. If this is the case, then we should count on the value of the virtual and improve its quality. Most anatomy textbooks are two dimensional and blindingly functional. Yet such functional anatomy remains the dominant fare in medical schools globally and reduces learning to rote methods. This not only demeans anatomy learning in the curriculum, but also demeans the beauty of the human body as this is reduced to mechanics and architecture, resisting appreciation of embodiment – the body in space and time as an expressive and uncertain or unpredictable body.

In the medical school in which I worked, Peninsula (Universities of Exeter and Plymouth), which opened to students in 2002, we had a particularly innovative anatomy section headed by John McLachlan (McLachlan et al. 2004) that pioneered the use of new technologies in teaching and learning. But these technologies and simulations were paired with medical humanities approaches as second stimulus to move students away from potential dulling by functional anatomy texts to aesthetic appreciation, as a "thinking otherwise". The general pedagogical rule again was 'appreciation before explanation'. The pedagogical question at play was: "how can we expand the object of the activity of anatomy teaching without increasing curriculum content space devoted to anatomy teaching?" We must be more precise about what students really do need to know, and more inventive about how such knowledge can be acquired (Regan de Bere and Mattick 2010). This, again, can be done through employing the medical humanities thoughtfully as second stimulus.

The medical humanities as second stimulus in double stimulation

1. The first pedagogical shift is to replace "body" with "expressive embodiment" as a conceptual shift in understanding the body as time-bound, contextualized, inscribed, social and a medium for art. This raises issues about

the political body and identity politics, such as ageing, gender, stigma and disability.

2. By introducing an aesthetic dimension to learning through the arts and humanities, the most important second pedagogical shift we can make is to place appreciation of the body prior to explanation. If a major problem of everyday clinical medicine is objectification of patients, then medical education must nip this in the bud to encourage appreciation of patients' dignity and worth. Anatomy learning – despite rituals such as formal recognition of those who have donated bodies for cadaver dissection (in schools, mainly North American, that continue this tradition) – can easily descend into a reductive and instrumental exercise, losing all sense of the worth and beauty of the body to functional explanations. A first step is to place an emphasis on living and surface anatomy. In resisting objectification of the body, students embrace authentic patient-centredness.

3. A third shift afforded by using the medical humanities as second stimulus is to frustrate the classical clinical gaze described by Foucault as individual and penetrating (also a male gaze), and to re-distribute that gaze as collective and feminized (Bleakley and Bligh 2009). This is achieved through collaborative meaning making and achievement of expertise such as inter-professional and inter-disciplinary teaching and learning. This is to realize authentic inter-professional clinical collaboration and inter-disciplinary teaching.

Below, I briefly consider a range of ways that anatomy can be collaboratively experienced, appreciated and learned beyond the functional classroom and formal dissection laboratory in medical education. Most of these methods (see Box 10.2) have been tried and tested at Peninsula Medical School (latterly Peninsula College of Medicine and Dentistry) UK between 2002 and 2013 in developing an innovative medical education programme for the undergraduate curriculum, where medical humanities acted as second stimulus in expanding the object of the activity system – optimal patient care and safety. Students are sensitized rather than de-sensitized to various presentations of embodiment, and they learn collaboratively. Projects developed within the medical school were often turned into public engagement projects with curated shows and associated educational events involving the Tate Gallery St Ives and the Newlyn Gallery Penzance in the UK, and the University of Alberta Gallery in conjunction with the Medical School, Edmonton, Canada. Literary events were also held at hospitals in Toronto, Canada.

The medical humanities act as second stimulus in learning anatomy

Attending an autopsy and surgery

While students do not get "hands on" interaction with a cadaver, they see fresh cadavers at post-mortem (autopsy) and live persons in surgery.

Peer learning of living and surface anatomy with sensitive peer examination

Students examine issues of consent and trust. Peer examination lays the ground for examining patients and offers ideal conditions for learning how to give feedback as a basis to peer assessment.

Life drawing

This is a tried and tested format for both observation of living and surface anatomy and representation through drawing. This is often the gateway project for an understanding of how the visual arts can be an ally of medicine. This can open the door to further explorations such as appreciating the historical value of Leonardo da Vinci's or Andreas Vesalius' anatomy drawings; Barbara Hepworth's drawings from surgical departments during WWII; Andre Serrano's photographs of bodies from the morgue; or the sketches of the cardiac surgeon Francis Wells, who works at Papworth Hospital in the UK, which help him to visualize prior to making surgical interventions (Kennedy 2004):

> His instrument is a pair of surgical forceps, his medium blood on sterilised white paper, and his inkwell is the opened human chest on which he is operating. … "it's a wonderful drawing medium," he said thoughtfully of blood. "It flows beautifully." As he explains, it is simply a question of practicality when teaching his students: the paper, in which the sterilised medical instruments come wrapped, is at hand, as are the forceps – an excellent substitute for a quill pen – and the blood. "No camera can rival drawing as a teaching aid. Only drawing can let somebody see what you are thinking." … Mr Wells admitted he had always wanted to be an artist: he received an art A-level and wanted to go to art college, but his mother urged a "proper" career.

Frank Wells was a keynote speaker at the AMH annual conference held at Peninsula Medical School, Truro centre, in 2005.

See also: https://jacsaorsa.wordpress.com/2016/05/10/heart-surgery-at-papworth-hospital/

Drama for embodied collaboration

Taking the workplace as theatre, doctors and medical students have worked with the Royal Shakespeare Company, Clod Ensemble, and with final year drama and performance students from Falmouth University to look at how the body is related to identity and how it performs in power-saturated settings such as patient consultations and inter-professional clinical teamwork settings. Such embodied self-presentation and impression management is linked to discussions about how the sick body is managed and presented by "patients". This issue is extended to questioning of traditional separation of the "sick" and "healthy" body and the "normal" and "pathologized" through working with (i) body based radical performance artists; (ii) body builders, male and female, who can isolate developed muscle groups; and (iii) gymnasts who can contort and extend the body.

Persons with disabilities such as wheelchair users

In contrast to the extended naturalistic social and isolated bodies above, students also learned from persons with disabilities about bodily limitations and adaptations, and about stigma.

Faced with a skeleton, what does an artist do?

We appointed visiting professors of Music and Medicine, the History of Medicine and Visual Arts and Medicine. The latter was Christine Borland, a high-profile visual artist who has been shortlisted for the Turner Prize and has an international reputation. Christine's career is unusual in that it has been dedicated to medical and forensic medical themes. She carried out an extended project on simulation learning at Peninsula that resulted in a public engagement exhibition at the Newlyn Gallery, Penzance, UK. Prior to this, and a scenario that was often used with medical students learning anatomy, was a project that Christine completed much earlier in Glasgow. Before an act came into law that forbids the buying, selling and storing of human organs, even for educational use, Christine noted that a company was still selling human skeletons as drawing aids for art schools or as educational models for medical schools. She mail ordered a female and a male skeleton. Her curiosity was piqued not by function (skeleton as a drawing aid) but by a moral question: "to which persons did these skeletons belong?" Drawing on the expertise of facial reconstruction practitioners, she was able to re-flesh and re-store dignity to the skulls, as a form of identity reclamation and an honouring of two lives of real people who had, in a very real sense, donated their bodies to science and art.

Radiologists using multiple images

The diagnostic visual imagination is particularly important to radiologists, dermatologists and histopathologists (Bleakley 2015), although medical imaging is used across a number of specialties, including ophthalmology, cardiology and radiation oncology. Where a key skill of radiologists is to read two-dimensional images in depth or as perceptually projected three-dimensionality, current use of multiple images from CT or MRI scans allows for ready three-dimensional reading. Contemporary radiology requires the doctor to scan a sheaf of images (multi-slice examinations) from computed tomography (CT) and magnetic resonance imaging (MRI) scans, where the scanner's imaging process is a rotation around the body, rather than looking at just a single image (as in ultrasound, projection X-ray images – e.g. bone, chest, mammography – and dynamic X-ray exams – e.g. fluoroscopy). Scanning and developing a composite picture from multiple images allows for a three-dimensional viewing. This radically challenges the penetrating gaze of modern medical diagnostics described by Foucault, now replaced by a "glance". Use of software to aid image interpretation also distributes the gaze.

A vocabulary of "looking" and "seeing": Medical metaphors

In an award-winning research project at Peninsula, as part of the medical humanities programme, we teamed up a radiologist, dermatologist and histopathologist (all senior consultants) with three visual artists and arranged exchanges of work visits – artists to clinics and laboratories, and doctors to studios and gallery spaces. Conversations and practices were videotaped and observed and cross-fertilizing ideas about "how to look" were distilled from these exchanges. A public engagement seminar was held at the Tate Gallery St Ives to disseminate findings. One outcome of the project was to develop a model of how medical metaphors are used in Type 1 (pattern recognition) diagnosis (Bleakley 2015).

Walt Whitman and a poetics of the body

A good example of the use of the medical humanities in double stimulation is to consider embodiment from the point of view of the poet rather than the anatomist or the doctor. The poet stresses appreciation before explanation and aesthetic approaches to the body. This approach has been considered in Chapter 3, with reference to the American poet Walt Whitman, who "sings the body electric". To refer back to that section: Whitman embodies an aesthetic form of political resistance to the dominant functionalism and conservatism of the anatomical text. He also democratizes the body, refusing to privilege kinds of bodies but rather celebrating ordinary function as extraordinary. An acutely observant journalist by training, Whitman had no need of learning anatomy through cadaver dissection. As a volunteer wound dresser or auxiliary nurse in Unionist field hospitals during the American Civil War, he saw many badly wounded soldiers, recovering and dying: "in one of the hospitals I find Thomas Haley, Company M, 4th New York cavalry – a regular Irish boy … shot through the lungs – inevitably dying". Whitman's gaze is not the penetrating medical glance, but a long, sinuous meandering that is reflected in his experimentation with long sentence prose poems.

Historical and cross-cultural mappings of the body (e.g. Chinese medicine)

Students study maps of the body across historical periods and differing cultures with some incredulity – for example, why do Chinese maps of the body show meridians for acupuncture when we know that such anatomy is a fiction? This is partly explained by the ban on dissection of corpses in China until relatively recently. In the absence of "opening up a few corpses" to develop a clinical gaze, Chinese anatomy was developed in the dark, through processes of psychological projection.

Non-manipulative and gender sensitive resources long used in human sexuality education

Educating medical students in conducting sensitive intimate examinations and discussions of sexual health requires making students feel at ease about discussing sexuality. Educators can draw on resources used in human sexuality courses, or for the education of sex therapists, such as explicit film.

In summary, anatomy teaching is reconceptualized through the second stimulus of the medical humanities. This does not decry traditional anatomy teaching as an activity but rather expands the scope and vision of that activity to a more holistic rather than partitioned view. In turn, this challenges and transforms the pedagogical basis for the clinical gaze, now both distributed and a glance, away from looking into the body to appreciating embodiment: the body in space and time as expressive and social. Such a pedagogical shift advertises a resistance to normative anatomy teaching that is aesthetic rather than functional, and undoes false roadblocks between disciplines to make anatomy an inter-disciplinary study.

The roles of contradiction

In double stimulation, a temporary resolution of contradictions raises another set of contradictions but at a new level of sophistication and meaning. I have laid bare in previous chapters' medicine's concurrent embrace and rejection of politics as contradictory. Medicine works generally in realms of ambiguity, uncertainty and contradiction, all the while trying to iron out such uncertainties through diagnostic and prognostic sureties. Tolerating such ambiguity is a central hallmark of a good physician. This is readily understandable by stating its opposite – the central feature of an authoritarian personality is intolerance of ambiguity. Authoritarians would continue to support hierarchical working patterns in medicine that have been shown to be a source of medical error, poor care and work dissatisfaction.

Medicine has been unable to deal with its own contradictions or paradoxes. Primarily, over three decades of research have shown that clinical outcomes and patient safety are improved where medical interventions are collaborative – team based – and inter-professional, as noted above, yet medicine is slow to democratize. A further paradox is that, while more women than men are now entering and working in medicine worldwide, the culture of medicine remains broadly patriarchal. Although change is evident globally, it is slow. These power, or political, contradictions demand to be addressed through a progressive medical education.

Other contradictions and paradoxes, however, do not simply offer blockage but also can act as resource. We can reframe power or political contradictions as potential resource, exploring this through a metaphor introduced by Helga Nowotny (2015): "the cunning of uncertainty". If we give uncertainty voice, we may find that it calls up previously unrecognized, or under-utilized, resources in medicine, such as the artistry and humanity that are central to good practice. Uncertainty's cunning is realized in "thinking otherwise". Brought centre-stage, such artistry and humanity can address some of medical education's current contradictions, turning them into resources. Those who are sceptical of the value of the medical/ health humanities may not have seen what is right under their noses – that medical science and practice are already art forms based on humanistic values. The pedagogical challenge is how to best mobilize such inherent resources. Where human biology boasts an extraordinary array of displays of anatomies and physiologies, we consistently crush this by insistence upon function before form. A pedagogical rule could be: "appreciation before explanation", the central teaching of the biologist Adolf Portmann.

The philosopher Immanuel Kant admitted: "Out of the crooked timber of humanity, no straight thing was ever made". This means two things – first, that humanity cannot be put into a common mould, where difference is far more important than forcing common identity through regulation. Second, all things, no matter what their moral claims, will have a twist or a contradiction inherent to their natures. This book is a story of the "crooked timber" of politics as medicine's concurrent ally and foe, filtered through aesthetics to parry the blunt functionalism and reductionism that can so readily dominate medical practices.

In subsequent chapters, I detail curricula interventions as judicious employment of a medical humanities perspective in response to the circumstance of medical education as an activity prone to reductionism. Central to this reductionism – advertised in the unreflective use of terms such as "training" and "competence" – is the compulsory mis-education of the senses in modern medical education, detailed in a previous book (Bleakley 2020).

Tolerance for ambiguity as a learning outcome

Peninsula Medical School was launched in the UK in 2002. It promised, and delivered, an innovative undergraduate medicine and surgery curriculum. The acid test would be how graduates from the school performed as junior doctors. We tracked the first two cohorts (2007/ 2008) after graduation (Brennan et al. 2010; Bleakley and Brennan 2011). Many of the Peninsula graduates remained to work as pre-registration and junior doctors in their UK local (South West) Deanery. They were joined by a roughly equal number of graduates from other medical schools around the UK. Serendipitously, we had a ready-made two cohorts' comparison design for our evaluation research: Peninsula graduates' performances compared with performances from graduates of other schools.

We used a variety of performance evaluation measures, including (i) self-report on technical and non-technical capabilities and skills (using a validated instrument that had been developed at Manchester University medical school); (ii) interviews; (iii) tutor reports; and (iv) audio diaries, over two consecutive cohorts each over Foundation Year 1 (FY1). Data were obtained well into FY1, so that graduates had a chance to see how well they were coping with their first real doctoring experiences.

The results showed that Peninsula graduates perceived and rated their clinical skills performances as well as, or in some cases better than, graduates from other medical schools (on the basis of questions such as "how well did your medical school prepare you for drug prescribing?") They also perceived and reported their communication capabilities (including teamwork) and confidence on the job (such as ability to seek guidance) as well as, or in some cases better than, graduates from other schools. So far, so good, as one of the common criticisms of more innovative medical schools is that they will produce graduates with less confidence in clinical skills and clinical medicine based on a lack of knowledge. Tutor reports confirmed these self-report claims. Our graduates were as adept clinically as graduates from other medical schools.

However, what was striking, and showed the greatest difference between the Peninsula group and the other graduates, was that Peninsula graduates perceived and rated themselves as showing significantly higher confidence in their abilities, and higher tolerance for ambiguity (DeForge and Sobal 1989; Weissenstein et al. 2014), than graduates from other schools. These two factors may or may not be linked. In short, graduates from other schools generally craved certainty and stability in clinical work, where Peninsula graduates had high tolerance for ambiguity and coped well with uncertain or unstable clinical contexts. This was particularly pleasing for those who had devised the original Peninsula curriculum, as one of the stated aims was to prepare medical students transitioning into their clinical roles as trainee doctors, and then registered doctors, for situations requiring high tolerance of ambiguity and uncertainty. Central to such perceptions included knowing one's limits to knowledge and skill, and when to ask for help. Even at this stage, after graduating from medical school, junior doctors can be afraid of exposing their vulnerabilities in calling for help, and male doctors in particular can overestimate their abilities, mistaking confidence for actual competence (Roland et al. 2015).

Medical practice is fluid, complex and shot through with uncertainty and contradictions. Young doctors, as they make life-changing decisions about specialty tracks, have to align the knowing, doing and valuing of medicine with *becoming* a specialist as an identity construction and entry into a prescribed community of practice (Gill 2013). They are simultaneously called upon to suspend emotional investment in carrying out "professional" practice, just as they must be interpellated, or "inserted", into series of specialty-specific rotations towards which affective-laden responses (likes and dislikes) are required. The capital produced from their emotional labour gradually becomes invested in preferred specialties as they come to inhabit the basement of the hierarchy. Investing their senses in career paths, they find that those senses are also claimed and shaped – in the name of a postgraduate medical education – by their seniors. Unlike Foucault's call for an aesthetic *self*-forming, the art of character building becomes a forming in the hands of the *other*. This is described as a necessary sacrifice. But of course medical education can be far more democratic than this, where apprenticeships are framed as much in terms of what apprentices bring as what masters offer.

Medicine's purpose of diagnosing, treating and managing illness and disability wherever possible continues, inevitably, in the face of ageing and death. Life is essentially contradictory where it is entropic, and perhaps humans are the only life forms able to appreciate disjunction between appetite for life and the inevitability of death. Medical advances mean that we live longer, but also perhaps suffer more in old age as a consequence. As medicine becomes more sophisticated, contemporary culture paradoxically produces "lifestyle illnesses" such as Type 2 diabetes linked to obesity, and associated cardiac problems linked to diet and lack of exercise; and mental illnesses such as body dysmorphias, self-harming, chronic depression and anxiety.

Poverty and hardship invite ill health, while economic models such as neoliberal capitalism produce structural inequalities that can lead to disadvantage, poor quality of life and associated ill health. Finally, medicine's major paradox is that it harms as well as cures (iatrogenesis) through medical error such as surgical mistakes, hospital-acquired infections and prescribing errors. Politics too harms by proxy – for example by withdrawing or freezing funds for health and social care, as occurred during the UK's near-decade of austerity from 2010 to 2019 after the global financial crisis of 2008; and, in the USA, Brazil, Sweden and the UK in particular, failing to rapidly initiate proper measures such as widespread testing and tracing during the coronavirus outbreak in February–March 2020.

Medicine, both somatic and mental or psychological, occupies the impossible territory of the immortal gods, with a mission to defy symptom. In many cases, medicine can claim victory or near victory – the eradication of smallpox; the drive to eradicate polio and malaria worldwide; the promise of AIDS/HIV eradication less than 40 years after outbreak; and so forth. Yet, due to shifting population profiles, new epidemics emerge such as dementia, Parkinson's disease and Alzheimer's, linked primarily to old age. New pandemics occur because of animal-borne viruses jumping the species gap, such as COVID-19. Symptoms are aggravated by environmental degradation such as air pollution causing respiratory disorders. While accidents are a main leading cause of death outside the influence of medical intervention, the relatively high rate of suicides, especially amongst younger people, might be reduced through mental health interventions. Led by the nose by Big Pharma, doctors may continue to prescribe opioid pain relief in the knowledge that treatments are potentially addictive. Here, medicine, a major profession for educating the senses, has lost its own sense, sometimes failing to notice the stink.

Medicine, like all institutions and cultures, displays symptoms. Ironically, medicine is poor at attending to its own wounds. Given its ideological stance and fervour – to cure disease at all costs – medicine has not been able to cure its own dysfunctions. It should be said that symptoms are inevitable in any organism, body or institution. The main issue is how we address symptom; eradication of symptom in institutions is often not a good idea or impossible. Rather, symptoms may be mobilized as a resource through transformation. Other disciplines, such as the social sciences related to medicine, study these symptoms and in some cases suggest how they may be addressed through cure, management or mobilization.

Medicine's symptoms are investigated by anthropology (through the methods of ethnography), studying medical culture as "other"; by sociology, looking at medicine as a hierarchical social structure mirroring to some extent the military, the fire service and the police; by auto-ethnography, where doctors and surgeons tell their own stories; by narrative-based medicine, where patients tell their stories; and by fiction, where stories are woven around medical themes, to include drama such as television medical soap operas and film. Such media stray into the post-human, such as artists' books and "flash fiction" representing illness experiences, often archived online and centred on building supportive online communities. Such symptoms can include:

- Medicalization of society (assimilation of non-medical affairs into medical models), including labelling of widely tolerated behaviours as mental disorders (Attention Deficit Hyperactivity Disorder). Medicine's symptoms here may be compulsion and arrogance.
- Avoidable deaths through medical error (fixation on individualism rather than collaborative responsibility).
- Over-diagnosis (compulsion).
- Over-prescribing (compulsion).
- Lack of self-care (arrogance or hubris).
- Objectification (emotional insulation).

A basic contradiction haunting medicine is that doctors and surgeons seek certainty in a world of uncertainty. In many cases, diagnoses are made, treatments such as drug therapies identified and prognoses set out, or surgical interventions conducted, with great confidence and accuracy. But, especially in the field of mental health, and where a high psychosomatic component affects illness, such as in gastro-intestinal disorders, uncertainty stalks medical practice. Uncertainties haunt the territory between surgical intervention and autopsy report. A Norwegian study suggested that one-third of reported causes of death may be changed after post-mortem investigations (Alfsen and Mæhlen 2012). In contrast, a post-mortem report may, for example, note cause of death as severe intra-abdominal bleeding, but does not record that this was due to a surgical mishap (https://www.ncepod.org.uk/2006Report/results_of_study_13.html).

So, we have plenty of inroads to medicine's symptoms, both as intended and unintended consequences of medical practice and the shifting structures of medical communities. Psychology, particularly psychoanalytic approaches, moves beyond description of medicine's symptoms to intervention. For example, James Hillman (1975) points out why we should celebrate "pathologizing", or the production of symptom, as gift rather than curse. The contradictions in symptom production can provide capital for development of medical culture once analysed and "revisioned", in Hillman's term. As medicine treats many debilitating symptoms and cures them or alleviates suffering, so some of medicine's symptoms can be "cured". But some remain incurable yet can act as valuable resources – once re-visioned or reconsidered for their paradoxical value – as we shall see. In short, we must not just wade in to eradicate medicine's symptoms, repeating the mistakes of "heroic medicine", but "think otherwise" to assess the paradoxical value of symptom. In psychotherapy, we do not eradicate symptom as first step, but rather ask: "what does the symptom want?" Does this approach work for medicine? This reflective pause is a consequence of the double stimulation provided by the weighty historical anchor of psychotherapy that is Freud's legacy.

The human body as a contradiction: The bio-illogical

Medicine's focus – the optimal functioning of the human body in a health-conscious social setting – is necessarily grounded in contradictions. Evolution – itself both ambiguous and contradictory, dependent upon chance mutations for species development and survival – has produced a range of complex individuals whose thought processes and languages in many ways transcend the limits of their bodies. Long after their deaths, Shakespeare's plays and sonnets, Marie Cure's discovery of radium, Lao Tzu's philosophy and Leo Tolstoy's novels continue to speak. A pessimist might say that the body has a relatively short lifespan and extending it only brings the possibility of multiple chronic illnesses. Even while "healthy" – much as it is a wonder – the human body is grounded in contradictions or evolutionary glitches, flaws and errors (Lents 2018).

For example, the evolution to bi-pedalism places excessive strain on the knee joints that are prone to injury; and where the abdominal cavity carries the guts in mesenteries – sheets of connective tissue – these are not suspended from the top of the abdominal cavity but from the back. This makes the mesenteries prone to tearing in persons with largely sedentary lifestyles. Our eyes are poorly designed for clearly focusing images – a major handicap where sight is our primary sense; our nasal cavities inconveniently drain upwards; and evolution has compromised between the size of a newborn's head and the mother's birth canal in relation to the size of the pelvis, resulting in humans being born too early and then experiencing a long period of vulnerability. Psychologically, too, our lives are grounded in contradictions. Cultural and social values drive us to believe anecdote over evidence, even to invest in anecdote as acts of faith. We then daily enact cognitive biases where we fit perceptions into preformed values, seeing truth in opinion and forming stories to confirm our prejudices.

Medical education as contradiction

To ground medicine and medical education in contradiction and uncertainty offers an opportunity to draw on the value of the arts and humanities as a resource for medicine and medical education and for medical students' identity formations. The arts and humanities are our primary media for education of tolerance of ambiguity and uncertainty. As noted above, Helga Nowotny (2015) suggests in the title to her book that *The Cunning of Uncertainty* must be recognized and harvested as resource and not impediment. We can apply the cunning of uncertainty – uncertainty's inherent value, for example as serendipity – to the development of medical students as doctors-in-training; and as "proto-professionals" learning how to enter the social world of medicine and to act professionally and ethically with patients and colleagues. This includes not just the ethics of medicine (making value judgements about interventions that are appropriate for context), but also the politics and aesthetics of medicine.

We have seen that the "cunning of uncertainty" is a paradoxical logic at work in uncertainty principles, such as the flow of a complex, dynamic adaptive system through time. Uncertainty can drive a surgeon to make a split-second life-and-death decision, or an oncologist to prescribe a highly toxic treatment for a cancer patient, where the decision adds "hunch" or "instinct" beyond consideration of guidelines and protocols. On closer inspection, "hunches", 'intuitions' and 'gut feelings' may be based on a "cognitive unconscious" (Reber 1993) that is composed of connections between bits of knowledge that do not quite become explicated. This may be a series of interacting "memory scripts" for certain illness configurations. Hunches are then not woolly, but may be developed cognitive process stored as tacit knowledge.

There is no doubt that much of our habitual practice such as driving a car or riding a bicycle operates at this border between tacit and explicit knowing, and it is no surprise that in a novel or out-of-the-blue critical situation, we suddenly find ourselves adapting, inventing and creating, where the "tacit dimension" (Polanyi 1966) is dynamic and adaptive, as a complex system that does not follow linear laws. How else would expertise reach new heights? Here, improvised actions are not entirely based on what is known – rather they produce new knowledge that can perhaps be articulated in retrospective deliberation: "The cunning of uncertainty may manifest itself in the choice of the right moment. Timing is also cunning" (Nowotny 2015: ix). The ancient Greeks knew this and termed such timing *kairos* or "opportunity", a cunning whose clinical implications are articulated by Arno Kumagai and Thirusha Naidu (2020b). In busy, pressing clinical circumstances, teaching "moments" are hard to find. Good teachers, however, are sensitive to timing and opportunity, finding just the right moment to engage with learners. This brings us back to Roland Barthes' sense of rhythm as central to community living and working activities.

Detienne and Vernant (1978: 3) note the origin of "cunning" in the ancient Greek *metis* combining both wisdom and cunning or strategy. The Greek goddess Metis, who personified these qualities, was said by Plato to have birthed a son – Poros – freely translated as "ingenuity", "resourcefulness" and "abundance". Metis embodies flair, wisdom, forethought, resourcefulness, vigilance, opportunism and subtlety in contexts that are shifting, disconcerting and ambiguous. Importantly, the cunning of uncertainty can offer an alternative to hubris or psychological inflation, a condition of excessive belief in one's abilities (or the power of a culture) that has haunted modern, heroic, masculine medicine.

The realism of the cunning of uncertainty can be the natural success to the idealistic dragon-slaying mentality that has dogged medicine and medical education. This requires medical culture (and then medical students and doctors) to recognize its limits, to embrace tolerance for ambiguity and calculated risk and to think in terms of fluid, complex, adaptive systems, where contradictions (as strange attractors in the system) can act as potential resources, especially where these fuel "boundary negotiations" and "boundary crossings" (Hannele and Engeström 2003) for the expansion of activities and the systems that express such expansions. In turn, a medical education grounded in contradiction is to be welcomed – but not as an excuse for sloppiness and obfuscation, or lack of clarity and direction.

Bibliography

Adams T. 2017. Henry Marsh: The Mind–Matter Problem is Not a Problem for Me, Mind is Matter. Neuroscience: *The Observer*, 16 July 2017. Available at: https://www.the guardian.com/science/2017/jul/16/henry-marsh-mind-matter-not-a-problem-inte rview-neurosurgeon-admissions

Alfsen GC, Mæhlen JP. The Value of Autopsies for Determining the Cause of Death. *Tidsskr Nor Legeforen*. 2012;132(2):147–51.

Allthusser L. 2008. *On Ideology*. London: Verso.

Baudrillard J. 1983. *Simulations*. Los Angeles, CA: Semiotext(e).

Bleakley A. 2015. *The Medical Humanities and Medical Education: How the Medical Humanities Can Shape Better Doctors*. Abingdon: Routledge.

Bleakley A. 2020. *Educating Doctors' Senses Through The Medical Humanities: "How Do I Look?"* Abingdon: Routledge.

Bleakley A, Bligh J. Who Can Resist Foucault? *Journal of Medicine and Philosophy*. 2009;34:368–83.

Bleakley A, Brennan N. Does Undergraduate Curriculum Design Make a Difference to Readiness to Practice as a Junior Doctor? *Medical Teacher*. 2011;33:459–67.

Brennan N, Corrigan O, Allard J, et al. The Transition from Medical Student to Junior Doctor: Today's Experiences of Tomorrow's Doctors. *Medical Education*. 2010;44:449–58.

Case A, Deaton A. 2020. *Deaths of Despair and the Future of Capitalism*. Princeton, NJ: Princeton University Press.

DeForge BR, Sobal J. Intolerance of Ambiguity in Students Entering Medical School. *Social Science and Medicine*. 1989;28:869–74.

Deleuze G, Guattari F. 2013. *A Thousand Plateaus*. London: Continuum.

Detienne M, Vernant J-P. 1978. *Cunning Intelligence in Greek Culture and Society*. Sussex: Harvester Press.

Dubin B. Innovative Curriculum Prepares Medical Students for a Lifetime of Learning and Patient Care. *Missouri Medicine*. 2016;113:170–73.

Engeström Y. 2018. *Expertise in Transition: Expansive Learning in Medical Work*. Cambridge: Cambridge University Press.

Foucault M. 1976. *The Birth of the Clinic: An Archaeology of Medical Perception*. London: Routledge.

Foucault M. 1977. *Discipline and Punish: The Birth of the Prison*. New York: Random House.

Fu D. Vygotsky and Marxism. *Education and Culture*. 1997;XV:10–17.

Gill D. 2013 *Becoming Doctors: The Formation of Professional Identity in Newly Qualified Doctors*. Available at: http://discovery.ucl.ac.uk/10020735/1/__d6_Shared%24_SU PP_Library_User%20Services_Circulation_Inter-Library%20Loans_IOE%20ETH OS_ETHOS%20digitised%20by%20ILL_GILL%2C%20D.pdf

Hannele K, Engeström Y. 2003. Boundary Crossing and Learning in Creation of New Work Practice: Creation and Re-creation of Routines During Tool Implementation. *Organizational Learning and Knowledge: The Annual Conference 2003*. Available at: https://pdfs.semanticscholar.org/9b31/4ad09fa90f5023950bee6d9f63b8b44708d4.pdf

Hattenstone S. The Dad Who Gave Birth: "Being Pregnant Doesn't Change me Being a Trans Man'". *The Guardian*, 20 April 2019. Available at: https://www.theguardian.c om/society/2019/apr/20/the-dad-who-gave-birth-pregnant-trans-freddy-mcconnell

Heidegger M. 1962. *Being and Time*. New York: Harper & Row.

Hillman J. 1975. *ReVisioning Psychology*. New York: HarperCollins.

Inui TS. 2003. A Flag in the Wind. Educating for Professionalism in Medicine. Association of American Medical Colleges. Available at: https://members.aamc.org/eweb/uploa d/A%20Flag%20in%20the%20Wind%20Report.pdf

Johnson D. 1992. *Jesus' Son: Stories*. New York: Farrar, Straus & Giroux.

Kennedy M. Doctor's Bloody Work on Show. *The Guardian*, 4 June 2004. Available at: https://www.theguardian.com/uk/2004/jun/04/arts.artsnews

Kierkegaard S. 1989. *The Sickness Unto Death*. Harmondsworth: Penguin.

Kumagai AK, Naidu T. On Time and Tea Bags: Chronos, Kairos, and Teaching for Humanistic Practice. *Academic Medicine*. 2020b; 95:512–17.

Lents NH. 2018. *Human Errors: A Panorama of Our Glitches, from Pointless Bones to Broken Genes*. Boston, MA: Houghton Mifflin Harcourt.

Leont'ev AN. 1977. *The Development of Mind*. Marxists Internet Archive. Available at: https ://www.marxists.org/admin/books/activity-theory/leontyev/development-mind.pdf

Mannino N, Pregler J. 2018. *Benefits of an Organ-Based Block Curriculum*. Available at: https://medschool.ucla.edu/body.cfm?id=1158&action=detail&ref=27

McLachlan JC, Bligh J, Bradley P, Searle J. Teaching Anatomy Without Cadavers. *Medical Education*. 2004;38:418–24.

Nowotny H. 2015. *The Cunning of Uncertainty*. Cambridge: Polity Press.

O'Doherty B. 1986. *Inside the White Cube: The Ideology of the Gallery Space*. Berkeley, CA: University of California Press.

Polanyi M. 1966. *The Tacit Dimension*. Gloucester: Smith.

Reber W. 1993. *Implicit Learning and Tacit Knowledge: An Essay on The Cognitive Unconscious*. Oxford: Oxford University Press.

Regan de Bere S, Mattick K. From Anatomical "Competence" to Complex Capability. The Views and Experiences of UK Tutors on How We Should Teach Anatomy to Medical Students. *Advances in Health Sciences Education*. 2010;15:573–85.

Roland D, Matheson D, Coats T, Martin G. A Qualitative Study of Self-Evaluation of Junior Doctor Performance: Is Perceived "Safeness" a More Useful Metric Than Confidence and Competence? *BMJ Open*. 2015;5:e008521.

Sannino A, Laitinen A. Double Stimulation in the Waiting Experiment: Testing a Vygotskian Model of the Emergence of Volitional Action. *Learning, Culture and Social Interaction*. 2015;4:4–18.

Steiner CJ, Reisinger Y. Understanding Existential Authenticity. *Annals of Tourism Research*. 2006;33:299–318.

Vygotsky LS. 1987. Lectures on Psychology. In *The Collected Works of L. S. Vygotsky. Vol. 1. Problems of General Psychology*. New York: Plenum.

Weissenstein A, Ligges S, Broiwer B, et al. Measuring the Ambiguity Tolerance of Medical Students: A Cross-Sectional Study from the First to Sixth Academic Years. *BMC Family Practice*. 2014;15:Article 6.

11 Thinking with curriculum

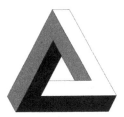

Thinking as doing

A familiar oppositional mindset that characterizes human behaviour is that of "thinking *vs.* doing" or "conceptual *vs.* practical". The psychologist Kurt Lewin heals this opposition through his 1946 maxim that "there is nothing as practical as a good theory". Lewin was the founder of "action research", a collaborative model that I return to in Chapter 14. Katherine McCain (2015) has looked at the contemporary influence of Lewin's maxim in social sciences articles and notes its increasing popularity. It is not a throwaway remark, but a description of how theory and practice can be fused as "praxis" – theory's enactment, embodiment or realization. Politics abounds with praxis – a local pressure group meets to discuss protest against plans to develop land for a factory that will not benefit local people, and devises three activities: writing to the local MP to register protest, asking for action such as questioning in Parliament; writing to the chief executive of the company concerned expressing concerns and asking for these to be answered; and actively protesting with banners and leaflets at the proposed site. The theory of socialism is enacted and embodied: concept-runs-into-percept-runs-into-activity.

Learning theory such as Cultural-Historical Activity Theory, as we have seen, draws together "activity" and "theory" as an unfolding process through time. The general theory of how the object of an activity is expanded, through addressing contradictions between differing aspects of the activity (learner; artefacts; community of practice, with its differentiated rules and division of labour; and outcome), is modulated through personal and collaborative theory-building (hypotheses) and testing (practices). A curriculum is built this way and, as a dynamic object, generates more theory about its purpose and trajectory as the curriculum itself can be used to "think with". To divide theory and practice and then to oppose them is a potentially destructive rather than instructive process, as John Dewey's pragmatism advertises.

Set in Vienna at the end of the Great War in 1918, Robert Musil's (1995) *The Man Without Qualities* describes a mathematician, Ulrich, who has no desire to "know" or "discover" himself, living like a leaf in the wind. Yet his peculiar lethargy, set against the impulse to activity that he so resents, leads Ulrich to pass judgement on the dominant education system of the time in America, which he sees as fixated upon *doing* at the expense of *thinking*: "Our age drips with practical energy anyway. It's stopped caring for ideas, it only wants action". Yet, continues Ulrich: "It's so easy to have the energy to act and so difficult to find a meaning for action!" (ibid.: 87). Such North American pragmatism, championed by Charles Sanders Peirce, William James and John Dewey, linked to masculinist heroic endeavour, or the ideal of the self-sufficient "frontiersman", describes the main value system underpinning Western medical education for most of the last century since the reforms initiated by Abraham Flexner in 1910, as discussed in previous chapters.

Medical education, following medicine as a hands-on practice, historically "drips with practical energy". Medicine curricula as a consequence have become instrumental, where "curriculum" is seen as a means to an end – a collection of content to be crammed and reproduced for assessment – and then no more than a bundle of syllabi. Curriculum, derived from the Latin *currere* meaning "to stay the course", is then no longer something to "think with", but rather a vehicle for cramming knowledge and skills. It is often claimed that medical students historically have craved training rather than education – "just tell me what to do!" – but this claim is grounded in a theory–practice opposition and divide, rather than meaningful dialogue or complex conversation.

The root of training, *trahere*, means "to drag behind", as in the trail of a wedding dress. Medical students – supposedly the brightest of us all – have, we are told, craved jumping on the coattails of their illustrious teachers rather than thinking for themselves. But this again is a medical education myth, reinforced by those who see themselves as "trainers" rather than educators. What the curriculum might promote in the wider sense – such as values, discrimination, a sensibility, a critical mind, the powers of innovation or "thinking otherwise", the ability to appreciate as well as measure – all of these may be masked or muddied in the race to meet "competences". Here, history ("how did we get here?") and future thinking ("where are we going?") may be collapsed into an obsession with the present so that education becomes, again, one-dimensional "training", reductive, instrumental and functional. Capability – what medical students, or any other learner, may be able to achieve in the future – is then ignored.

Curriculum reconceptualization

The curriculum reconceptualization movement encourages us to not simply implement curricula, but also to *think with and about* curricula. Curriculum is both a message and a medium, framed as "conversation" (Applebee 1996) and varieties of "texts" (Barone 2000; Pinar 2006, 2011, 2012; Pinar and Reynolds 2015; Doll 2019). In turning the noun *curriculum* into the infinitive *currere* – literally "to run the course" – we turn an ahistorical thing into a historical flow, a procession. William Pinar's method of learning *from* curriculum study, rather than just planning a curriculum, involves four steps towards an identity construction as a learner:

1. The regressive: returning to, or reactivating, the past to chart how I have developed.
2. The progressive: imagining the future – how will I adapt and innovate, or will I stagnate or crystallize?
3. The analytic: understanding myself and not simply enacting a role; this means coming to know oneself reflexively – for example, what values drive and shape me and how does this affect others?
4. The synthetic: how might I develop and what qualities in learning may enhance this?

The woven curriculum

By stressing the importance of thinking with and about curriculum, again I am not ignoring the importance of practice and action. Like Musil's Ulrich, we recognize, and tire of, an age that "drips with practical energy" and has "stopped caring for ideas" where "it only wants action". At the risk of stereotyping, this characterizes "can do" doctors who become educators, always seeking a "route 1" pragmatism. "Thinking with curriculum" leads, however, to more deliberate action often requiring travel by side-roads and circuitous routes.

Again, curriculum, or course of study, is a written, spoken and enacted – or performed – text. "Text" and "texture" have the same linguistic root. "Text" is derived from the Latin *textus*, meaning the style or texture of a work, or a thing that is woven, braided, interweaved, fabricated or constructed. This emphasis shifts focus from the common reading of text as something cerebral and written. Rather, a text is a series of actions performed over time and knitted together in a meaningful way – a "co-configuration".

A text is then an artefact having a written record and a spoken history, providing a medium through which activity is modulated and potentially expanded. Texts are made and re-made, sometimes badly so that they fall apart, and sometimes well so that they form a basis for expansion. Texts are made for re-invention, re-interpretation and reconceptualization. To return to Musil's Ulrich above, texts are something to think about, to think with and to enact – they "drip" with praxis, or theory in action. Woven texts, like blankets and rugs, are patterned on the upper side, but turn them over and they are loose threads. A woven text is necessarily contradictory, speaking two languages simultaneously.

Medical education's primary texts are curricula. We can then describe curricula as woven and interwoven, or fabricated. But the hands of the fabricators are to a great extent tied – to historical antecedents, traditions and cultural patterns. In medicine, this is amplified where the consequences of a poor education may potentially be an unsafe or incompetent practitioner. But this too can lead to conservatism rather than innovation. We must again distinguish between curriculum content, or syllabus; and the way that content is learned, or medical pedagogy. It is not the syllabus or content that produces good or poor practitioners, but rather quality of engagement with the curriculum as a whole – the lifelong *currere* or track of learning – combined with the learner's emerging capabilities and the facilitators' abilities to draw out such capabilities in a learner. This must be set against a background of a culture (medicine) that can simultaneously be a supportive and an absent parent.

A fabrication is both an invention and a lie – the word offers a dual meaning like the Greek *pharmakon* – a "healing poison". A curriculum is a fabrication, both a fact and a tissue of lies. It appears to offer a guide, but in any decent curriculum this is sometimes guidance to a cliff-edge. This is why, in the 1960s, Jerome Bruner described meaningful learning as "scaffolding". The learner is helped to step out of her comfort zone into the unknown, but a scaffold – expert tutoring and facilitation – is always present. Innovation in learning is partly unpredictable and necessarily collaborative to include others' minds and actions, and facilitating media or objects. Scaffolding is a gloss on Lev Vygotsky's zone of proximal development (ZPD) – the territory delineated by what is known and can be done independently, and what can be achieved with facilitative help.

As noted, the Latin etymology of "curriculum" – a course of study – refers to running a racetrack, as the Roman chariot race, but this can be readily extended to running the course of life, where what is made or achieved is identity. By "identity" (better in the plural, as we shape and re-make multiple identities) I do not mean a stable, core, subjective "self" that is a heroic fiction. Rather, I take identity to be the natural consequence of the recognition of difference. Identity is achieved not by looking into a mirror and seeing a self-reflection, but by looking at another as a mirror and source of difference. As I look into the worlds of the "other" I recognize myself in difference to them, but I also remain deferent to them as I acknowledge their value and worth, and what I can learn from them. This is the basic democratic gesture.

At the same time, I can reflect on and improve my own value through self-education, forming myself as an art. Finally, my identity is shaped through identification with cultures into which I have been socialized, such as family, ethnic groups, friendship groups and work groups such as healthcare and medicine. This does not mean that I cannot enter such cultures with eyes wide open, ready to critique and help to transform such cultures. Multiple identities can then develop according to context or varieties of curricula as organized modes of learning.

A curriculum is not restricted to content for learning, and ways of learning and assessment. Again, this is a syllabus. Curricula embrace process as well as content as they move through time and respond flexibly to change and opportunity. Even if it is carefully documented and archived, much curriculum process is necessarily transient or intuitive as it is characterized by spontaneous and improvised adaptation to learning, teaching and assessment contexts. Typically in medicine, work-based learning, even where it is well planned to include briefing, de-briefing and in situ scaffolding of learning, presents ambiguous and complex contexts where improvisation is necessary.

The syllabus here might describe, say, a dozen learning outcomes that a fourth-year medical student must achieve at a certain level of competence to pass an assessment, but a curriculum also includes a host of factors – such as identity construction (as explained above), communication with patients, team working with colleagues, managing self-care, tolerating ambiguity, responding to contexts beyond one's current level of competence to address capabilities or what is possible, dealing with emotional changes, facing ethical dilemmas, thinking out of the box and so forth – that may not be captured by the syllabus focus. We might think of this complex, fuzzy and fluid background as a "backstage" curriculum, where the front stage is the more crystallized and instrumental syllabus.

Curriculum as varieties of text and values orientations

Let us now return to curriculum and politics. The focus of this book is not primarily on the relationship between medicine and politics, but medical *education* and politics, with a specific theme of the undergraduate or preparatory medicine curriculum as both political and aesthetic text. Of course medical education and medicine are necessarily entwined, where medical education traditionally serves three purposes:

1. Preparation for, and ongoing deepening of, the practice of medicine in terms of knowledge and skills, to include an education of sensibility for clinical diagnostics.
2. The formation of "professionals" through values clarification and reflexivity, to include communication capabilities such as sensitivity, close attending, listening and dialogue; establishing democratic habits and habits of lifelong learning.
3. The socialization of medical students into medical culture and the formation of the identity of "doctor".

   To this triad of outcomes we must now add two more:
4. The psychologically astute doctor who recognizes signs of psychological wear and tear – such as incipient burnout and longer term anxiety and depression – in herself and in others, and is capable of intervening therapeutically.
5. The formation of the "medical citizen" – the upstream medical student and doctor who can engage publicly with issues related to heath such as the climate emergency, and is politically aware, and not blinkered as a downstream doctor only dealing exclusively with clinical patients. (I say this with awareness of how pressured doctors are in clinical contexts, with the view that all in medicine and medical education must look at the structural bigger picture of health and social care to make radical changes, such as the introduction

of longitudinal integrated clerkships [LIC] with inter-professional practice at the core into all undergraduate medicine curricula [Worley et al. 2016]. See for example the Dundee medical school Year 4 clerkship at: https:// sites.dundee.ac.uk/discovermeded/2017/06/02/longitudinal-integrated-cler kship/; the Hull-York medical school Year 4 clerkship scheme at: https://ww w.hyms.ac.uk/medicine/tailoring-your-experience/longitudinal-integrate d-clerkship.)

The notion of the curriculum as a form of text is, again, common parlance within the curriculum reconceptualization movement. Here, the purpose is not primarily pedagogical – putting an educational plan into operation through appropriate pedagogies (that relates more to syllabus as content and process of learning than to curriculum as the course of study) – but theoretical. How can we explain and explore curriculum theoretically in order to better appreciate and explore the values that shape and drive curricula, and are necessarily transmitted to students as a "hidden curriculum"?

Curricula must be reconceptualized, or more deeply understood, before they can be re-designed. It sounds blatantly obvious, but is rarely followed as a rule: curricula must be developed by "thinking with" curricula. Paradoxically, "curriculum" acts as second stimulus in double stimulation of "embodying and enacting curriculum with curriculum in mind". The curriculum reconceptualization movement is grounded in democratic principles, so that any curriculum is designed simultaneously to express democratic values and to advertise democracy at work in its design, implementation, evaluation and progression. As medicine realizes patient-centredness (Little et al. 2001), so curricula realize student-centredness. A curriculum is necessarily a performed manifesto.

A starting point for understanding curricula is to ask what values they primarily express and what values might shape them. Eduard Spranger (1914), a German philosopher and psychologist, wrote a book on personality types – *Types of Men* – expressing seven values. In little over five years, by the end of 1920, the book had sold 28,000 copies, remarkable for a psychology text. Spranger's types were:

(i)   The theoretical (expressing truth through knowledge).
(ii) The economic or utilitarian (what is of practical use).
(iii) The aesthetic (interest in form, beauty and sense impressions).
(iv) The individualistic (interest in self-sufficiency and identity).
(v)   The social (interest in collaboration).
(vi) The religious (interest in spirituality).
(vii) The political (interest in power).

A student of Spranger, the American psychologist Gordon Allport (1955), updated his mentor's work to publish a personality typology of values with an associated scale to measure this in individuals. Interestingly, Allport and colleagues removed "individualism" from Spranger's original list, presuming that individualism or self-sufficiency was intrinsic to the American type. Allport's descriptors were:

(i)   The theoretical (discovery of truth).
(ii)   The economic, instrumental or functional (what is most useful).
(iii) The aesthetic (form, beauty and harmony).
(iv)   The social (seeking love of people).
(v)   The religious (unity).
(vi)   The political (power).

We can apply Spranger's and Allport's categories to curriculum, as differing texts. A medicine curriculum could embrace all seven of Spranger's value orientations, although in reality, the aesthetic, religious and political dimensions would generally be seen as forming a "hidden" curriculum and then not made explicit in curriculum design. The religious might be touched upon in considering end of life care.

Spranger's and Allport's categories can be expanded to embrace the ecological, historical, ethical, gendered, international (and neo-imperialist/ neo-colonialist), autobiographical, phenomenological and educational, as shown in Table 11.1. These are all topics covered in the rapidly expanding field of curriculum reconceptualization studies. Can, and should, a medicine undergraduate curriculum be reconceptualized to embrace all the texts in Table 11.1?

To summarize the discussion so far, the main contributions of the curriculum reconceptualization movement are:

i.   To see "curriculum" not as content – a body of knowledge to be learned (a "syllabus") – but as process and embodied performance. This recovers curriculum as a verb – *currere* – to run not only a course of study, but also the

Table 11.1 Curriculum as text – a variety of inflections

Text type	Focus
Ecological	Nature and sustainability/ climate emergency
Scientific	Knowledge and evidence as fact, and appreciation of quantities in judgement and proof
Historical	Conditions of possibility for the emergence of phenomena
Economic	Utility and worth
Ethical	Values across contexts: both universal and context-specific
Spiritual	Meaning in life and facing death
Gendered	Respect for gender orientations
International	Respect for difference and resistance to neo-colonialism
Autobiographical	Self-forming and care of self
Phenomenological	Felt experience and authenticity
Aesthetic	Developing the senses and appreciation of qualities
Political	Understanding kinds of power and developing resistance
Educational	Curriculum understood reflexively and used to think with

course of a life (within which there are many racetracks to navigate both competitively and collaboratively).

ii.   To see the many life "courses" one runs serving to develop identity (or multiple identities), or sense of self as autobiography and auto-ethnography. This is similar to a "making" of self, described by Michel Foucault (1988) as aesthetic and ethical "self-forming". In previous chapters, we saw that Foucault describes the origins of practices of "self-care" and "self-improvement" from late Greek and early Roman times as ways that power is exercised. Self-forming is both a kind of politics (uses of power as self-informing) and aesthetics (a self-forming or identity sculpting, and modes of expression). In our current era (the Anthropocene), the pressing ecological crisis demands that we frame our self-forming not as an ego-logy (psychological insight) but as an existential eco-logy (how will selves be formed in the face of potential environmental stress and possible extinction of the species?) In contemporary medicine, since the patient-centred and inter-professional "turns", medical education does not focus on masculinist heroism and self-help, but on feminine collaboration and other-directedness.

iii. To see curricula as a bundle of interwoven texts with particular value interests and foci. The weave of the texts reveals a pattern on one side and a bunch of loose threads on the other, as productive contradiction.

Point (iii) above is the main focus for this part of the chapter. In the following chapter, I develop a concept map to better understand curriculum inflections and to lead to a discussion in particular about the neglect within medical education of the curriculum as both political and aesthetic texts. This leads to a practical example of how an innovative undergraduate medicine curriculum can be planned that realizes the value of a range of texts. This is the "top layer" of organization of a curriculum at the level of values. The next layer down deals with particular syllabi, to include factors such as content, appropriate learning processes and assessment issues.

Why is this mapping essential in curriculum planning? The code, script or text by which a curriculum is organized may fundamentally shape a student's cognitive process. For example, an organ- or bodily systems–based curriculum teaches students from the outset to think in terms of specifics and not holistically, and is an invitation to objectification of patients and reduction of complex processes to linear explanations. The origin of the words "organize" and "organ" are the same – the Greek *organon* and Latin *organum* meaning "an instrument" or "a tool". "Organs" are cast as functional and an organ/systems-based curriculum as instrumental.

Having taken the person out of his or her historical, cultural and social contexts, and then after biologizing the person and breaking him or her down into disparate systems, how do we put such systems back into context and treat the patient as a whole, rather than continue to reduce patients to presenting symptoms, or case them in population statistics? In other words, how do we develop a curriculum true to the descriptor "biopsychosocial" (this might be extended to the cumbersome "biopsychosocialimmunological") (Kusnanto, Agustian and

Hilmanto 2018); or one grounded in the (again cumbersome) "psycho-somato-socio-semiotic" (Pauli, White and McWhinney 2000), rather than just reductive "biomedical" promising objectification of persons-in-communities?

Developing a patient-centred curriculum with multiple patients and no centre: A Longitudinal Integrated Clerkship/ Curriculum

A century after the Flexner Report and in response to the intervening century of medical education, a new "Carnegie Report" was published (Cooke, Irby and O'Brien 2010). This encouraged medical schools to develop a longitudinal, integrated clerkship (LIC) as a key, work-based, curriculum component. Medical students are attached to a group of patients and follow them over a period of time, thus gaining experience by shadowing patients' journeys through physical and mental medical diagnoses and treatments and, importantly, varieties of community-based social care. But what is more, they get to know how patients live with symptoms in a non-medicalized way, thus seeing patients as persons and citizens first. The student observes and learns from a range of family-, community- and clinically based experiences and is able to contextualize these in the wider knowledge of patients' lives. Naturally, the number of patients seen will be limited, and understanding of their treatments and care must be supplemented by other activities based in classroom or laboratory learning. A blueprint can be made to itemize what essential knowledge and skills have not been gained from the LIC experience, so that these gaps can be addressed. Students learn about prevention as much as cure.

Safety requirements mean that students cannot carry out certain clinical interventions *in vivo* before these have been practised to a set level of competence *in vitro*. Even with the most sophisticated LIC curriculum, it will be necessary for medical students to learn to relate to "patients" beyond flesh-and-blood, "authentic" patients in clinics, consulting rooms, at the bedside, in operating theatres, in the emergency department, undergoing adjunct treatments such as physiotherapy or radiology or in the community. The "patient" also appears as cadavers for dissection and prosection, or inspection during autopsy; anatomical specimens; actor-patients; "paper patients" in problem-based learning scenarios; basic anatomical models; complex manikins such as SimMan; plastinated specimens; online virtual bodies; medical images; paper or electronic records; specimens in laboratories (blood tests, biopsy); anonymized in pharmaceutical trials or in research activity and subsequent reporting; online patient forum activity; a member of an expert advisory group; representations through public engagement projects such as art exhibitions; media representations including television soap operas, memoirs and fictions; and as a population statistic. It is in the mirrors of the mix of such *in vivo* (authentic and simulated) and *in vitro* (dead, alive but simulated, and informational) patient presentations that the identity of the proto-doctor is formed to displace the identity of the novice medical student.

Examples of how the "patient" (the object of learning) can appear

- Flesh-and-blood real life.
- A "case" in a multi-disciplinary team meeting or a grand round.

- A subject of "corridor conversations" between clinicians.
- A constantly re-constructed set of narratives.
- Cadavers for dissection, or inspection during autopsy.
- Anatomical specimens.
- In intensive care.
- Confused, in psychiatric care.
- Actor-patients.
- "Paper patients" in PBL scenarios.
- Basic anatomical models.
- Complex manikins such as SimMan.
- Plastinated specimens.
- Online virtual bodies.
- Medical images.
- In "recovery" at a substance and alcohol abuse support group.
- Augmented patients with a variety of technological enhancements.
- Paper or electronic records.
- Specimens in laboratories (blood tests, biopsies).
- Anonymized in pharmaceutical trials or in research activity.
- Online patient forum activity.
- Member of an expert advisory group.
- Representations through public engagement projects such as art exhibitions.
- Media representations including television soap operas, memoirs and fictions.
- A population statistic.
- In the imaginary, or archive, of medical education as textbook "cases", where they may even be canonized in medical eponyms.

However and wherever the "patient" appears, a curriculum text bias will directly affect the quality of learning. For example, as noted already, the curriculum is commonly treated as an instrumental or functional text, stripped back to a list of learning outcomes as "competences" and assessed unimaginatively, failing for example to provide opportunities for criteria-based self- and peer-assessments. This readily leads to objectification of patients and a well-documented pattern of empathy decline requiring compensatory education (Batt-Rawden et al. 2013), paralleled by a rise in intolerance of ambiguity, emotional detachment and cynicism ("tough minded" pessimism mistaken for realism). The medical student is "good enough".

Here, *in vitro* and *in vivo* patients may be subject to a common gaze that reverts back to conservative tradition and a will-to-stability in learning ("please don't rock the boat", "if it ain't broke, don't fix it"). The curriculum is crystallized, reduced to building blocks of syllabus chunks, often based on organs- or systems-thinking and a crude distinction between the "normal" and the "pathological", rather than a more integrative and holistic model such as a life-cycle approach. Patient-centredness (Stewart et al. 1995; Stewart 2001) is now impossible as traditional medical hierarchies are conserved and strengthened.

Such conservatism may be blamed on lack of resources rather than on lack of pedagogical imagination, where the curriculum as an economic text interweaves with curriculum as an instrumental text. This is not to deny or decry curricula as either economic or instrumental texts – funding and functionalism are central parts of all curricula. Rather, we must note how other influences – such as curriculum as aesthetic, ethical and political texts – are engaged. "Tradition" too is often invoked as a justification for conservative curriculum planning (curriculum as a historical text), with a plea for maintaining "continuity". But history here is treated literally as an unbroken lineage rather than seen as a messy series of events open to interpretation, where curricula can be read genealogically, the central question being: "what are the conditions of possibility for the curriculum to take shape in this way?"

In a competitive, free market, neo-liberal economically centred society, we can see why the major values driving curriculum development are economic instrumentalism and functionalism, leading to an obsession with immediate outcomes (competences) rather than long-term possibilities ("horizon" capabilities). The curriculum is subsumed within the "organ-ization". In a climate of deep social inequality, contemporary medicine curricula can so readily mirror this condition through an intake profile that bears little resemblance to the general population. There have, of course, been some values shifts such as intake that was once almost wholly male now showing a 60:40 bias to women, yet little attention has been paid to how the medicine undergraduate curriculum advertises its qualities as a gendered text.

If we shape a curriculum as highlighting an interweaving of aesthetic, ethical and political texts, we are more likely to address the deadening effects upon learning of instrumentalism – to give the curriculum life, vitality and vision without losing essentials for developing a medical student into a junior doctor. For example, reading the curriculum as a political text necessarily asks fundamental questions about how a curriculum addresses issues of equity, equality, social justice and democracy. Here, conservatism is challenged as learning is framed in terms of opportunity and experimentation. Again, curriculum planners must "think otherwise" by thinking with curriculum theory.

For example, framing a curriculum in terms of an authentic democratic experiment would lead to patient-centredness without a centre, or to patient-directedness. This is the ability for medical students to learn that a professional encounter with a patient is not necessarily a justification for the exercise of knowledge and technique as power over the patient, but rather a platform for empowering the patient in a collaborative act of resistance against traditions of conservative authority. Here, medicine is explicitly political. In turn, the dialogue with a patient refreshes the doctor's understanding of clinical medicine and the social contexts for health and illness. Framing the curriculum as an aesthetic text demands that we place high value on educating the senses for close noticing in diagnostic work (Bleakley 2020). Here, developed sensibility (particularly developing diagnostic acumen) and sensitivity (developing empathy for patients, collaborative capabilities for working in flexible teams, and self-care) become primary learning outcomes.

It is often hard for medical students not to reduce patients to objects when seniors frequently model this. Meeting "patients" *in vitro* reinforces this, where, by definition, "they" have no feelings (even as actor-patients), such as anatomical models and animations, SimMan, paper PBL cases, laboratory tests, paper patient records or classic textbook cases. The curriculum as an aesthetic text would work to animate such patients as tutors develop the senses and aesthetic capabilities of students. For example, patient records, PBL cases, classic cases and so forth can be read as narratives rather than reduced to scientific "reports", focusing on the patient's chief concern rather than chief complaint (Schleifer and Vannatta 2013). There is a burgeoning literature on how to develop narrative thinking and techniques as a means of resisting reductive scientific thinking. This expands to ethics "cases" that can be read as narratives or medical fictions pretending objectivity, but larded with rhetoric (Chambers 1999). Working with actor-patients brings about greater appreciation of medicine as performance, where narratives are enacted. A dramaturgical model would describe "frontstage" and "backstage" performances where a variety of "masks" are adopted as appropriate to context. Professionalism and communication have long been taught through role-play.

Importantly, if students learned the basics of actor-network theory (ANT) and object-oriented ontology (Harman 2018), they would grapple with the idea that we can afford equal ontological status to humans and objects or artefacts. This would cut through the characteristic objection to working with simulations, that they do not reflect "real life". This might orient medical students to view, say, a patient on life support in intensive care as one element in a round of circulating objects (such as ventilators and patient notes) with, during treatment, equal ontological status.

Another view is to reject the object-oriented ontology for one that brings objects to life, or animates them. I have already outlined how the medical humanities can be used as the second stimulus in double stimulation learning, to expand the objects of medical education. Typically, for example, living and surface anatomy learning has been enhanced through the arts and humanities as second stimuli in dual stimulation. At Peninsula Medical School (UK), noting that students felt displaced and even disgruntled in learning invasive clinical skills *in vitro* on a manikin (albeit a sophisticated one), our visiting professor of Visual Art, Christine Borland, set up a project to explore and enhance the aesthetics of learning by simulation, culminating in a public engagement exhibition. As an example, Borland animated and aestheticized SimMan, re-contextualizing and vivifying the manikin through film, and also asking critical questions about gendering manikins through producing a one-off "simWoman" (https://vimeo.com/60543571; Richardson and Borland 2015). Paradoxically de-sensitized by the simulation setting, double stimulation set out to re-sensitize students through aesthetic appreciation and re-gendering of what is basically a plastic manikin.

In the following chapter, I set out in detail a curriculum reconceptualization experiment for an undergraduate medicine and surgery curriculum at a UK medical school.

Bibliography

Allport, GW. 1955. *Becoming: Basic Considerations for a Psychology of Personality*. New Haven, CT: Yale University Press.

Applebee A. 1996. *Curriculum as Conversation*. Chicago, IL: University of Chicago Press.

Barone T. 2000. *Aesthetics, Politics, and Educational Inquiry*. New York: Peter Lang.

Batt-Rawden SA, Chisolm MS, Anton B, Flickinger TE. Teaching Empathy to Medical Students: An Updated, Systematic Review. *Academic Medicine*. 2013;88:1171–17.

Bleakley A. 2020. *Educating Doctors' Senses Through The Medical Humanities: "How Do I Look?"* Abingdon: Routledge.

Chambers T. 1999. *The Fiction of Bioethics: Cases as Literary Texts*. London: Routledge.

Cooke M, Irby DM, O'Brien BC. 2010. *Educating Physicians: A Call for Reform of Medical School and Residency*. San Francisco, CA: Jossey-Bass.

Doll MA. 2019. *The Reconceptualization of Curriculum Studies: A Festschrift in Honor of William F. Pinar*. Abingdon: Routledge.

Foucault M. 1988. Technologies of the Self. In: L Martin, H Gutman, P Hutton (eds.) *Technologies of the Self: A Seminar with Michel Foucault*. London: Tavistock, 16–49.

Harman G. 2018. *Object-Oriented Ontology: A New Theory of Everything*. London: Pelican.

Kusnanto H, Augustian D, Hilmanto D. Biopsychosocial Model of Illnesses in Primary Care: A Hermeneutic Literature Review. *Journal of Family Medicine and Primary Care*. 2018;7:497–500.

Little P, Everitt H, Williamson I, et al. Preferences of Patients for Patient Centred Approach to Consultation in Primary Care: Observational Study. *British Medical Journal*. 2001; 322: 468–72.

McCain KW. 2015. "Nothing as Practical as a Good Theory" Does Lewin's Maxim Still Have Salience in the Applied Social Sciences? *ASIST 2015 Computer Science*. Available at: https://dl.acm.org/doi/10.5555/2857070.2857147

Pauli HG, White KL, McWhinney IR. Medical Education, Research, and Scientific Thinking in the 21st Century. *Education for Health: Change in Learning & Practice*. 2000;13;15–26 (part1)/13:165–186 (parts 2 and 3).

Pinar WF. 2006. *The Synoptic Text Today and Other Essays: Curriculum Development After the Reconceptualization*. New York: Peter Lang.

Pinar WF. 2011. *The Character of Curriculum Studies: Bildung, Currere, and the Recurring Question of the Subject*. New York: Palgrave Macmillan.

Pinar WF. 2012. *What is Curriculum Theory?* 2nd ed. London: Routledge.

Pinar WF and Reynolds WM. 2015. *Understanding Curriculum as Phenomenological and Deconstructed Text*. New York: Educator's International Press.

Richardson C, Borland C. Talking About a Christine Borland Sculpture: Effective Empathy in Contemporary Anatomy Art (and an Emerging Counterpart in Medical Training?) *Journal of Visual Art Practice*. 2015;14:146–61.

Schleifer R, Vannatta JB. 2013. *The Chief Concern of Medicine: The Integration of the Medical Humanities and Narrative Knowledge into Medical Practices*. Ann Arbor, MI: University of Michigan Press.

Spranger E. 1914. *Types of Men*. Bel Air, CA: G. E. Stechert Company.

Stewart M. Towards a Global Definition of Patient Centred Care. *British Medical Journal*. 2001; 322: 444–5.

Stewart M, Brown JB, Weston WW, et al. 1995. *Patient-Centred Medicine Transforming the Clinical Method*. Thousand Oaks, CA: SAGE.

Worley P, Couper I, Strasser R, et al. A Typology of Longitudinal Integrated Clerkships. *Medical Education*. 2016;50:922–32.

12 Curriculum reconceived

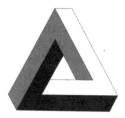

A medicine and surgery undergraduate curriculum for the future

UK medical schools enjoy a good deal of latitude over curriculum content and process while monitored for quality by the General Medical Council (GMC 1993, 2015, 2018a, 2018b). Graduates from these schools, however, must gain a common profile of competences before entering their first year of junior doctoring, the Foundation Programme – Foundation Year 1 (FY1). At the end of this year they are registered as doctors and enter the second year of the Foundation Programme (FY2), where they are prepared for either specialist training routes or general practice. A review of studies suggested that on graduation from medical school and entry into FY1, "trainees lack appropriate knowledge and skills in providing immediate care in medical emergencies (especially when things don't go according to plan) and areas where the evidence is mixed (e.g. learning and working effectively in a multidisciplinary team)" (Monrouxe 2014). This makes sense in view of the analysis in previous chapters of the importance of learning tolerance for ambiguity in undergraduate settings, and adapting to fast-moving and open-ended fluid "teeming" in early clinical work.

Maulin Sharma, Ruth Murphy and Gillian Doody (2019) have recently scoped the literature on UK undergraduate medicine provision from 1996 to 2019 to discover trends. Surprisingly, almost shockingly, the literature revealed only 31 articles published since 2002 describing core curriculum recommendations, less than two articles per year. There are 33 medical schools recognized by the GMC in the UK. The focus of such literature (18 papers) was on the way in which clinical specialties, such as surgery, general practice, pathology, radiology, ENT, urology and dermatology, fed thinking from the specialty Royal Colleges into the medical school curriculum as blueprints. Four papers were related to foundation subjects such as anatomy and pharmacology, and four papers were related to professionalism, focusing on communication skills provision. Consensus statements were available for inclusion of medical ethics and communication, providing curriculum blueprints. The reality of such provision, however, was that it focused on syllabus (content) rather than the broader curriculum (course of study and processes of learning) to include process.

The paper notes that one regional medical school developed a core curriculum for the medical humanities. This was Peninsula Medical School (Universities of Exeter and Plymouth), and I was instrumental in developing that curriculum in particular with Dr Robert Marshall, a consultant pathologist and medical educator (Bleakley, Marshall and Brömer 2006). I was also involved in wider curriculum planning beyond medical humanities provision, prior to that I had developed several full curricula at postgraduate level in psychotherapy, clinical psychology and education. It is from these experiences that the curriculum model in this chapter is developed.

Sharma, Murphy and Doody (2019) note a large variation in structure and content provision that has led the GMC to set out a framework of standards for medical school graduates. Further, the GMC plans to introduce a common Licensing Exam by 2022. Sharma and colleagues (2019: 6) further note: "How individual providers of medical education map curriculum content, learning outcomes and assessments for specialties is not explicit". What is perhaps more surprising is that "content", "learning outcomes" and "assessment" should be assumed to form a "curriculum". This is a "lean" and instrumental reading of what is a complex educational process. Such a reading does not recognize that a curriculum is process as well as content – primarily that it is the process of constructing an identity or a self-forming; and that a curriculum serves a wider historically and culturally contingent process of conserving a culture (in our case, medicine) as it expands that culture, creating the conditions for innovation. Curriculum is first a verb rather than a noun; second, it is not a list of things to do, but rather a way of thinking about the doing.

Where Sharma and colleagues summarize what UK medical schools offer, there is little indication of how content may be best taught or learned, or in what locations this may best happen (such as classroom, anatomy laboratory, simulation laboratory, clinic, community or patients' homes). Reference is made to "multidisciplinary" approaches and to a "longitudinal integrated clerkship" that would presumably involve students following patients or patient groups over time. This hints at the curriculum as unfolding narrative, although any mention of "story" would seem incongruous in such a functional account. Content rather than process thinking again dominates where the authors suggest: "curricula could be split into essential, desirable and nice to know categories to help prioritise areas of teaching and learning" (ibid.: 6).

Pressures on medical schools for curriculum reconceptualization come from

1. Consumers through changing patient demographics. This includes a growing number of elderly patients with multiple chronic conditions, requiring

complex cross-specialty care in the community; a growing number of mental health-related issues such as treatments for anxiety and depression; and a changing profile of disease manifestations such as a sharp rise in cardiac conditions.

2. Royal Colleges promoting specialties interests, based partly on perceived future needs and partly on vested interests (for example, medical schools may have successful research interests in particular specialties, raising significant income and affording prestige).

3. Iatrogenesis – a recognition that a significant number of patient deaths occur through avoidable errors – has led to interest in providing patient safety input to the curriculum, especially around quality of intra- and inter-team communication.

But we must ask: who is the curriculum designed for – teachers, administrators, learners or patients? What might an authentic patient-centred undergraduate medicine curriculum look like? Here, I am not inquiring into specifics such as what could be taught in molecular biology, genetics, artificial intelligence, health economics, statistics, or best design of quantitative research and so forth. Rather, I concentrate on principles that shape a curriculum as ways of re-thinking what a medical education serves.

The Peninsula curriculum experiment

An undergraduate medicine and surgery degree for a new UK institution – Peninsula Medical School – was planned from 2000 and launched in 2002, but had been envisaged since the 1990s. The 1990s afforded a unique climate for the progress of medical education in the United Kingdom. The UK General Medical Council (GMC) published *Tomorrow's Doctors* in 1993, promoting a radical re-think of the core undergraduate medicine and surgery curriculum (GMC 1993). Students would learn a holistic, patient-centred approach and appreciate the impact of social and cultural contexts on health, where clinical experience would embrace community as well as hospital practice.

The curriculum set out a fundamental humanistic aim: to educate for democratic habits. This would form a basis to developing patient-centred practice, working with colleagues in inter-professional team settings, and engaging with social justice issues such as health inequities. Central to curriculum implementation was to educate for tolerance of ambiguity (hereafter "ToA") in the knowledge that ToA helps eventual transition to the complexities of clinical work (including the value conflicts this often entails), while intolerance of ambiguity is associated with authoritarian traits and inflexibility. DeForge and Sobal (1989: 869) described intolerance of ambiguity as "the perception of ambiguous situations as a threat" rather than a challenge, while Geller, Faden and Levine (1990: 619) argued that "If medical schools admitted students who possess a high tolerance for ambiguity, quality of care for ambiguous conditions might improve".

Disappointingly, more recent research shows that ToA remains characteristically low among medical students (Weissenstein et al. 2014). Central to curriculum planning was to develop medical humanities provision in particular as media for educating ToA and democratic habits. As Mark Slouka (2010: 168) notes: "The humanities are a superb delivery mechanism for what we might call democratic values". Students, for example, ran a decision-making student parliament that fed back into curriculum development groups.

The medical humanities aspect to the curriculum – both process and content – served, as noted in previous chapters, the important purpose of acting as a second stimulus in medical students' learning. Where (i) basic and applied sciences (including anatomy), (ii) clinical skills and (iii) work-based placements (with briefing and debriefing) formed the core curriculum and first stimulus, the medical humanities and ethics provided the second stimulus through which the core learning could be reconceptualized or creatively progressed, as a "thinking otherwise".

Content was learned in years 1 and 2 through small group, problem-based learning (PBL) settings and was based on a life cycle of normal development from conception to death. Anatomy was learned as surface and living modes, not through dissection. Clinical and communication skills were learned *in vitro* (simulation settings) with inter-professional staff groups such as nurses and actor patients. Work-based clinical placements were introduced from week one, and small group learning contexts allowed for reflection and de-briefing on these experiences, including communication aspects. In years 3 and 4, work-based clinical placements dominated, and the spiral curriculum progressed again through the life cycle but on this cycle focusing on disease and symptom from conception to death. Small group activities focused on clinical reasoning, and clinical and communication skills were mainly learned *in vivo* on clinical placements. Year 5 was an intensive work-based set of rotations with a shadowing of junior doctors built in. Assessment included regular progress tests for knowledge, Integrated Structured Clinical and Communication Examinations (ISCEs) and portfolios reflecting learning experiences. There were no "big bang" written examinations. The cumulative assessments allowed for profiling of strengths and weaknesses so that feedback and mentoring could be tailored to individual needs. Personal tutors were assigned for pastoral care. Emphasis was placed on the language used with and about patients – for example, students were encouraged to think of not "taking" a history, but rather "receiving" a history.

In 2013, Peninsula Medical School, due to political differences between the previously collaborating university hosts, was dissolved and two new schools were formed: the University of Exeter Medical School and the University of Plymouth Peninsula School of Medicine and Dentistry. The former was made part of the University of Exeter College of Medicine and Health, while the latter was recently absorbed into a larger interdisciplinary Faculty of Health at the University of Plymouth. Peninsula Medical School developed a School of Dentistry in 2006 and was re-named Peninsula College of Medicine and Dentistry. Peninsula – probably the most innovative of UK medical schools

– would also be the most short-lived due to a wholly political decision and not an educational one. Where many faculty members were previously in denial about the close relationship between medical education and politics, now they woke up to its consequences.

When five new UK medical schools were established in the early 2000s, despite the promise of *Tomorrow's Doctors*, medical education was highly instrumental, still in the grip of the model blueprinted by Abraham Flexner's 1910 report – with little meaningful patient contact prior to Year 3. Flexner's legacy was a rigid anatomy and science training for the first two years, to socialize medical students as bench scientists before they became clinicians. The new pedagogical climate promised in the wake of *Tomorrow's Doctors* would encourage early and sustained contact with patients through work-based learning, and more intensive learning of clinical and communication capabilities through safety-conscious simulation. This invited patient-centred pedagogical innovations influenced by a new wave of studies of workplace activity outside medicine, collectively termed "social learning" and "new apprenticeship" theories (Bleakley 2002). Cultural-Historical Activity Theory (CHAT) had already been at the cutting edge of these approaches to learning and work for some time (Engeström 1987; Cole 1989; Cole, Engeström and Vasquez 1997; Daniels et al. 2010).

What kinds of doctors do patients want?

The first question we asked ourselves in planning an innovative curriculum was "what do patients want from their doctors?" We turned to an emergent literature discussing and evaluating authentic patient-centred approaches (reflecting patients' views and not what doctors think patients want). While the descriptor "patient-centred" was first introduced into medicine in the mid-1950s, the *practice* did not gain traction until the 1980s (Stewart et al. 1995; Bleakley 2014). Patient-centred medicine advertised a paradigm shift of enormous consequence, best understood "for what it is not – technology centred, doctor centred, hospital centred, disease centred" in Moira Stewart's words (Stewart 2001: 444). But it was not until the 1990s that patient-centred pedagogies acquired traction in medical *education*.

The research literature on the topic is now mature and repeats the same message offered by the foundational study of Paul Little and colleagues (Little et al. 2001) on what patients want from their consultations in primary care. In short, they seek mutual understanding of, and attention to, their presenting symptoms in the wider context of their worlds, including emotional needs. This should strengthen the professional relationship between patient and doctor as a platform for future consultations. Later evidence adds: patients want doctors who are not just technically efficient but also trustworthy (Bleakley 2019), often generating trust through appropriate touch (Kelly et al. 2019); and can empathically "inhabit" patients' stories where "More empathetic physicians are more likely to achieve higher patient satisfaction, adherence to treatments, and health outcomes' (Costa et al. 2014: e89254).

This profile of the ideal doctor has, however, been compromised by two contexts: health services that are over-burdened and under-resourced, and a medical education system that reproduces debilitating habits. The latter includes communicating relatively poorly with patients and colleagues despite bespoke undergraduate training; cognitive empathy decline and objectification of patients as symptoms of increasing levels of cynicism; and deteriorating self-care associated with increasing incidence of anxiety, anomie, depression and burnout. These symptoms were already noted in the early 2000s and – despite the hope for a culture change in medical education that emerged out of the early 1990s – are seen by many to have returned with a vengeance in the current era of over-zealous regulation (patient safety trumping patient care) and standardization (with associated competences and over-determined assessments).

Returning to the era post-*Tomorrow's Doctors*, if that climate of innovation were summed up in one word it might, again, be "democracy". Medicine had, historically, functioned hierarchically with an over-zealous work ethic and a punishing socialization. The culture was also overtly masculine and valued the heroic individual. Now, a paradigm shift was at work valuing democratic habits such as patient- and colleague-centredness (or inter-professional collaboration). The increase in women entrants to medical schools, outnumbering their male colleagues, invited the development – without being essentialist – of a more "feminine" medicine that can be characterized as collaborative and "tender-minded" (optimistic and open) rather than "tough-minded" (pessimistic and closed, or cynical). Research evidence began to support the practical turn in this pedagogical vision. For example, hospitals with strongly democratic teamwork cultures outperformed those with more hierarchical cultures in terms of patient outcomes and safety, and staff work satisfaction (Borrill et al. 2000).

In the knowledge that medical education typically reduces cognitive empathy and increases cynicism, we set out to counter this trend. A key curriculum innovation in response to these issues was to develop the medical humanities as core and integrated provision. Drawing on the arts, humanities and liberal social sciences can generate a curriculum climate for humanizing, and promoting democratic habits (Bleakley 2015). First, what innovative pedagogical framework should be drawn on to design and implement the curriculum?

A pedagogical framework fit for purpose

Medical education had been dominated by learning theories focused on the individual's acquisition of knowledge and skills (often in simulated settings) applied to work contexts as transfer of learning (Bleakley 2002). This model is not fit for purpose in contemporary medical education, where doctors work largely within fluid, multi-team contexts demanding skills and knowledge co-ordination deepening to social co-operation and collaboration (Engeström 2008). Social learning frameworks, such as CHAT, promote a quite different view of knowledge, skills and values acquisition. The gradual adoption in medical education of such frameworks over two decades has created another paradigm shift paralleling authentic

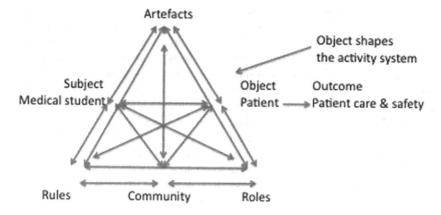

Figure 12.1 Initial learning in medicine as an activity system

patient-centredness, inter-professional learning and engagement with social justice issues.

Where individualistic learning theories are grounded in a Western ideology that promotes self-sufficiency, social learning theories have their origins in Marxist dialectical materialism. "Dialectic" describes negotiation among competing positions, where "materialism" describes how concrete goods are produced and consumed. Production, distribution and exchange of goods and services (including knowledge) necessarily involve negotiation between contradictory positions in a network of power. CHAT describes how multiple, historically contingent forces, material objects and humans interact around complex tasks in ways that utilize such contradictions as drivers for learning rather than seeing them as hindrances. Learning is conceived as the development or expansion of activities, where learners are encouraged to take risks and step out into the unknown while they are "scaffolded" by what they already know and can do, and by the presence of trusted teachers or facilitators. This expansive front-line of scaffolded learning – the zone of proximal development (ZPD) – is characterized by the value of dialogue, making it a radically democratic model.

The adoption of CHAT as our guiding framework for curriculum design and implementation is summarized in Figure 12.1. Each element of the activity system was equally important in curriculum planning, while the object of the activity system – in this case the "patient" – shapes activities.

Medical humanities as core and integrated curriculum provision

How then to develop ToA, sensibility and sensitivity – to humanize our students and inoculate them against empathy decline, cynicism and burnout – when much of their early "patient" contact is necessarily *in vitro* (actor patients, manikins, models) rather than *in vivo*? At the time of conceiving the medical school, the chief medical officer (1991–98) for England was Sir Kenneth Calman. He was a passionate advocate of the new wave of thinking behind *Tomorrow's Doctors*, and of the "rounded" doctor who does not oppose science/technology and the arts/ humanities but rather seeks to bring them into fruitful conversation. Our students were encouraged to appreciate medicine as an art as well as a science.

A main purpose of the arts is to encourage creative "thinking otherwise"; and of the humanities, to promote democratic habits and tolerance of difference, as noted. The medical humanities had been established for some time particularly in North American medical schools but not in UK schools, and nowhere as core, integrated and assessed curriculum content and process (Bleakley, Marshall and Brömer 2006) where they can authentically provide gravity of curriculum presence to act as second stimulus in double stimulation.

As discussed earlier, Lev Vygotsky and associates described experiments where children were asked to solve problems that were essentially contradictory. Faced with high levels of uncertainty about how to proceed, a second stimulus would be introduced that in itself was ambiguous, but also would offer a means to both understand and interfere with the first stimulus. The children would be moved on to an expanded level of involvement with the problems or tasks at hand through double stimulation, but the outcome would not be predictable – these were not controlled "experiments" but self-generative activities. They describe what happens too when adults shift problem-solving contexts into problem-stating contexts. In the face of a wave of interest in medical schools in problem-based learning (PBL) in small groups with limited teacher input but rather hands-off facilitation, we capitulated in naming our learning process PBL. However, we insisted with students that patients should not be framed as "problems" (although of course diagnostic work requires problemsolving in principle).

Our double stimulation experiment employing the medical humanities suggested to us that clinical learning could encompass aesthetic self-forming, or the generation of qualities as the heart of the learning process. Later, as described in the following chapter, our curriculum overhaul or reconceptualization would introduce PPBL – patient- and population-based learning – as we realized that a key deficiency in our curriculum model was lack of emphasis upon political and social justice issues set in community-oriented, public medicine that refused medicalization in promoting medicine's accommodation to a variety of other approaches.

In designing and implementing the original curriculum, four approaches were developed: (i) anatomy and biomedical sciences; (ii) clinical and communication skills (including applied social sciences); (iii) hands-on work placements with briefing and debriefing; and (iv) medical humanities and ethics (with some law input). As chair of the latter curriculum development group, I engaged in a good deal of footwork, brokering, and staff development input, moving between the four groups. Students worked with anatomy, science and clinical skills faculty committed to educating with ethical, aesthetic and political values and dimensions to their work. "Boundary crossings" (Kerosuo and Engeström 2003) were achieved through staff development programmes realizing "perspective taking". For example, a biomedical scientist would look at her work from the point of view of an ethicist and a visual artist, considering wider issues such as transparency and public engagement.

Informing curriculum planning, a developing evidence base suggested permeating value for the medical humanities in educating for democratic values and practices. Subsequent studies have confirmed such value. A systematic review by Batt-Rawden and colleagues (2013) notes that arts- and humanities-based interventions (such as immersion in patients' narratives) are as successful as more instrumental interventions (such as communication skills training) in developing empathy in medical students. There is also a well-documented correlation between medical humanities curriculum provision and increases in ToA (Mangione et al. 2018). Medical students who are more "open to experience" are also less prone to develop cynicism (O'Tuathaigh et al. 2019), while ToA and engaged empathy are closely linked in preventing doctors' burnout (Kim and Lee 2018).

Medical humanities "spearheads" as a zone of proximal development

The curriculum was then developed in a unique climate of medical education innovation. The primary potential of CHAT rested with articulating trajectories for practice innovations, described by Yrjö Engeström (2018) as deliberate steps away from "tradition" (as a "will-to-stability") towards "possibility knowledge" or learning for change, where the loci for learning are fluid forms of collaboration. In maintaining a traditional "will-to-stability" curriculum, medical education is in danger of reproducing intolerance of ambiguity, empathy decline, emotional insulation, cynicism and poor self-care.

Specific innovative learning trajectories marked a shift from an older, individual-heroic medicine to a more collaborative and dialogue-based practice as a paradigm shift from "masculine" to "feminine" values embracing a more optimistic and less cynical medicine ("tender-minded" rather than "tough-minded"). Each of these innovations affords what Engeström (ibid.) terms a "spearhead" (Figure 12.2), to represent a focused ZPD for expansive learning. This articulates the creative momentum hinted at in Figure 12.2, serving to radically widen the horizon of possibility for the curriculum.

CHAT provided an indispensable model in focusing ideas about curriculum design and, during implementation, developing practice innovations. The main drivers were multiple interactions between mediators for learning (dialectic) and multi-voiced activity (dialogue). In both dialectical and dialogical activities, learning occurs as events are turned into experiences – or, events become meaningful to those who purposefully participate in them. This involved innovative pedagogies such as consented peer-examination for learning surface and living anatomy; actor-patients facilitating communication; nurses teaching clinical skills; ethics-focused ward rounds; a student parliament; expert-led briefed and

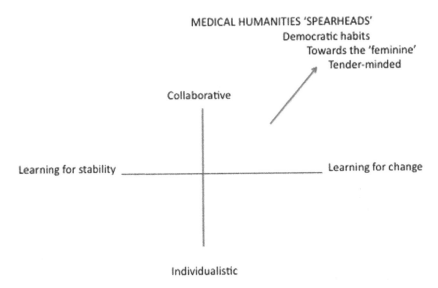

Figure 12.2 Three innovations, as medical humanities "spearheads", form a ZPD for expanding learning

debriefed work-based learning placements; and pervasive medical humanities curriculum process and content.

CHAT inspired both planning and implementation of the curriculum based on a variety of responses to the question "what do patients want from their doctors?" The curriculum was designed, implemented, evaluated and adapted through cycles of expansion of the primary object of activity – kinds of "patients" (both *in vivo* and *in vitro*) and modes of patient care. Tensions and contradictions between medical students developing identities as doctors-in-training or proto-professionals and medicine's historically dependent norms and mediating artefacts served as energizing forces for possibility learning through democratic process. The medical humanities can provide media through which such possibility learning is realized, and offers a second stimulus to "jump start" learning into an expanded vision. CHAT proves to be an approach that embraces and celebrates opportunism and serendipity as much as rational design.

The first model of the Peninsula curriculum had many interesting innovations, but also several blind spots to expansion that created opportunities dressed as contradictions. For example, due to logistical reasons, we were never able to develop a longitudinal integrated clerkship (LIC) model, where students were matched with a panel of patients, and would follow these patients wherever they were: in clinics, hospitals, GP practices, with carers, in physiotherapy and so forth, over a period of time (Cooke, Irby and O'Brien 2010). Our PBL "cases" were still "paper" cases in Years 1 and 2. Many of the faculty warmed to an LIC model and to converting PBL cases to live patients, but this was one area in which the curriculum showed a lack of imagination. However, through use of the medical humanities as second stimulus, we had addressed the issue of curriculum as aesthetic text. In the following chapter, I describe a radical overhaul of the curriculum described here to embrace curriculum as political text, where medical education could engage with health inequalities, social justice issues and health eco-literacy.

Bibliography

Batt-Rawden SA, Chisolm MS, Anton B, Flickinger TE. Teaching Empathy to Medical Students: An Updated, Systematic Review. *Academic Medicine*. 2013;88:1171–17.

Bleakley A. Pre-Registration House Officers and Ward-Based Learning: A "New Apprenticeship" Model. *Medical Education*. 2002;36:9–15.

Bleakley A. 2014. *Patient-centred Medicine in Transition: The Heart of the Matter*. Dordrecht: Springer.

Bleakley A. 2015. *The Medical Humanities and Medical Education: How the Medical Humanities Can Shape Better Doctors*. Abingdon: Routledge.

Bleakley A. Invoking the Medical Humanities to Develop a #MedicineWeCanTrust. *Academic Medicine*. 2019; 10: 1422–24.

Bleakley A, Marshall R, Brömer R. Toward an Aesthetic Medicine: Developing a Core Medical Humanities Undergraduate Curriculum. *Journal of Medical Humanities*. 2006;27:197–213.

Borrill C, West MA, Shapiro D, Rees A. Team Working and Effectiveness in Health Care. *British Journal of Health Care Management*. 2000;6:364–71.

Cole M. Cultural Psychology: A Once and Future Discipline. *Nebraska Symposium on Motivation*. 1989;37:279–335.

Cole M, Engeström Y, Vasquez O. 1997. *Mind, Culture and Activity*. Cambridge: Cambridge University Press.

Cooke M, Irby DM, O'Brien BC. 2010. *Educating Physicians: A Call for Reform of Medical School and Residency*. San Francisco, CA: Jossey-Bass.

Costa P, Alves R, Neto I, et al. Associations Between Medical Student Empathy and Personality: A Multi-Institutional Study. *Public Library of Science One*. 2014;9:e89254.

Daniels H, Edwards A, Engeström Y, et al. 2010. *Activity Theory in Practice: Promoting Learning Across Boundaries and Agencies*. London: Routledge.

DeForge BR, Sobal J. Intolerance of Ambiguity in Students Entering Medical School. *Social Science and Medicine*. 1989;28:869–74.

Engeström Y. 1987. *Learning by Expanding: An Activity-theoretical Approach to Developmental Research*. Helsinki: Orienta-Konsultit Oy. Available at: http://lchc.ucsd.edu/mca/Paper /Engestrom/Learning-by-Expanding.pdf

Engeström Y. 2008. *From Teams to Knots: Activity-Theoretical Studies of Collaboration at Work*. Cambridge: Cambridge University Press.

Engeström Y. 2018. *Expertise in Transition: Expansive Learning in Medical Work*. Cambridge: Cambridge University Press.

Geller G, Faden RR, Levine DM. Tolerance for Ambiguity Among Medical Students: Implications for Their Selection, Training and Practice. *Social Science & Medicine*. 1990;31:619–24.

General Medical Council (GMC). 1993. *Tomorrow's Doctors*. London: GMC.

General Medical Council (GMC). 2015. *Promoting Excellence: Standards for Medical Education and Training*. Available at: https://www.gmc-uk.org/-/media/documents/

Promoting_excellence_standards_for_medical_ education_and_training_0715.pd f_61939165.pdf

General Medical Council (GMC). 2018a. *Outcomes for Graduates*. Available at: https:// www.gmc-uk.org/-/media/documents/dc11326-outcomes-for-graduates-2018_pdf-7504 0796.pdf

General Medical Council (GMC). 2018b. *Medical Licencing Assessment*. Available at: https://www.gmc-uk.org/education/standards-guidance-and-curricula/projects/medic al-licensing-assessment

Kerosuo H, Engeström Y. Boundary Crossing and Learning in Creation of New Work Practice. *Journal of Workplace Learning*. 2003;15:345–51.

Kim K, Lee Y-M. Understanding Uncertainty in Medicine: Concepts and Implications in Medical Education. *Korean Journal of Medical Education*. 2018;30:181–88.

Little P, Everitt H, Williamson I, et al. Preferences of Patients for Patient Centred Approach to Consultation in Primary Care: Observational Study. *British Medical Journal*. 2001;322:468–72.

Mangione S, Chakraborti C, Staltari G, et al. Medical Students' Exposure to the Humanities Correlates with Positive Personal Qualities and Reduced Burnout: A Multi-Institutional U.S. Survey. *Journal of General Internal Medicine*. 2018;33:628–34.

Monrouxe L. 2014. *How Prepared Are UK Medical Graduates for Practice? Final Report from a Programme of Research Commissioned by the General Medical Council*. Available at: https://www.gmc-uk.org/-/media/gmc-site-images/about/how-prepared-are-uk-medical -graduates-for-practice.pdf?la=en&hash=1D87E30FB8A260AB20D662629D0F65 4FB64695FA

O'Tuathaigh CMP, Idris AN, Duggan E, et al. Medical Students' Empathy and Attitudes Towards Professionalism: Relationship with Personality, Specialty Preference and Medical Programme. *PLoS One*. 2019;14:e0215675.

Sharma M, Murphy R, Doody G. Do We Need a Core Curriculum for Medical Students? A Scoping Review. *BMJ Open*. 2019;9:e027369.

Slouka M. 2010. *Essays From the Nick of Time: Reflections and Refutations*. Minneapolis, MI: Graywolf Press.

Stewart M. Towards a Global Definition of Patient Centred Care. *British Medical Journal*. 2001;322:444–5.

Stewart M, Brown JB, Weston WW, et al. 1995. *Patient-Centred Medicine Transforming the Clinical Method*. Thousand Oaks, CA: SAGE.

Weissenstein A, Ligges S, Broiwer B, et al. Measuring the Ambiguity Tolerance of Medical Students: A Cross-Sectional Study from the First to Sixth Academic Years. *BMC Family Practice*. 2014;15:Article 6.

13 Democratic gestures

Language as power: A curriculum teaching medical students to democratize talk in the consultation

As noted earlier, a medicine curriculum, suggest Pauli, White and McWhinney (2000), is "psycho-somato-socio-semiotic" as well as biological. The "semiotic" refers to signs and symbols for communication, extending written and spoken language to use of objects, media and the non-verbal. The "curriculum as conversation" (Applebee 1996) then embraces the semiotic, acting as a primary artefact for expanding activity. Semiotically, "curriculum as conversation" connotes both dialogue and emotional entanglement with warmth, engagement and what linguists and anthropologists refer to as "turn-taking" (Drew and Heritage 2006), a universal conversational pattern (Sidnell 2007).

Also, an important development in medicine has been the technological revolution, where instruments or artefacts such as scopes and scanners, and their subsequent images, mediate diagnostic and treatment interventions. These provide a range of specialist technical semiotics – medical signs, symbols, images and metaphors that need to be translated by doctors into lay terms in consultations with patients.

In its third historical phase of development (Engeström 2018), Cultural-Historical Activity Theory (CHAT) has moved from intra-community of practice mediation of learning by artefacts and collaboration – with particular emphasis on the tension between horizontal sharing of resources and interpellation through vertical power structures or hierarchies – to communities of practice intersections between activity systems with potentially shared objects. This introduces issues of boundary keeping and boundary crossing, as noted in previous chapters. In contemporary medicine, "patient-centredness" would indicate shared objects and facilitation of boundary crossing. Language – signs and symbols – are important media for facilitation of boundary crossing.

Where healthcare has become increasingly focused on multiple disciplinary provisions around individual patients, for example with an elderly population displaying multiple chronic conditions, co-ordination of such provision has become a priority. But for such provision expertise to develop, co-ordination must progress to collaboration and communication – in other words, a wholesale democratizing of care. As this book argues, this is a political as much as a therapeutic challenge. Authentic democracy promises to be the shared, facilitative sign and symbol that signifies a new horizon for healthcare, while issues of boundary crossing for practitioners are at the core of its fulfilment. Such a vision describes the progress of Hegelian spirit (the realization of community) in healthcare through "the dialogic imagination" (Bakhtin 1982) and historical-dialectical process.

However, historically, medical language, signs and symbols have served to create boundaries between doctors and their patients and frustrate moves to transparency (Bleakley 2017). The communication issues of boundary crossing embrace, for example, the range of semiotics associated with diagnostic testing, such as the visual languages of sophisticated technological imaging, where, ironically, radiologists notoriously work as isolated figures rather than in collectives. However, radiologists have always contributed to inter-disciplinary clinical meetings, and are increasingly asked to meet face-to-face with patients (Bleakley 2020).

Medical education continues to find ways to encourage medical students to learn patient-centredness almost as a virtue, but unreflective and habitual use of specialist language and semiotics can stifle such ambitions. A co-ordinated effort is needed in medical education to bring about productive collaboration between patients, carers, doctors, other health- and social care professionals and students to transcend even "inter-professional" ambitions, and a common language and semiotics are central to such a vision. More, this is neither an idealistic nor an optimistic hope – one of a "happy families" vision. Rather, tensions, sticking points and contradictions will be the all-too-familiar terrain greeting a radical collectivist healthcare, but this can be re-visioned as Prospero's Island (in Shakespeare's *The Tempest*) seen through the eyes of the wise councillor Gonzalo, who scans a fertile common wealth, where sceptics see scrubland and furze.

How can we, through curriculum work, de-centre doctors' power and recast the clinical exchange as both a dialogical and dialectical conversation mediated by sign and symbol that develops patient-centredness and expands the possibilities of fruitful boundary crossing? Here, we must again treat the curriculum as conversation, with a view to reconceptualizing medicalized language to offer conversational and dialogical patient-centred care without a centre.

Following the critique of the medicalization of society as an assimilative strategy, discussed in Chapter 6, what would authentic patient-centred clinical talk look like as medical students can learn this, and how would this work as a dialectical strategy of resistance to longstanding structures of medical authority? This is not to say that medical students should not learn a technical language. Rather, it is to use technical language as the first stimulus within medical education (serving a socialization function), and to use lay language (now the stranger, or Other) as second stimulus through which patient-centredness is achieved.

Language as common property

While much of the Earth's natural resources such as land, minerals, oil and coal have been either privatized or are owned by governments or nations, we might think that language has remained uniquely free as common property. But of course this is not the case where specialist languages, such as medical jargon, have evolved as ways of providing inclusion for professionals and exclusion for laypersons. Language is political, or, as Nietzsche argued, language is expression of forces, intensities and differences. Language uses can then be resisted.

How can the curriculum exert influence as a political text in a simple gesture, such as democratizing medical talk by drawing on lay language or developing a shared language between doctor and patient? As noted previously, this can start with the simplest but also one of the most used (and abused) phrases in medical consultation: "taking a history" from a patient. As this is changed to "receiving a history" from the patient, this is not just a linguistic trick, but also a highly symbolic gesture of subscription to patient-centred practice.

As introduced in the previous chapter, at Peninsula Medical School (UK), a planning group set out to blueprint a curriculum fit for the 21st century with a view to future iterations. The broad brushstrokes of that planning are outlined below. However, as noted, political concerns intervened resulting in Peninsula, then a joint venture between two universities (Exeter and Plymouth), being dissolved as two new medical schools were formed. The curriculum blueprint (Bleakley 2012) was shelved.

I have returned to the archives to reconstruct the essence of that thought experiment to illustrate how curriculum can be used as a medium for re-thinking medical education. The important thing here is the set of principles that guided the shaping of that curriculum blueprint as a set of "ways of thinking". While our initial curriculum – developed from 2000 and applied first in 2002 – was widely considered as highly innovative, we promised that we would overhaul the curriculum at regular intervals, and this blueprint would have been our first major overhaul. It can now serve as a second stimulus for curriculum planning in medical education as the current curriculum, almost certainly riddled with inconsistencies and contradictions, is reframed or reconceptualized. Readers can obviously freely adopt the ideas here for reconceptualizing curricula in their own medical schools.

Again, socialization into medicine understandably involves learning a specialist technical language. This serves the dual purpose of allowing ease of communication between professionals and identity construction through identification with a common tongue that excludes the layperson. Such specialist language in all walks of life offers shorthand for conceptual understanding and remembering. This tongue is grounded in collapsing and translating what a patient suffers as "illness" into what a medical student and doctor understand as a "disease". The complex and contextualized narrative of the patient (the "chief concern") is collapsed into specifics and technical details (the "chief complaint") (Schleifer and Vannatta 2013). Classificatory schemata (e.g. "carcinomas of the skin" include "squamous cell" and "basal cell" types) aid diagnoses in medicine.

Of course sensitive doctors adapt to their patients' languages and semiotic cultures, but even the simplest of medical distinctions – for example between the workings and effects of a bacterium and a virus – can readily confuse and exclude patients. Thus, a patient demands an antibiotic for a sore throat, but the doctor knows this is an inappropriate treatment. However, simply pointing out the distinction between bacterial and viral infections may not help the patient and may end up causing confusion. A semiotic solution is necessary within the consultation. A large-scale study in Holland (Eggermont et al. 2018) showed that where female general practitioners met with women patients to discuss options for treating a sore throat, prescribing antibiotics was less frequent than in other gender mixes. It was the way the women doctors communicated that mattered. Semiotics is important in the consultation, where collaborative symbol production and metaphor use both oil and expand the dialogue. It is likely that the women-to-women meetings produced, in terms of talk, more dialogue and less of monologue (doctors' talking), affording an opportunity for informed negotiation of treatment.

This balance of talk, however, is symbolic of a gendered world. The same complex of language and semiotics (a dialogical imagination at work) underpins effective curriculum design. Metaphorically, as we saw in Chapter 8 and borrowing from Roland Barthes' semiotics, a curriculum may have an overall shape and rhythm, say that of a swell at sea producing land-bound waves. If you are all at sea planning a curriculum or implementing it, striving for innovation, do not panic but let the currents and waves bring you ashore and learn from what they afford.

A further example of taking medicine to patients through language: take the psychiatric label "attention deficit hyperactivity disorder" or ADHD, now enshrined as a treatable cognitive and behavioural condition in the Diagnostic and Statistical Manual of Mental Disorders (DSM). This is a readymade example of obfuscation (and, following Illich's and Szasz's arguments, of medicalization). The parent might say "Billy finds it impossible to concentrate, or stay at one thing for any length of time". If we cheekily recast this as a gain rather than a loss, we might say that Billy has "multiple attention possibilities and boundless energy". The parents might say "you try living with Billy", so I am not trying to be smart here. But the technical descriptor is like a straitjacket or an anchor.

The words are not actually even that technical – it's the way that they are put together and the smugness in which they form a label that captures a huge range of activity and, again, both medicalizes and negatively judges such activity. An assimilative medicine follows this model, where an accommodative medicine challenges such medical imperialism. The pharmaceutical companies add to the potential misery of patients with their semiotics, such as selling

Dexmethylphenidate under the brand name "Focalin" – a symbolic promise that the drug will reduce attention deficit and produce "focus".

Any sociologist of medicine (or any other profession) will tell you that exclusion through specialist language operates as a political tool, a form of power. The use of specialist language affords legitimate authority, but such authority may be wielded in ways that maintain exclusion rather than invite some inclusion, and that maintain hierarchy rather than inviting collaboration through democratic habits. As a democratic gesture, in order to bridge from doctor to patient and redistribute power and sensibility, could common "translational" terms be used? This would also embrace the curriculum as a phenomenological text, drawing on the lived experience of the patient.

Here are some examples:

<u>Patients' words: both physical and psychological symptoms</u>

Billy's just exhausting
I feel tired all the time
I feel depressed a lot of the time
It's like living in a fog or a bubble
I have uncontrollable anger
I get aches and pains all over
I drink a lot
I use drugs a lot
I don't feel safe a lot of the time
I'm homeless with no hope
I'm getting forgetful
I'm always reaching for painkillers
I have constant headaches
I have a lot of muscle pains
Food makes me feel sick
My body doesn't look right
I'm too fat
My skin's bad
I don't want to talk to anybody
I don't trust myself
I have no confidence
I'm frightened of sex
I'm lonely
I watch porn all the time
I always feel inferior
I don't like to go out
My skin's really flaky
I can't stop smoking
My breath smells
I have bad body odour

In turn, the doctor may be thinking about the patient's descriptions not in specific technical terms, but in general terms, as "semantic qualifiers" that aid clinical reasoning by sharpening up possibilities for a diagnosis from options presented by symptoms. The doctor's thinking process diverges from the patient's experience as the story told by the patient is represented medically at the generalized level of opposing pairs such as acute/chronic, proximal/distal, tender/non-tender, sharp/dull, insidious/abrupt. Such "semantic qualifiers" combine with an evolving tacit store of "illness scripts" that are prototypes or typical cases; for example, here is a script for croup:

1. Epidemiology: Infants and toddlers (6 months to 3 years). Usually late fall and early winter
2. Pathophysiology: Parainfluenza virus. Swelling/edema of the subglottic area (laryngo-tracheo-bronchitis)
3. Clinical Presentation:
    a. Viral URI prodrome followed by fever, barky cough, stridor and retractions usually ill appearing.
    b. Worse in middle of night.
    c. Gets better with warm steam or cold air.
    d. Steeple sign on AP soft tissue X-ray of neck.
4. Management: Dexamethasone p.o. × 1.

Except for 3b and 3c, we have now drifted away from the patient's world into the doctor's world. Here is a recent example of a COVID-19 diagnosis in the *British Medical Journal* (2020):

> An 80-year-old man has a dry cough. This has been present for five days and is getting worse. He also says he feels very tired and unwell. He is quite short of breath and is unable to speak a full sentence without taking a breath. On examination, he has a tachycardia and a fever. He also has conjunctivitis. Chest x-ray shows bilateral lung infiltrates, and computed tomography of the chest reveals multiple bilateral lobular and subsegmental areas of ground-glass opacity. ... This man had no previous illnesses.

The case is written for a medical audience, so I am not criticizing the language per se, and in introducing a cognitive aspect such as semantic qualifiers informing clinical reasoning (a widely taught strategy in medical education), I am reminding the reader that thought and language are of course intimately linked. But imagine you were talking to the patient in question (a phenomenological text). The first half of the case would make perfect sense, but the second half is riddled with technical clinical terms that would need to be translated in consultation. These mix technical language with semiotics such as the descriptors of X-ray and CT images that conjure visual signs and metaphors ("ground glass opacity").

    The thinking has now strayed far from "patient-centredness" (that is a deterritorializing tactic affording power to the patient) to reintroduce the boundary that denotes "medical territory: do not enter". Thus:

1. *Tachycardia* is a condition that makes your heart beat more than 100 times per minute: "your heart is racing".

2. A *pulmonary infiltrate*, observed on the chest X-ray, is a substance denser than air, such as pus, blood or protein, which lingers within the lungs: "your lungs are clogged, stopping you from breathing easily".

3. *Ground-glass opacity* is a metaphor or resemblance used to shortcut to an instant diagnosis (technically referring to an area of increased attenuation in the lung with preserved bronchial and vascular markings). While it is a non-specific sign with a wide aetiology including infection, chronic inter-stitial disease and acute alveolar disease, here it is linked with a COVID-19 infection. The patient could readily identify with this resemblance ("ground glass" as opaque) giving him (in the example above) a strong image for relating to his illness. Resemblances, often used as rapid diagnosis in medicine ("strawberry tongue" – possibly scarlet fever) can readily be related to by a layperson.

Typical generic medical words are sometimes already patient-friendly and so can be used readily in consultations:

Generic medical words with crossover potential for patients

Organ damage
Balance (as homeostasis)
Defence
Risk
Error
Safety
Life cycle, growth, maturation
Ageing
Damage and repair, regeneration
Control
Movement
Investigation
Diagnosis
Treatment
Decision-making
Prevention
Cure
Uncertainty
Ambiguity
Complexity
Change
Communication
Teamwork
Resource management

Rights
Responsibilities
Professionalism
Governance
Prevention
Treatment

Fundamental principles shaping the curriculum

Let us now move away from language and semiotics to broader pedagogical issues concerning curriculum design and implementation. In developing the Peninsula curriculum, we were guided by five primary issues:

1. We drew on curriculum reconceptualization models, where the curriculum is viewed as a verb (*currere*) – literally to "run the course". This switches the focus from content to process, where the curriculum is *embodied* and *performed*.
2. Conceptualization is vital – for example: "biomedical" is reductive, where "biopsychoimmunosocial" and/or "psycho-somato-socio-semiotic" are expansive. But how do we translate these baroque descriptors into everyday terms? Is "holism" as a generic descriptor more acceptable?
3. We preferred thinking with an issue (for example, damage and repair) rather than with an organ (for example, liver function), where the issue offers self-limitation or cramps capability and potential (otherwise labelled as "illness" or "disease"). Where "organ" or "body systems" curricula bind the medical student into, for example, the "circulatory system" or "the reproductive system", it is easy to forget or shelve the patients who, for example, are suffering from heart failure, or are HIV positive and whose intimates, family, friends and work colleagues are implicated. A more encompassing way of using curriculum "to think with" is conceiving of it as "life cycle" (at Peninsula, our first model was a "life cycle" curriculum with "normal" as first year and "pathological" as second year). But how can we be sure that this is inoculated against medicalization, so that, for example, "ageing" does not become an illness, or "deafness" a loss and stigma? A wider view is needed, moving from text to context. The curriculum as a political text is enacted in a variety of power contexts – for example, the patient reporting with symptoms of anorexia and self-harming is living in a dysfunctional family situation. The medical student suffering harassment through rolling micro-aggressions from a senior doctor on a work-based learning placement can be read as a political text suggesting inappropriate use of power. However, the wider context may be that the supervising doctor is suffering from work-related stress and has not been able to see how he or she has been displacing this onto the student. This may reflect a lack of psychological insight that can be addressed.
4. We preferred "limiting conditions" to "disease".

5. We preferred "complexity" to "linearity" (patients are persons; persons cannot be reduced to symptoms, diseases or organs without loss of quality in the clinical encounter; shorthand is not an excuse for objectification).

Medicine curricula are impoverished by poor design, such as:

1. Lack of theoretical understanding: curriculum is treated as a syllabus (content focus) and not as a variety of texts to think medicine with.
2. Who is the curriculum designed for? Teaching faculty and administration or patients and learners?
3. Curricula are conservative, focused on a will-to-stability, rather than innovative and progressive, focused on possibility knowledge, inquiry and meta-cognition.

(1)–(3) form resistance to conventional outcomes and competence based curricula, focused rather on process and capabilities (what is possible). This is also a transformative pedagogy.

Curriculum reconceptualization: A thought experiment

We began defining an undergraduate medicine curriculum through "sacred" principles, but this is necessarily an arbitrary list. These came out of a series of expert group meetings between clinician-educators and academics in medical education, where participants also responded as patients and consumers of health services. We generated a long list of themes from medical school faculty across disciplines, advertising a curriculum reconceptualization to change our current problem-based learning (PBL) curriculum to a patient- and population-based learning (PPBL), where patients and their illnesses are not cast as "problems" but as "limiting conditions", and community healthcare matters as much as hospital practice. Here is an example from a psychologist on the faculty (Table 13.1). Our initial list of themes serves as prompts, but participants were free to add their own themes, as this person did.

Through several meetings, we boiled curriculum themes down to a manageable number. This is to some extent arbitrary of course. We were happy for the list to be a "rough guide" to generate forward thinking. Our list is also biased to our interests in curriculum reconceptualization models, *currere*, and the curriculum as text. We thought of these principles as interacting, or, drawing on Deleuze and Guattari (2013), as territories without borders. The final, distilled, principles were:

1. Core holistic science.
2. What is "normal" and what is "pathological"?
3. Anatomy.
4. Democracy (patient-centredness without a centre).
5. Clinical reasoning.

Table 13.1 Generating illustrated themes for PPBL curriculum development

PPBL Curriculum Development (Example)

Your name (optional) _____
Area(s) of expertise Communication, psychology, psychotherapy, medical education, medical humanities _____

Thank you for agreeing to contribute to the development of the PPBL curriculum.
This questionnaire is designed to help us develop the content of the curriculum – the PPBL "cases".
We have decided to start this process with a set of "themes". These have been selected, following discussion with a number of clinicians and academics, to reflect the broad roles of doctors today. So that the PPBL cases represent the needs of patients and populations, we are asking you to identify examples for each of the themes that, in your speciality, discipline or area of interest, are **common** and/or **important**. As the number of PPBL cases is limited, we would like you to identify just one or two suggestions for each theme, not a comprehensive list. If you can briefly comment on the reasons you have chosen these examples, this is also helpful. We also ask you to add themes that you think are important.

At this stage we are purposefully not using the traditional medical systems approach. Rather we would like the themes to act as triggers for thinking about cross-specialty and inter-disciplinary approaches. It is important when making your responses to keep the medical student in mind rather than the faculty. What is important for students to learn and how should they learn?

THANK YOU VERY MUCH FOR YOUR TIME

THEME	1 or 2 common and/or important example (s) or scenarios from my area of expertise	Rationale/comment as to why chosen
Organ damage	Disability/poor quality of life	Psychological/emotional consequences of organ damage
Homeostasis & balance	Maximum complexity at the edge of chaos	Systems view of life is important/systems are inherently unstable
Feedback/feed forward Control	As a form of assessment of learning Excessive authority Intolerance of ambiguity	Feedback is essential for learning Intolerance of ambiguity is the mark of the authoritarian style
Defence	Defence mechanisms of the ego	Students must learn about the psychodynamics of encounters with patients & colleagues
Safety	Patient safety	70% of medical error grounded in systems based miscommunication (e.g. team)

		Greater support for carers
Life cycle, regeneration & ageing	Economic burden of an ageing population on younger members	
Damage & repair	Emotional damage e.g. from abusive relationships Support for victims of abuse	Knock-on effects of anxiety and depression GPs working with social workers & counsellors
Growth	Tumours grow as well as healthy bodies and minds Economists and bankers use terms like growth, development, trusts, bonds and securities as well as psychologists	Terms like "development" and "growth" should be treated critically
Storage and retrieval	Memory – dementia	An ageing population needing more care Resources needed for therapies such as reminiscence Psychological effects
Movement	Restricted movement e.g. chronic joint disorders	
Investigation	Taking/receiving a history Use of the senses Over-testing/unnecessary investigations	Why are doctors still so relatively poor at listening to patients? Are we losing physical examination acumen as we rely more on imaging and test? Is fear of complaint driving over-testing?
Diagnosis	Misdiagnoses account for 15% of medical errors Diagnostic acumen learned through hands-on encounters with more patients	Students need to know about autopsy findings Early and sustained patient contact to improve pattern recognition
Treatment	Many conditions are medicalized e.g. light anxiety and depression Patients not compliant – traces of antidepressants in the ground water	Driven by drug companies? Lack of time in consultations Treat the culture, not the patient
Learning	Any encounter with patients and colleagues implies learning with, from and about patients or colleagues Learning is where an event is turned in to an experience – the magic ingredient is imagination	Medical culture needs to be democratized Teachers need to be imaginative
Decision making	Holy Grail of medical education is "hot housing" clinical reasoning	We know how to do it, but the curriculum gets in the way! Early and sustained contact with patients, integrated with basic science.

(Continued)

Table 13.1 (Continued)

Prevention *vs.* cure	Self-care – doctors need to be more involved in prevention, starting with their own lifestyles	We need to learn how to do therapy on the culture, not on individuals (e.g. treating our mania)
Diversity	Tolerance of difference is the mark of the democratic person – people should be treated with respect and difference celebrated	Democratic literacy should be at the heart of the curriculum
Uncertainty and certainty	Admitting uncertainty is important in the consultation Educating for uncertainty is the function of the arts & humanities	Medical humanities should be core and integrated, as a way of educating for tolerance of ambiguity/uncertainty
Complexity	Human–artifact–languages interactions are necessarily complex	Students need to learn complexity science
Change	Medicine is a complex, adaptive system	Students need to learn complexity science
Systems	As above	As above
Mind body interaction	50% of presenting symptoms in a typical GP's practice are psychological/psychosomatic	Students need to learn psychological medicine
Communication	70% of medical error is grounded in miscommunication, mainly in team settings with colleagues	Students need to learn to communicate effectively with patients and colleagues
Teamwork	As above	As above
Resource management	Bullying in any setting lowers morale	Humans are resources Students need to learn about professional interpersonal communication
Ethics	Should I treat the person or the "numbers"?	Medical interventions have ethical dimensions
Self-management	Unacknowledged, chronic and disabling psychological patterns are repeated without challenge from others	Self-insight is the first step to psychological health
Quality improvement	Quality also means beauty, elegance and style	Professions have an aesthetic as well as an instrumental and ethical dimension
Law	My patient is sexually active but underage legally, and requires advice	What are the doctor's responsibilities?
Patient centredness	Patient-centredness is a work in progress	The evidence base suggests that medicine is yet to achieve authentic patient-centred status
Health v illness v disease	If a culture is ill and symptomizing, how can we judge the relative quality of individual "health"	Medical students must be able to contextualize patients historically, culturally and socially
Population health	If television is a barometer, the population is neurotic	How can students diagnose and treat social ills?

Individual and society	Narrative-based medicine (single patients) and evidence-based medicine (population) are in conflict	How do we square narrative-based and evidence-based practices?
Caring	"That's for nurses"	Whither inter-professional education?
Governance	Protocols should guide, not smother	We can educate into writing better protocols
Humanities	Empathy is key to patient-centred practice but empathy decline is a persistent phenomenon	Medical humanities provided as core and integrated in the curriculum can provide a vehicle for maintaining empathy
Culture	Medical provision and practice are culture-bound	Cross-cultural experience is essential for students
Structure	Complexity and systems thinking dissolves the structure–function opposition	Structures can be thought of as processes
Function	Medicine sometimes treats structures without regard for wider function e.g. Benign Prostatic Hyperplasia (BPH) treatments relieve urinary symptoms but ruin quality of sex life as a side effect	More informed conversations are needed between doctors and patients
Personal and professional development	Humans are vulnerable and liable to make mistakes	How can we develop a culture of support and education rather than blame and shame?
A good doctor	Is role modelling redundant as "professionalism" is institutionalized?	Is "character" part of professionalism?

PLEASE ADD ANY THEMES YOU FEEL ARE MISSING BELOW

Gender	Woman are better listeners than men	Why are women not well represented in senior positions in medical education?
Confrontation	Doctors are poor at handling confrontation. "Angry" patient incidents are on the increase	Students need to learn about confrontation
Sex and eroticism	Managing erotic transference and counter-transference between professionals and patients, and between colleagues	Students need to learn the difference between private and professional encounters, and manage erotic dynamics
Money	Doctors are now relatively highly paid	Are doctors worth their wages in an age of austerity?
Leadership	Should doctors lead multi-professional clinical teams?	What do we mean by "leadership"?

6. Complexity.
7. The idiographic and the nomothetic.
8. Location (where medicine happens).
9. Continuity (following patients over time).
10. Psychology.
11. Team players or collaborators (inter-professionals).
12. Authenticity.
13. Integration.
14. Identity.
15. Innovation.
16. Risk and safety.
17. Globalization.
18. Health eco-literacy

Some of these are set as contradictions or tensions. We then fleshed these out, as in Table 13.2.

A Question-Based Curriculum

We also mapped curriculum as text types against the principles (above), to generate questions – developing a "Question-Based Curriculum", where contradictions and questions form the springboard for inquiry. Here are some examples (Table 13.3).

We also mapped text types against most common illness presentations, to generate questions (Table 13.4). **This table has purposefully been left blank so that readers can draw on the template to generate their own questions.**

Most common illness presentations (limiting conditions):

1. Structural constraints on health (inequalities: economic, social, gendered, ethnic).
2. Ageing.
3. Cancers.
4. Obesity and diabetes.
5. Heart conditions.
6. Mental health, particularly depression and anxiety.
7. Respiratory conditions.
8. Medical error.
9. Road traffic accidents (RTAs), shootings and stabbings.
10. Domestic violence.
11. Gastric ulcer.
12. Addictions.
13. Headaches/migraines.
14. Inflammatory bowel disease.
15. Hypertension.
16. Rheumatoid arthritis.

Table 13.2 Curriculum territories without borders

Principle	Description	Curriculum shorthand
Science	The biomedical extended to THE BIOPSYCHOIMMUNOSOCIAL. While core science is essential, doctors are not primarily scientists, but as "science using" practitioners who also embrace the morality, artistry and humanity of medicine and its public duties Core science must include leading-edge issues such as artificial intelligence (AI), personalized medicine, genetic engineering, neuroscience and neuropsychology	HOLISM
Normal and pathological	A neat way of dividing form and function that has limitations in application Universal categories often fail in local settings Difficult to apply to mental health It may be better to think about LIMITING CONDITIONS	LIMITING CONDITIONS
Anatomy	Anatomy is essential to medical learning but may be best learned in view of how it will be used by most graduates – as surface and living anatomy Cadaver dissection is more a rite of passage and less a learning experience for human anatomy Bodies are best thought of in terms of embodiment, to resist objectification and view bodies as active Embodied persons are appreciated before they are explained	EMBODIMENT: SURFACE AND LIVING ANATOMY
Democracy	Medicine promises patient-centredness and inter-professional team care Medicine necessarily intersects with policy and politics.	DEMOCRATIZATION
Clinical reasoning	Conceptualizing or "thinking with" is vital to this model: thinking with an issue (damage and repair) or with an organ (liver function) is embedded in thinking with a person	"THINKING WITH" AS DIAGNOSTIC
Complexity	Closed systems are best understood through linear thinking The body is an open, complex, dynamic system best understood through complexity models	COMPLEXITY/DYNAMIC SYSTEMS

(Continued)

Table 13.2 (Continued)

Principle	Description	Curriculum shorthand
Idiographic and nomothetic	"Upstream" hospitalism is extended to "downstream" community health; patient- and population-based learning (PPBL) are given equal prominence	PATIENT- AND POPULATION-BASED LEARNING (PPBL)
Location	Wherever patients appear with health issues is where medicine happens	PATIENT PANELS
Continuity with patients	Patient panels extend to longitudinal attachments	LONGITUDINAL ATTACHMENT
Psychology	Relationships, communication and self-awareness extend to mental health Co-counselling educates for self and peer assessment, self-help and mentoring of peers; basics of psychodynamic psychology inform co-counselling outlook Facilitator skills and styles	COMMUNICATION/SELF HELP/ HELPING OTHERS
Team players or collaborators	Teams are multiple and dynamic and work better where hierarchies are flattened and leadership is distributed Doctors must become effective collaborators	NEGOTIATED KNOTWORKING
Authenticity	While medicine is performative, this does not negate the need for authenticity as a defence against cynicism	AUTHENTICITY
Integration	Medicine is a series of inter-dependent dynamic, complex, adaptive systems with emergent properties	INTEGRATION
Identity	Identity is conceived as process: not being, but becoming	BECOMING DOCTORS
Innovation	Creativity, imagination, thinking on your feet Dual stimulation through the medical humanities	POSSIBILITY KNOWLEDGE
Risk and safety	Holding the contradiction Patient care is extended to safety	CONTRADICTION AS RESOURCE/PATIENT SAFETY ESSENTIALS
Globalization	The local and the global Pandemics Collaboration	GLOBALIZATION
Health eco-literacy	Ecological consciousness Activism	HEALTH ECO-LITERACY

Table 13.3 Examples of potential questions raised by matching a curriculum text type with a curriculum principle

Principles

	Core science	Normal/ pathological	Idiographic/ nomothetic	Complexity	Clinical reasoning	Democracy
Text type						
Instrumental					When might clinical guidelines be over-ridden?	
Ecological	How can science address the issue that the NHS is a major polluter?					
Scientific				What is the best way to learn complexity science?		
Historical		Are there historical reasons to question a sharp divide between the normal & the pathological?				Were Flexner's interventions fair?

(*Continued*)

Table 13.3 (Continued)

	Core science	Normal/ pathological	Idiographic/ nomothetic	Complexity	Clinical reasoning	Democracy
Economic						Is a national health service affordable?
Ethical					Should clinical judgement incorporate social justice?	
Spiritual	Can we reconcile science & faith?					
Gendered	Can tough-minded science become tender-minded?					How can we intervene to provide equal opportunities for women?
International						Should students learn about imperialism before international placements?
Autobiographical		What can we learn from auto-pathographies in both physical and mental health?				

	Location	Authenticity	Integration	Continuity	Identity	Innovation
Phenomenological					Will we lose use of the senses in bedside medicine where technology dominates?	
Aesthetic					Can visual artists educate "how to look"?	
Political						How can medical students learn to work democratically?
Text type						
Instrumental		Is professional communication best learned through formulaic methods in simulation?		How do you timetable a longitudinal integrated clerkship curriculum?		

(Continued)

Table 13.3 (Continued)

	Location	Authenticity	Integration	Continuity	Identity	Innovation
Ecological						How will medicine help to reduce carbon emissions?
Scientific					Are doctors primarily "scientists"?	
Historical		Can the history of medicine be trusted?				
Economic						How should pharmaceuticals be costed?
Ethical	Should postcode decide life expectancy?					
Spiritual					How do doctors of faith square medical science with religious beliefs?	
Gendered						How can we best address the needs of Muslim women in general practice?

International — How will medical education refrain from imposing Western educational ideas & methods?

Autobiographical — How can medical students best reflect on changing identity constructions?

Phenomenological — Can we learn anything about doctors' lived experiences from TV medical soap operas?

Aesthetic — How will the art, humanity & science of medicine be integrated?

Political — Should politics enter the clinical encounter?

Table 13.4 Limiting conditions mapped against curriculum text types to generate questions

Limiting condition

Text type	Structural	Ageing	Cancer	Obesity/ diabetes	Cardiac
Instrumental					
Ecological					
Scientific					
Historical					
Economic					
Ethical					
Spiritual					
Gendered					
Global					
Autobiographical					
Phenomenological					
Aesthetic					
Political					

Text type	Mental health	Respiratory	Medical error	RTAs	Domestic violence
Instrumental					
Ecological					
Scientific					
Historical					
Economic					
Ethical					
Spiritual					
Gendered					
Global					
Autobiographical					
Phenomenological					
Aesthetic					
Political					

Text type	Gastric ulcer	Addiction	Headache	Inflammatory bowel disease	Hyper tension
Instrumental					
Ecological					
Scientific					
Historical					
Economic					
Ethical					
Spiritual					
Gendered					
Global					
Autobiographical					
Phenomenological					
Aesthetic					
Political					

(Continued)

Table 13.4 (Continued)

	Rheumatoid arthritis	Dental hygiene	STDs	Influenza	Broken bones
Text type					
Instrumental					
Ecological					
Scientific					
Historical					
Economic					
Ethical					
Spiritual					
Gendered					
Global					
Autobiographical					
Phenomenological					
Aesthetic					
Political					

	Pandemics	Racism	Sexism	Micro-Aggressions
Text type				
Instrumental				
Ecological				
Scientific				
Historical				
Economic				
Ethical				
Spiritual				
Gendered				
Global				
Autobiographical				
Phenomenological				
Aesthetic				
Political				

17. Dental hygiene.
18. STDs.
19. Influenza and common cold.
20. Broken bones.
21. Pandemics.
22. Racism.
23. Sexism.
24. Micro-aggressions.

Table 13.3: Examples of potential questions raised by matching a curriculum text type with a curriculum principle.

These mapping exercises may seem a little formulaic, but the point is not to provide answers but to raise questions. This should be envisaged as a mapping without borders.

Bibliography

Applebee A. 1996. *Curriculum as Conversation*. Chicago, IL: University of Chicago Press.

Bakhtin M. 1982. *The Dialogic Imagination: Four Essays*. Houston, TX: University of Texas Press.

Bleakley A. The Curriculum Is Dead! Long Live the Curriculum! Designing an Undergraduate Medicine and Surgery Curriculum for the Future. *Medical Teacher*. 2012;34:543–47.

Bleakley A. 2017. *Thinking With Metaphors in Medicine: The State of the Art*. Abingdon: Routledge.

Bleakley A. 2020. *Educating Doctors' Senses Through The Medical Humanities: "How Do I Look?"* Abingdon: Routledge.

Deleuze G, Guattari F. 2013. *A Thousand Plateaus*. London: Continuum.

Drew P, Heritage J (eds.) 2006. *Conversation Analysis*. London: SAGE Ltd.

Eggermont D, Smit MAM, Kwestroo GA, et al. The Influence of Gender Concordance Between General Practitioner and Patient on Antibiotic Prescribing for Sore Throat Symptoms: A Retrospective Study. BMC *Family Practice*. 2018;19:175.

Engeström Y. 2018. *Expertise in Transition: Expansive Learning in Medical Work*. Cambridge: Cambridge University Press.

Pauli HG, White KL, McWhinney IR. Medical Education, Research, and Scientific Thinking in the 21st Century. *Education for Health: Change in Learning & Practice*. 2000;13;15–26 (part1)/13:165–186 (parts 2 and 3).

Pinar WF. 2015. *Understanding Curriculum as Phenomenological and Deconstructed Text*. New York: Educator's International Press.

Schleifer R, Vannatta JB. 2013. *The Chief Concern of Medicine: The Integration of the Medical Humanities and Narrative Knowledge into Medical Practices*. Ann Arbor, MI: University of Michigan Press.

Sidnell, J. Comparative Studies in Conversation Analysis. *Annual Review of Anthropology*. 2007;36:229–44.

14 Effective collaboration

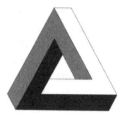

Medicine as close noticing – but not too close

In the previous chapters, I have considered many implications of power dynamics in medicine and medical education, suggesting that practice should be artful: thoughtful, cultured, graceful and, above all, ethical and authentic. In this final chapter, I elaborate on what "authentic" communication in medicine might mean. It is important that medical education invests in ways of expanding the capacities of medical students for relationships that are equally caring, thoughtful, transparent and frank, because the body of research on how medical students develop into junior doctors continues to show a pattern of decline of empathy – from openness to cynicism (including emotional distancing or insulation, and objectification of patients). And many doctors (particularly surgeons) continue to find horizontally structured inter-professional team communication a challenge, despite the fact that collaborative teams have been shown to have better patient outcomes, develop a better safety climate and promote work satisfaction (Borrill et al. 2000).

Medical education has, historically, been complicit in the decline of medical students into patterns of cynicism, where it commodifies students' emotional labour (Hochschild 1983) as "communication skills". Medical schools buy in to this commodification following the habit of instrumentalizing that most difficult and complex of human affairs – affect-laden human exchanges. As medical students are stripped of their natural emotional capital, so this is re-distributed in terms of communication-by-numbers under the guise of "professionalism". This may explain the paradox that while medical schools have invested in empathy training, studies show that empathy continues to decline usually from the third year of medical school onwards.

"Empathy" is a complex and contested notion (Marshall and Bleakley 2017), particularly as "emotional empathy" and "cognitive empathy" are different psychological traits. Empathy scales usually measure cognitive empathy (being conscious and deliberate in setting up and maintaining a relationship, involving close listening and reflexive awareness leading to adaptation to the patient, and not being overwhelmed by feelings but able to maintain some free attention). However, again, studies consistently show decline in both cognitive and affective empathy across cohorts of medical students' careers.

Carefully designed and controlled studies show the benefits of empathy to patient health outcomes. For example, Hojat and colleagues (2011) looked at the clinical outcomes of 891 diabetic patients treated by 29 family physicians (usually the most empathic of doctors along with paediatricians and psychiatrists) over a period of three years in a North American setting. They found that the patients of doctors with the highest empathy scores were significantly more likely to show good control of haemoglobin A1c and LDL-C than patients of doctors with the lowest empathy scores, having controlled for factors such as patients' and doctors' genders and ages, and standing of patients' health insurance. Del Canale and colleagues (2012) carried out a similar study in Italy with the outcome measure as number of acute complications – such as coma and ketoacidosis – experienced by a cohort of nearly 21,000 diabetic patients treated by 242 primary care doctors. The more empathic doctors' patients experienced significantly fewer adverse events.

Empathy decline and growth of cynicism has to be nipped in the bud, yet 30 years' worth of combined patient communication skills and clinical team training (usually incorporated into clinical skills) has failed to do this (Bleakley 2020). Something is wrong – we need a different approach to educating for capabilities needed for effective communication with patients and collaboration with healthcare colleagues (Peterkin and Bleakley 2017; Allard, Wilson and Bleakley 2020). One of the key problems with such training is that it is largely conducted in simulation settings rather than live clinical work placements where briefing and debriefing can be incorporated. Such simulation carries through to assessment (usually by communication scenarios with actor patients, again in simulation), in objective structured clinical examinations (OSCEs). Such settings invite students to dissimulate or fake communication and then breed inauthenticity (Gillett 2017). Students are taught checklist, instrumental approaches to patient communication – such as use of acronyms like ICE – ideas, concerns and expectations – that fail the tests of transfer of learning to actual, messy and emotion-laden patient encounters, often in fluid contexts, and sometimes with little privacy (Snow 2016). Rosamund Snow (ibid.) says:

> I saw a doctor who I felt had gold standard communication skills. Afterwards I thought about what she had done to make me feel so able to talk to her. Instead of probing my feelings with ICE-based questions, her primary focus

was answering the questions I had asked, so I felt she was listening, and that we were working together. If she needed information I had not yet volunteered, she made clear why she was asking each question. She shared her thoughts as we went along, so we could discuss them, rather than putting me on the spot – and that made it much easier for me to share my thoughts and worries with her, too. It didn't take long. I had already started to trust her in the first 15 seconds.

Snow queries the claim that such formulaic communication skills training will necessarily transfer to clinical reality to build rapport with patients, raising more questions than answers. She ponders: "Did anyone ask patients how these questions make them feel?" (ibid.). Her question is addressed by Curtis and colleagues' (2013) study of the effect of skills training on how well doctors and nurses communicate with patients about end-of-life care, one of the most challenging aspects of medical and healthcare work. In a randomized trial including 391 doctors, those who had undergone skills training were reported by patients and family members as no better at communication than the control group who received no intervention. The authors note that the findings raise serious issues about "skills transfer from simulation training to actual patient care". Of course, it may have been that the training offered was unusually poor or dysfunctional in some way, but this is not the likely explanation.

Lack of transfer to real work contexts is the key issue. In a damning account of communication skills training for medical students, George Gillett (2017: unpaginated), a medical student, describes losing the "authentic human voice", where applying rote tools and scripts is not a good educational tactic. Gillett talks of medical students entering a medical education with good intentions to find that they have to "learn to feign that we cared", where "The supposed virtues of a doctor – integrity, transparency and empathy – had been side-lined by a customer service approach to medicine", a damning conclusion. Again, emotional capital is open to commodification.

The way forward, says Gillett, is to learn (and assess) communication capabilities in real work settings, using triangulated feedback from patients, supervising doctors as medical educators (or psychologists who have expertise in communication) and students themselves: in other words, a structured pedagogy in real life and real time. Communication can range from casual conversations to taking histories to breaking bad news. Harvard Medical School has trialled a more innovative approach based on double stimulation with an arts intervention as second stimulus (Atluru 2016).

Drawing on improvisational comedy – a performance technique – Anu Atluru, an ER doctor, bemoans medical education's reliance on formulaic communication training where "There's still no algorithm for patient interaction". Ironically, such supposedly personalized medicine, where students are supposedly "oven ready" for practice after simulation training, is de-personalized. Structures, scripts and roles replace the realities of noisy work contexts heavy with body odours and the smell of cleaning fluids, inhabited by shaky hands, tentative skin on skin, sudden interruptions, a misplaced comment, a wry smile, a nervous cough, a flicker of recognition, a wink, an unwanted face-off. Atluru (ibid.: unpaginated) continues:

> Traditional educators view improvisation as a risk. Yet, the practice of medicine is spontaneous and, often times, risky. And, if educators teach students to tread carefully even in simulated encounters, how can physicians be expected to form genuine relationships with their patients?

Improvisational theatre teaches you to be "firmly rooted in the instinctive". Life experience has already prepared you for communication exchanges – does professional behaviour really differ so much from everyday authenticity, discretion and codes of honour such as confidentiality and careful monitoring of self-disclosure?

Common decency and existential authenticity (Steiner and Reisinger 2006) may be uncommonly hard to achieve, however. Isn't that why, relatively, so many doctors are fatigued at best and close to burnout at worse? This is not just physical – long hours and short breaks, arduous tasks – but emotional. Straining to do good work – "Above All, Do No Harm! (Smith 2005) – doctors may snap. Like all other forms of medical education, we need to work hard on our collaborative intentions. Like democracy, this is a "horizon" project, always in development. And conditions change, so that collaborative capabilities needed for today's workplace are not the same as those needed "yesterday". Look at "teamwork" for example, as discussed at length in Chapter 8. Only three decades ago, healthcare was set on establishing "stable" teams, where members get to know the idiosyncrasies of other members. But such teams get stale and habitual too, as the airline industry began to recognize quite some time ago. This can lead to the formation of bad habits and a kind of blindness ("this is the way we do things around here") that can lead to errors, sometimes catastrophic.

Back to communication demands – above I said: "'Common' decency and authenticity may be uncommonly hard to achieve". Returning to Sartre's waiter and his existential dilemma of "bad faith" discussed earlier and described in *Being and Nothingness*, faced with a life that could be seen as meaningless, how do you introduce meaning? The waiter is offered as a model of inauthenticity, where meaning is drained from the occasion through play-acting. The waiter could grasp the nettle and make choices rather than slipping out of his own skin and occupying the role that is set for him as parody.

The same conditions apply to doctors in terms of upholding the Hippocratic injunction to "first, do no harm" and to extend this to consistent ethical and professional behaviour. This ethical injunction does not invite doctors to step out of their own skins and inhabit some angelic ethical territory. Rather, it asks doctors to be inquiring about their own unique approaches to authentic interactions with patients in the face of recognized contradictions. This is to grasp the nettle of responsibility for the consequences of interventions. Good faith demands artistry in developing a personal style of responsible actions. Bad faith would be acting into the role of the doctor as an ideal while failing to tolerate what Donald Schön (1983) calls the "swampy lowlands" of clinical practice – full of uncertainty and values conflict where technical solutions are never the full story.

While authentic relationships demand a level of suffering and uncertainty, they mean something: there is love, connection, friendship, admiration, exchange – all qualities with emotional substance, rather than the void that Sartre's waiter occupies. Yet a shadow side of slippage – perhaps from exhaustion, temptation of a biblical kind, erotic transference of a Freudian kind, end of tether days, and creeping cynicism of the sort that seems to grip many doctors in mid- to late-career in particular – may creep in.

I have stressed throughout this book the importance of the imperative of "patient-centredness" not as an ideal but as a lived reality, shifting even to a patient-directed medicine. In the 1950s, the American psychologist and psychotherapist Carl Rogers developed a non-interventionist "client-centred" approach in which the therapist or counsellor follows the lead of the client without compulsive intervention or analysis. This was the basis to patient-centred care, developed by Moira Stewart and Ian McWhinney amongst others in the 1990s (Stewart et al. 1995; Stewart 2001; Bleakley 2014). Rogers placed Sartrean authenticity ("congruence" or "genuineness") as one of the three pillars of client-centredness along with unconditional positive regard and empathy. But Rogers was "human, all too human" (to borrow from Friedrich Nietzsche) and showed ethical slippage later in his life and career.

In Timothy Thomason's (2016) "The Shadow Side of the Great Psychotherapists", we learn that Rogers, the great promulgator of "trust" as the key to a therapeutic alliance (Bleakley 2014), in later life broke trust by having an affair with one of his clients. Later in this chapter, in discussing co-counselling as a democratic technique for teaching medical students how to communicate well with patients, we find that the founder of "re-evaluation counselling", the original model of co-counselling, Harvey Jackins, like many male charismatic and cult figures, fell foul of (unproven) allegations of sexual misconduct with younger women trainees, and also disgraced himself by expressing negative views about homosexuality. Authenticity requires moral courage.

But such relationships are particularly ethically fraught because of the power imbalance. It is vital that doctors, as with psychotherapists and counsellors, are aware of the potential damage they can cause by exploiting the power differential between them and patients. It is rare for doctors to have relationships with their patients, and ethical guidelines globally are clear about the dangers, often seeing such relationships as abusive. Roger Collier (2016) notes:

> Simon Holmes … a 59-year-old family doctor in the United Kingdom … got to know his first wife … while treating her for depression. And he got to know his second wife … while counselling her over relationship troubles with her former husband. After these details eventually came to light, a medical disciplinary panel suspended Holmes from practising for three months for failing to maintain professional boundaries.

Collier notes the remark of Dr Carol Leet, former president of the College of Physicians and Surgeons of Ontario, that "There is no such thing as a consensual sexual relationship between a doctor and a patient ... There is a power imbalance that makes it impossible for a patient to actually be consenting to having that relationship". In fact, such relationships are treated as sexual abuse. Leet notes "a lack of consensus regarding how to educate medical trainees and physicians with regard to sexual boundaries", and that there is "a need for greater attention to this critical topic within medical education curricula".

If we are in agreement that the emotional life of doctors is important, that psychological insight and psychotherapeutic acumen are key to effective practice, that self-care is vital in such a demanding job and that current "communication skills" approaches linked with resistance to the psychological aspects of medicine are inadequate, then what can be done? In this chapter, I suggest that learning basic psychotherapeutic models, skills and interventions that can also be used reflexively and can be "practiced" in pairs and small group settings is essential to contemporary medicine and could replace much of the instrumental "communication skills" training currently offered. In part, this is a political issue, but it also draws in the aesthetic, where communication is an art, and style is central to effective human encounters.

The fundamental basis for the model I suggest here is an education in democratic encounters grounded in collaboration. Democratizing medicine is in the hands of the current and following generation of medical students. These students can learn reflexivity and psychotherapeutic acumen for later clinical encounters and interprofessional healthcare work by learning:

i.   Basic understanding of psychodynamics: transference and counter transference, resistance and counter resistance, and defence mechanisms of the ego – for it is here that resilience to burnout can be fostered.
ii. Capability across a range of intervention skills and styles that foster dialogue and debate rather than monological or authority-led styles, careful listening and narrative appreciation.
iii. Self and peer assessment, including criteria setting for judgements.

A balance is achieved between the social (professional relationships with patients and colleagues, or other-awareness) and the psychological (self-awareness).

Co-counselling

Harvey Jackins – a member of the Communist Party of America – first developed "re-evaluation counselling" in North America in the 1950s. He was born in Idaho and later went to university and worked in the Pacific North West. In 1954, after prominent activism in unions, Jackins was brought before the House Un-American Activities Committee (famed for witch-hunting left-wing activists and labour leaders).

Later, re-evaluation counselling was re-named "co-counselling". After complaints about Jackins' ethical behaviour and a sense that re-evaluation counselling, now an international network, was defying its own code of values by becoming internally authoritarian, a British national, John Heron, broke from the movement in 1974 and started an independent co-counselling network – first in the UK and then in New Zealand and other countries. Heron was a co-director of the British Postgraduate Medical Federation in the 1970s, when he worked with GP networks to introduce co-counselling and other psychological methods. But this work never stuck, and GP practices, following psychiatrists, largely took up Schwartz group techniques such as Schwartz Rounds. These are described by the UK General Medical Council (GMC) as "group reflective practice forums giving staff from all disciplines an opportunity to reflect on the emotional and social aspects of working in healthcare" (https://www.gmc-uk.org/education/s tandards-guidance-and-curricula/guidance/reflective-practice/schwartz-rounds).

Co-counselling is grounded in the assumption that everybody, no matter what their physical or mental condition, has unrealized potential, but such potential is often frustrated by cumulative chronic patterns of distress throughout life development. An authentic life consists of a genuine desire to help others wherever possible to achieve capabilities – a model that is also espoused by Amartya Sen (Dang 2014) and Martha Nussbaum (2011). Humans are existentially vulnerable and prone to fall short of potential unless they collaborate, and learn how to use artefacts, languages and symbols in ways that open up new horizons of possibility. But once basic needs are met – food, shelter, company, friendship and emotional life, a living wage – people differ in what they wish to achieve.

Capabilities define what people want from life after baseline inequities and inequalities are addressed. But psychotherapists point to chronic patterns of distress masking full understanding of individual capability. All of us carry distress from early life traumas and everyday social insults such as cumulative microaggressions, much of which remains unconscious because of defence mechanisms such as repression, denial and displacement. Such distress can be overt, such as those stemming from historical-structural religious, ethnic and racial intolerances. Capabilities are then not so easy to define unless each of us has the opportunity to do some soul searching, therapeutically or educationally.

In order to address chronic patterns of distress or other blocks to achieving potential, historically we have looked to teachers or spiritual guides as wise others, and this has become institutionalized in secular psychotherapy, counselling and psychiatry. But these professional arrangements go against the grain of democratic collaborative structures, where they are based on power differentials reproducing parent (therapist) – child (client) authority structures. Indeed, Freudian psychoanalysis is based on the model of therapist as substitute (good) parent against whom the client can rail without reprisal – first as cathartic "cleaning out" followed by insight into patterns of psychological defence. The resolution of the transference – where analyst counts as good parent – signals the end of a therapeutic encounter.

Harvey Jackins was sceptical of such power structures, suggesting that therapeutic encounters could occur in horizontal power arrangements where transference was negligible. Adults without acute psychological symptoms could pair up and counsel each other after a period of education into basic theory and skills of healthy psychological exchange. The basic model would involve a pair working over time, where one acted as counsellor and the other as client, for, say, an hour session, and then the pair would swap roles; in other words, a "co"-counselling. Absolutely key to the educational value of the exercise is that the client gives authentic feedback (say ten minutes) to the counsellor after the session. This should include strengths and limitations.

The important assumptions surrounding the sessions are:

1. Democracy and collaboration are agreed as the binding principles behind the practice.
2. The person who is "client" always states the terms of, and guides, the session – they can contract at any time for a less or more intense engagement from the "counsellor" in terms of intensity of intervention, from passive listening and presence to more active interventions, including confrontation, catharsis and interpretation.
3. The client must always have some "free attention" available to gain insight into what is happening in the session, to make rational and coherent decisions even if engaged in catharsis or release of emotions, and then to be able to stop the session at any time or to ask for a different level of engagement with the counsellor. Should the client sink into, or be overwhelmed by, a cathartic episode (such as extreme anger or sadness), without availability of free attention, the session should be terminated.
4. Counsellors act as facilitators of learning and not as teachers, gurus or substitute parents.
5. After a full co-counselling session (say one hour each way), it is useful to debrief. In any case, as noted above, the client can give the counsellor feedback at the end of the session (say ten minutes).
6. Content of sessions is confidential to participants.

Co-counselling also draws on the ideas of the psychoanalyst Karen Horney, who attempted to democratize psychoanalysis by introducing the idea of a "barefoot psychoanalysis" (Southgate and Randall 1978). Critics of co-counselling say "what is different about this arrangement and a good talk with a close and trusted friend?" Well, if you have a quasi-therapeutic and educational relationship with a close friend, then this is to be applauded. But even a friendship can be distorted by inability on both sides to listen closely without interruption or "taking over the wheel" ("you know, the same thing happened to me the other day … blah de blah"), to know how to be present for a cathartic episode (sadness, anger, fear – leading to crying, sobbing, outbursts of shouting and swearing, regression and so forth). Besides, there is the all-important confidentiality clause.

Teaching co-counselling frameworks and skills to medical students could readily be substituted for current instrumental and reductive "communication skills"
training. This can happen within the undergraduate medicine curriculum, where
trusted friendship groups have developed certainly by Year 2. A more radical
model would be to introduce co-counselling as the basis for an inter-professional
"buddy" and support group model from Year 1. A small, mixed inter-professional
group of students from a Faculty of Health and a medical school could meet first
as a support group and then more formally as a Schwartz Rounds group, split-
ting off into co-counselling sessions. It is not necessary to maintain the same
co-counselling partner over time. Indeed, it may help to refresh the arrangement
through new partnerships as long as confidentiality rules are maintained. As
with all therapeutic relationships, should mutual attractions or erotic feelings
enter the encounter, these should be worked through therapeutically as potential
transference effects. If confidence is broken, then the co-counselling relationship
should cease.

Six Category Intervention Analysis

Co-counselling is a way that medical students and doctors can provide each other
with mutual support while practicing and improving their therapeutic capabilities. The method is based on the understanding of a comprehensive repertoire
of intra-personal and inter-personal interventions addressing every kind of
encounter. These interventions have been articulated and systematized by John
Heron (1977a, 1977b, 1988, 1999, 2001) for, first, a one-to-one setting (Six
Category Intervention Analysis); and, second, a facilitated group-based setting
(Dimensions of Facilitator Style). Such categorization of course is in danger of
falsely systematizing what are often messy and complex human interactions in
medicine: doctor–patient, and doctor–team(s). The latter often involves boundary crossing across several clinical teams working around patients, where rapid,
"pulsating" and loose exchanges and encounters occur, largely as routine events
(quickly forgotten) rather than significant experiences (long remembered).
Heron's work is not an invitation to formulaic training but should be seen as a
natural history of communication in which species and their varieties are identified as a basis to taxonomies, but their behaviours are best appreciated in the wild.

In the 1960s, two management and organizational theorists, Robert Blake and
Jane Mouton, developed a category model of human interaction and intervention, shaped by contemporary leadership theory. Management theory was undergoing a revolution, shifting from interest in leadership as authority dictating to
others, to leadership as facilitative, drawing out qualities in others. Also, there
was growing interest in the role of affect in communication, as well as cognition.
Characteristically, professionals' weak spots are in developing varieties of "emotional intelligence" (the identification, tracking and management of feelings or
affect) to include an understanding of the vicissitudes of emotional exchange
through "emotional labour" (Hochschild 1983).

Heron places great emphasis on emotional capability – the vicissitudes of affect, surely the legacy of Freud and psychoanalysis whose tenet was the bringing to consciousness of repressed episodes saturated with feeling. In medical communication, "professionalism" demands that emotions are kept under a lid, or expressed mildly. Yet medical students and doctors work in highly charged environments where affect builds.

An American sociologist, Arlie Russell Hochschild (1983), would spearhead a movement that linked personal emotional life to public issues, coining the term "emotional labour" to describe work that people carried out with a high input of affect, such as in professional care work, social work, healthcare and medicine, but also in unqualified care work such as family help. Here, the personal became the charged and often troubled political, where emotional labour was often carried out by the unpaid or the poorly paid as unqualified carers, often as immigrant labour, leading to what Hochschild called "global care". Medical students and doctors of course engage centrally with emotional labour, yet medical schools do not educate students in the energetics or politics of emotional labour. Hence, the performance of so-called "professionals", educated in "professionalism" and "communication skills", often turns out to be no better than the unqualified, but life experienced, layperson.

Recall that medical students learn "communication skills" in pre-packaged formats and in simulated settings. We might see this as an aspect of neo-liberal capitalism engaging with an "emotion economy". A commodity – "communication skills" - is packaged as consumer product that Illouz (2007) calls, as a family, "cold intimacies". These include "self-help" (see Chapter 6), and "self-realization" programmes that stand outside authentic relationships but can be bought in the marketplace as "emotionologies" (Fineman 2010: 27). There is then a danger in what the rest of this chapter sets out – that is not taken as a pre-packaged consumer product, but rather is treated reflexively and critically, as guidelines and contemplation on authentic relating.

Against this background, let us consider Six Category Intervention Analysis. John Heron was born in 1928. He studied psychology and philosophy, and learned co-counselling within the Harvey Jackins model. As noted, he later broke from Jackins and set up his own international co-counselling network. He also developed a research programme at the University of Surrey, UK, looking at participatory research paradigms such as co-operative inquiry (also termed "collaborative inquiry") based on his early work (1968–69) on the phenomenology of social encounter and the democratizing of social science research. Heron directed the Human Potential Research Project at the University of Surrey from 1970 to 1977, developing an innovative programme of research, and subsequently award-bearing courses in humanistic and transpersonal psychology, the first in the UK.

From 1977 to 1985, Heron was assistant director of the British Postgraduate Medical Federation at the University of London, and it is here that he developed the first education courses for doctors in holistic communication and collaborative inquiry into practice. Later, he set up research and training centres in Italy and New Zealand. Six Category Intervention Analysis was the first of several models developed by Heron that described a comprehensive account of human encounters and how these could be developed, or how they could degrade to become manipulative or even perverted. The purpose of the model was to provide a clear guide for how professionals working with people – such as healthcare practitioners, social workers, carers, educators, managers, counsellors and psychotherapists – could develop communication capabilities. Later, he progressed the one-to-one model to a group form, as Dimensions of Facilitator Style.

The six categories of intervention for one-to-one encounters

AUTHORITATIVE
Prescribing
Informing
Confronting

FACILITATIVE
Cathartic
Catalytic
Supportive

The categories describe verbal and non-verbal communications between two people, or on oneself as reflexive awareness. While each category can be logically separated from any other category, in practice they interact, overlap and can be confluent or contradictory. The point about the system is that it offers a powerful post hoc analysis, as well as a prelude to encounters as an educational framework. But the system is auto-therapeutic: once introjected it can provide an internal "second stimulus" running commentary on one's behaviour, for the purposes of constant monitoring and adaptation – a critical awareness affording self-scaffolding of learning.

Heron suggested two broad styles of communication: authoritative and facilitative. An authoritative intervention comes from me to you and sets out to shape your response. I can tell you what to do (prescribing), inform you about something (informing) or challenge you about something (confrontation). All of these can be legitimate, helpful interventions. If there is an emergency, or information has to be passed quickly, or I need to challenge somebody's manipulative behaviour, then it is perfectly legitimate to engage in authoritative interventions. But what if these become habitual, the most common way that somebody communicates? And what if prescribing, informing and confronting degenerate into dictatorial habits, or bullying? It is apparent from a number of contemporary studies that cumulative micro-aggressions are the most common ways in which those who seek control treat others in healthcare settings, as habitual behaviour, especially through ageism (Segal 2020), sexism and racism (Gonzago et al. 2019).

Facilitative interventions on the other hand do not come from me to shape your response, but explicitly invite you to take the lead in the conversation, or exchange. Thus, I provide a listening and empathic ear that allows you to release feelings and perceive that this is safe to do (cathartic). Or, I open up a conversation or dialogue by asking questions, not giving answers (catalytic). Here, I act as catalyst to your thought process, enabling but not interfering. And, throughout the exchange, I offer explicit support – empathy, warmth and encouragement (supportive) (Table 14.1).

Each intervention – and they will entangle and inter-twine in exchanges – can be appropriate to context, but can also degenerate or become inappropriate, for example as manipulative, insincere, purposefully deceitful, overly sarcastic and so forth. The worst degenerations can become perverse – for example, somebody who gains pleasure from telling people what to do, or belittling them, or constantly pointing out faults in others while not recognizing faults in oneself, often called "micro-aggressions", as noted above. These are perversions in human communication, best treated therapeutically. This applies particularly to compulsive controlling types (authoritarians), but there are also people who facilitate compulsively but can never take the wheel when direction is necessary.

In consultations, medical students must learn the vocabulary of appropriate facilitation and authority where necessary. Research shows that exchanges with patients veer towards authoritative rather than facilitative interventions, where monologue is more characteristic of doctors' styles than dialogue (Waitzkin 1991; Livingston 2005); and within inter-professional team settings, especially marked in surgery, the same pattern obtains (Bleakley 2014). Surgeons characteristically, even habitually, tell and inform (monologue) rather than create conditions for dialogue and exchange, or democratic settings.

Table 14.1 The six categories explained

Authoritative	
Prescribe	On a continuum, to suggest at one end and to demand at another (including acting urgently where the other is incapacitated, in danger or endangering another).
Inform	To give information that is accurate and not knowingly misleading; question and answer exchanges.
Confront	To challenge appropriately; on a continuum from gently reminding through to insistently demanding. Facing up to bullying or harassment by challenging back.
Facilitative	
Cathartic	To be present when another is emotional, or to encourage emotional release (of fear in trembling, of sadness in crying, of anger in shouting or banging, of joy in weeping and so forth). Staying present with someone as they gain insight following a cathartic release.
Catalytic	Question and answer, clarification, developing conversation but not taking over the wheel of another.
Supportive	Being present, warm and caring.

Dimensions of Facilitator Style

After mapping Six Category Intervention Analysis, John Heron (1977a) turned his attention to interventions in group settings, mapping Dimensions of Facilitator Style. This was first mapped as transposing Six Category Intervention Analysis onto group settings, and offering these as sliding scales where facilitators may choose to intervene or remain present and non-interventionist. The six dimensions are:

Directive – Non-directive
Interpretative – Non-interpretative
Confronting – Non-confronting
Cathartic – Non-cathartic
Structuring – Non-structuring
Disclosing – Non-disclosing

The dimensions pretty much shadow the six categories of intervention, except that the "Supportive" category underpinning all other interventions is expanded to give the facilitator the choice of level of disclosure to any group of her own process or issues.

In later publications, *The Facilitator's Handbook* and *Group Facilitation*, Heron gradually developed a different category system to his original *Dimensions of Facilitator Style*. These two books were fused in *The Complete Facilitator's Handbook* (1999), which gives a full theoretical justification for the choices of categories. Heron now said that an effective facilitator for group settings should be able to balance "purposes" and "intentions". Purposes invoke planning ahead, making meaning of what happens and confronting or challenging where obstacles, difficulties or potential miscommunication, unethical practice or hurt is perceived. Intentions are less clear-cut and take into account uncertainty, change and contradiction.

Here, it may be that the best intervention is one of sensitivity, or creating a climate of support. However, if there is lack of clarity around an issue, the facilitator may structure, suggesting ways in which issues might be analysed or reviewed, looked at differently. Finally, the facilitator should set and maintain a supportive climate through valuing. The final set of dimensions to facilitator style is summarized below. The sliding scales of the original set of dimensions are now transformed into a set of questions about setting group climates and aims, sense-making, raising consciousness and widening remits, expressing feelings that may aid or block expansion of activities, structuring and planning and, above all, setting a tone that is supportive.

Six dimensions to facilitator style

PURPOSES
Planning
How shall the group/team achieve its aims?

Meaning
How shall the group/team make sense of experiences?
Confronting/ challenging
What are the challenges of raising consciousness, widening remits or innovating?

INTENTIONS
Feeling
How are emotions handled? What can be expressed?
Structuring
How will planning occur?
Valuing
Setting up a supportive climate

Again, as with Six Category Intervention Analysis, while each category can be logically separated from any other category, in practice they interact, overlap and can be confluent or contradictory.

Medical students learning co-counselling will be increasingly exposed to working in group settings such as clinical teams, but more, in complex cross-team settings. Heron describes their "teemings" and "negotiated knotworkings" across such liquid settings in a more traditional psychological lingo. As they progress through their clinical careers, trainee doctors will take on leadership roles (for example, looking after several wards as a junior doctor on night shifts). It is important that facilitative roles are acquired and practiced in these contexts in order to democratize inter-professional team settings. Such approaches are mandatory in some areas of clinical work, such as the World Health Organization Surgical Safety Checklist team briefing prior to surgery; and expected in others, such as a handover debriefing and briefing on a ward.

A politics of learning

In facilitating communications, Heron encourages striving for democratic encounters. This does not mean lack of intervention, indeed it may mean more vigorous intervention, but that interventions are grounded in a desire for inclusion and to address inequities and inequalities. Thus, a "politics of learning" (Heron 1999: 20–21) is present in every encounter in one-to-one or group settings, where (1) a facilitator/doctor can lead; (2) a facilitator/doctor can share decisions with others (patients, colleagues); (3) a facilitator can be present but power is handed over to the patient or colleagues. The politics of learning will shift according to whether the focus is task or process. A task may invite specialist input such as skill or knowledge, or guidance on procedures. Process may be more open-ended and call for collaborative structures, and may be reflexive – inquiring into the nature and process of the communication itself.

The reader may ask: why do we need separate category systems for one-to-one and group facilitation? Surely Six Category Intervention Analysis can be applied to group contexts? This is indeed the case, where the framework is highly adaptable. But Heron is thinking on two levels. Dimensions of Facilitator Style and "Complete" facilitation do exactly what they say on the tin: they deal with a "second order" of facilitation that is to do with the meeting of aesthetics and politics. The question here is, in professional communication, how can politics or power issues be elegantly and stylishly performed? A "first order" of facilitation invokes the six categories as the more instrumental workhorse, the groundwork that is extended, used creatively, and re-invented through the lens of group facilitation. This addresses the awkward problem of one approach for individuals and another for groups or teams, an unnecessary and indeed misleading division.

To return to employment of Six Category Intervention Analysis in co-counselling for medical students or inter-professional pairs, it is likely that democratic politics of learning will obtain, where the "counsellor" acts as "present facilitator", intervening only when the "client" asks or when the facilitator needs clarification. This arrangement can lead to co-counsellor facilitators beings stuck in supportive and valuing mode without the opportunity to practice the full range of interventions. Hence, it is common, if such an arrangement becomes habitual, that the co-counselling pair decides to move to "open" sessions where the counsellor is invited to utilize the full range of the six categories. This too is a democratic, mutual decision. It can be revoked at any time, with the client framing the nature of the session.

Most importantly, we must not become slaves to these typologies and category systems – they are analytical tools to be brought to complex, synthetic social situations. Rather, we should approach them as ways of developing habits of the heart, where politics, ethics and aesthetics are invoked in the ongoing venture to democratize medical practice through medical education. Our claims of authentic "patient-centredness" and "inter-professionalism" are premature. There is much work to be done.

Bibliography

Allard J, Wilson M, Bleakley A. 2020. Doctors Need Safe Confessional and Cathartic Spaces: What We Learned from the Research Project "People Talking: Digital Dialogues for Mutual Recovery". In: A Bleakley (ed.) *Routledge Handbook of the Medical Humanities*. Abingdon: Routledge, 410–18.

Atluru A. What Improv Can Teach Tomorrow's Doctors: Thinking Quickly and Occasionally Abandoning the Medical-School Script Are Critical for Quality Patient Care. *The Atlantic*, 24 August 2016. Available at: https://www.theatlantic.com/education/archive/2016/08/what-improv-can-teach-tomorrows-doctors/497177/

Bleakley A. 2014. *Patient-centred Medicine in Transition: The Heart of the Matter*. Dordrecht: Springer.

Bleakley A. 2020. *Educating Doctors' Senses Through The Medical Humanities: "How Do I Look?"* Abingdon: Routledge.

Borrill C, West MA, Shapiro D, Rees A. Team Working and Effectiveness in Health Care. *British Journal of Health Care Management*. 2000;6:364–71.

Collier R. When the Doctor–Patient Relationship Turns Sexual. *CMAJ: Canadian Medical Association Journal*. 2016;188:247–48.

Curtis JR, Back AL, Ford DW, et al. Effect of Communication Skills Training for Residents and Nurse Practitioners on Quality of Communication With Patients With Serious Illness: A Randomized Trial. *Journal of the American Medical Association.* 2013;310(21):2271–81.

Dang A-T. Amartya Sen's Capability Approach: A Framework for Well-Being Evaluation and Policy Analysis? *Review of Social Economy.* 2014;72:4.

Del Canale S, Louis DZ, Maio V, et al. The Relationship Between Physician Empathy and Disease Complications: An Empirical Study of Primary Care Physicians and Their Diabetic Patients in Parma, Italy. *Academic Medicine.* 2012;87:1243–9.

Fineman S (2010) Emotion in Organizations – A Critical Turn. In: B. Sieben and Å. Wettergren (eds.) *Emotionalizing Organizations and Organizing Emotions.* Basingstoke: Palgrave Macmillan, 23–41.

Gillett G. 2017. *"Communication Skills" and the Problem with Fake Patients.* 11 May. Originally published in Student BMJ. Available at: https://georgegillett.com/2017/05/11/communication-skills-and-the-problem-with-fake-patients/

Gonzago AM, Ufomata E, Bonicaino E, Zimmer S. "Microaggressions: What Are They? How Can We Avoid? How Can We Respond? *Slide Show,* 2019. Available at: https://www.chp.edu/-/media/chp/healthcare-professionals/documents/faculty-development/microaggressions.pdf?la=en

Heron J. 1977a. *Dimensions of Facilitator Style.* London: British Postgraduate Medical Federation.

Heron J. 1977b. *Catharsis in Human Development.* London: British Postgraduate Medical Federation.

Heron, J. 1988. Assessment Revisited. In: D Boud. (ed.) *Developing Student Autonomy in Learning.* London: Kogan Page, 77–90.

Heron J. 1999. *The Complete Facilitator's Handbook.* London: Kogan Page.

Heron J. 2001. *Helping the Client: A Creative Practical Guide,* 5th ed. London: SAGE.

Hochschild AR. 1983. *The Managed Heart: Commercialization of Human Feeling.* Berkeley, CA: University of California Press.

Hojat M, Louis DZ, Markham FW, et al. Physicians' Empathy and Clinical Outcomes for Diabetic Patients. *Academic Medicine.* 2011;86:359–64.

Illouz E. 2007. *Cold Intimacies: The Making of Emotional Capitalism.* Cambridge: Polity Press.

Livingston M. 2005. *Listening in Medicine: The Whiplash Mystery and Other Tales.* Victoria, BC: Trafford.

Marshall R, Bleakley A. 2017. *Rejuvenating Medical Education: Seeking Help from Homer.* Newcastle: Cambridge Scholars Publishing.

Nussbaum MC. 2011. *Creating Capabilities: The Human Development Approach.* Cambridge, MA: Harvard University Press.

Peterkin A, Bleakley A. 2017. *Staying Human During the Foundation Programme and Beyond: How to Thrive After Medical School.* Baton Rouge, FL: CRC Press.

Schön D. 1983. *The Reflective Practitioner.* New York: Basic.

Segal J. 2020. Ageism and Rhetoric. In: A Bleakley (ed.) *Routledge Handbook of Medical Humanities.* Abingdon: Routledge, 163–75.

Smith, C. M. Origin and Uses of Primum Non Nocere – Above All, Do No Harm! *Journal of Clinical Pharmacology.* 2005;45:371–77.

Snow R. I Never Asked to Be ICE'd. *BMJ.* 2016;354:i3729.

Southgate J, Randall R. 1978. *The Barefoot Psychoanalyst: An Illustrated Manual of Self Help Therapy.* London: Association of Karen Horney Psychoanalytic Counsellors.

Steiner CJ, Reisinger Y. Understanding Existential Authenticity. *Annals of Tourism Research.* 2006;33:299–318.

Stewart M. Towards a Global Definition of Patient Centred Care. *British Medical Journal.* 2001;322:444–5.

Stewart M, Brown JB, Weston WW, et al. 1995. *Patient-Centred Medicine: Transforming the Clinical Method.* Thousand Oaks, CA: SAGE.

Thomason TC. 2016. The Shadow Side of the Great Psychotherapists. *Counseling & Wellness Journal,* 5. Available at: http://openknowledge.nau.edu/2346

Waitzkin H. 1991. *The Politics of Medical Encounters.* New Haven, CT: Yale University Press.

Index

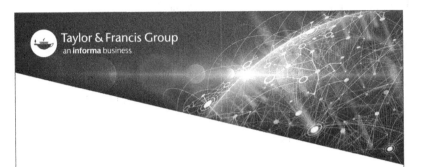

Printed in the United States
By Bookmasters